Effective Management of Coding Services

Third Edition

Edited by

Lou Ann Schraffenberger, MBA, RHIA, CCS, CCS-P

Lynn Kuehn, RHIA, CCS-P, FAHIMA

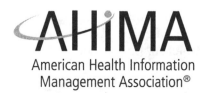

AHIMA
American Health Information
Management Association®

ISBN 1-58426-169-2
AHIMA Product Number AC100007

Claire E. Blondeau, MBA, Project Editor
Melissa Ulbricht, Editorial/Production Coordinator
Ken Zielske, Director of Publications

All information contained within this book, including Web sites and regulatory information, was current and valid as of the date of publication. However, Web page addresses and the information on them may change or disappear at any time and for any number of reasons. The user is encouraged to perform his or her own general Web searches to locate any site addresses listed here that are no longer valid.

*AHIMA strives to recognize the value of people from every racial
and ethnic background as well as all genders, age groups,
and sexual orientations by building its membership and leadership
resources to reflect the rich diversity of the American population.
AHIMA encourages the celebration and promotion of human diversity
through education, mentoring, recognition, leadership, and other programs.*

American Health Information Management Association
233 North Michigan Avenue, Suite 2150
Chicago, Illinois 60601-5800

http://www.ahima.org

Contents

Acknowledgments

We acknowledge with thanks the work of those individuals who authored or contributed to the first and/or second editions of *Effective Management of Coding Services* and lent their interest, enthusiasm, and helpful suggestions to the project.

About the Editors and Authors

Lou Ann Schraffenberger, MBA, RHIA, CCS, CCS-P, is manager of clinical data in the Clinical Information Services Department of Advocate Health Care in Oak Brook, Illinois. Schraffenberger manages systemwide HIM and clinical data projects, clinical coding education, data quality improvement, and coding compliance issues. In 1997, Schraffenberger was awarded the first AHIMA Volunteer Award. She has served as chair of the Society for Clinical Coding (2000) and is a former member of the AHIMA Council on Certification and the Certified Coding Specialist (CCS) Examination Construction Committee. Additionally, she has authored the AHIMA publication *Basic ICD-9-CM Coding* since 1999.

Lynn Kuehn, RHIA, CCS-P, FAHIMA, is president of Kuehn Consulting in Waukesha, Wisconsin. Previously, she was director of office operations for Children's Medical Group in Milwaukee. Additionally, she has served in HIM and coordination positions in a variety of healthcare settings. In her volunteer role, Kuehn served as secretary and chair of the Ambulatory Care Section of AHIMA and the chair of several national committees. She has been a member of the AHIMA Board of Directors for 2005–2007. Moreover, she has presented at numerous meetings and seminars in the field of physician office management, coding, and reimbursement. Kuehn has been the recipient of the AHIMA Educator-Practitioner Award and the Wisconsin HIMA Distinguished Member Award. Additionally, she has authored the AHIMA publication *CPT/HCPCS Coding and Reimbursement for Physician Services* since 2001.

Nadinia A. Davis, MBA, CIA, CPA, RHIA, FAHIMA, is an assistant professor of HIM at the College of Natural, Applied, and Health Sciences at Kean University in Union, New Jersey. She has worked as a coding consultant and auditor in acute settings and as director of medical records at a rehabilitation institute. Prior to her HIM career, Davis worked in the financial services industry, most recently as an internal auditor. Davis is former president and a Distinguished Member of NJHIMA, as well as a former member of the AHIMA Board of Directors. She was editor of and contributor to *Essentials of Health Care Finance: A Workbook for Health Information Managers* and contributed to *Health Information Management Technology: An Applied Approach,* 1st and 2nd editions.

Donna M. Fletcher, MPA, RHIA, is the manager of data quality for the Child Health Corporation of America (CHCA) in Shawnee Mission, Kansas. At CHCA, Fletcher developed and manages the data quality management program, facilitates member forums, monitors data quality, develops or identifies standardized guidelines, identifies best practices that result in improved data quality, and provides resources to improve data quality. Before joining CHCA in 1999, Fletcher was a professional practice manager at AHIMA providing professional practice support for products and member services including seminars, publications, and video-based training content development. Prior to that, Fletcher served as director of HIM at Wesley Medical Center in Wichita, Kansas, and at the Veterans Affairs Medical Center in Leavenworth, Kansas. Fletcher has 28 years of experience in HIM, has been a contributing author for several AHIMA publications, has published numerous articles in *Journal of AHIMA* and other HIM and information management periodicals, and has chaired several AHIMA national task forces/groups.

Marion K. Gentul, RHIA, CCS, is an independent HIM consultant in Parsippany, New Jersey. She is also an adjunct faculty at Kean University, Union, New Jersey. Previously, she was the director of HIM at Barnert Hospital, Paterson, New Jersey. Gentul has more than 30 years of experience in the HIM industry. She is a past president of the New Jersey HIMA and a recipient of its Distinguished Member award. It was during Gentul's presidency that NJHIMA established a scholarship fund for students enrolled in HIT and HIA programs. In addition to her many years of service to NJHIMA, Gentul has served on the board of the Society for Clinical Coding in chair and co-chair positions. In 1999, Gentul was the recipient of an AHIMA Triumph Award, Mentor.

Cheryl L. Hammen, RHIT, is the vice president of HIM for Community Health Systems, in Brentwood, Tennessee. Hammen has more than 26 years of experience in HIM and has been involved in coding on a national level since 1990. She also has expertise in healthcare compliance, documentation issues, HIM operations, case-mix analysis, and medical staff documentation education. Hammen has contributed to professional healthcare publications including the *Journal of AHIMA* and has addressed national and state HIM conferences. Cheryl served as a member of the American Hospital Association's Editorial Advisory Board for *Coding Clinic for ICD-9-CM* in 1995 and 1996. She also served as a member of the AHIMA Coding Policy and Strategy Committee (1998 and 1999), chair of the AHIMA Compliance Task Force (1999 and 2000), and co-chair of the SCC Data Quality/Compliance Committee (2000 and 2001).

Mia M. Isbell, CPC, CCS-P, ACS-EM, is the HIM supervisor for Texas Oncology in the Bone Marrow Transplant Clinic at Baylor Health Care System, Dallas/Fort Worth Metroplex. She has more than 16 years of experience in HIM including coding and billing compliance issues, training and education, and medical records auditing. Isbell currently is in charge of the HIM coding compliance program for four transplant clinics throughout Texas. Isbell has contributed to internal publications for US Oncology, parent company for Texas Oncology, on various topics ranging from coding to billing and A/R issues. In 2002, Isbell taught medical insurance billing at a local community college in Georgia. Isbell is currently attending Texas State University to finish her bachelor's degree in HIM. Mia has served as a book reviewer for AHIMA publications.

Erica M. Leeds, MIS, RHIA, CCS, CCS-P, is the coordinator for charge integrity and revenue realization for Clarian Health Partners in Indianapolis, Indiana. She has held positions as coding manager, chargemaster consultant, clinical auditor and various other IT roles in her career. She has served on several local and national committees for Society for Clinical Coding, including CCS job analysis and CCS-P expert panel, and has been a speaker at numerous educational workshops. She is a past president of the Indiana and Central Indiana HIMA.

Desla R. Mancilla, MPA, RHIA, is an assistant professor in the HIM program at Texas State University in San Marcos, Texas. She teaches courses in information systems, legal issues, and finance. Prior to joining Texas State University in 2004, Mancilla served as the regional director of information protection services at Community Healthcare System in northwest Indiana. Throughout her career, Mancilla also held the positions of IT staff development manager, EHR project manager, and Y2K project manager. Mancilla served as president and in many other roles for the Indiana HIMA. Additionally, she served on the RHIA Exam Construction Committee, the Virtual Lab Academic Council, and in several other roles throughout her 23-year career as a HIM professional.

Anita Orenstein, RHIT, CCS, has more than 20 years of experience in HIM and 5 years of experience working in a clinical laboratory. Orenstein is currently the corporate HIM compliance coordinator for Intermountain Health Care in Salt Lake City, Utah. She has primary responsibility for oversight of the HIM compliance program including the auditing and monitoring of coding functions and coder education for Intermountain's 20 acute care facilities. Orenstein has served as a member of the Editorial Advisory Board for *Coding Clinic for ICD-9-CM* and has been a contributing author for several AHIMA publications. She has presented numerous audio conferences and seminars and currently serves on AHIMA's Council on Certification as chair-elect.

Ann H. Peden, MBA, RHIA, CCS, is an associate professor of HIM in the School of Health Related Professions at the University of Mississippi Medical Center in Jackson, Mississippi. She currently serves on the Commission on Accreditation for Health Informatics and Information Management Education (CAHIIM), an 11-member commission that accredits health informatics and HIM degree granting programs across the country. Peden's HIM career spans 30 years. Prior to joining the faculty at the University of Mississippi Medical Center, she was director of the Medical Record Department at St. Francis Medical Center in Monroe, Louisiana. She taught for 11 years at Louisiana Tech University, where she also served as assistant director of the medical record administration program and director of the medical record technology program. Peden has been active in national and state HIM organizations throughout her career, including several AHIMA committees. Peden was president of the Louisiana Medical Record Association from 1983–1984, the Northeast Louisiana Medical Record Association from 1987–1988 and the Mississippi HIMA from 1995–1996.

Rita A. Scichilone, MHSA, RHIA, CCS, CCS-P, CHC, is director of clinical data standards for AHIMA. This unit of professional practice provides clinical terminology, clinical data management, and related e-HIM products and services. Before joining AHIMA in 1999, Scichilone served as director of the HIM Consulting Division at Professional Management Midwest. Prior to that, she served in numerous HIM roles, including director of health information services, clinical data manager, HIM program instructor, and medical assistant. Scichilone has authored several books and book chapters, and has conducted presentations for healthcare audiences nationwide. She has participated in various leadership positions throughout her career and has received several distinguished service awards. Scichilone completed a graduate certificate in biomedical informatics and holds a masters degree in health services administration from St. Joseph's College in Windham, Maine; a bachelor of science degree in HIM from the College of St. Mary in Omaha, Nebraska; and a medical assistant diploma from Southeastern Community College in Burlington, Iowa.

AHIMA wishes to acknowledge all of the above authors for their contributions to this work. In addition, AHIMA thanks Joan Usher, RHIA, of JLU Health Record Systems in Pembroke, Massachusetts for her work in editing the home health and hospice sections of chapter 3 of this book.

Preface

The effective management of coding services has never been more crucial to the stability of healthcare organizations than it is today. Healthcare organizations depend on timely and accurate coded data for a variety of reasons. The products of a coding department—coded health data and abstracted medical information—once produced a clinical database for healthcare statistics and research. Although this clinical database, now often combined with financial information, is still valuable, the products of a coding department now supply the healthcare organization with many more resources for making sound business decisions.

Using Codes for Reimbursement

ICD-9-CM and CPT codes are required on all insurance claims submitted to third-party payers. Government payers, including Medicare and Medicaid, use codes to determine actual reimbursement. Other insurance companies use the coded data to determine medical necessity and the benefits covered for each individual patient. Essentially, the coded data determine if and how much the healthcare organization will be paid for its services.

For years, the focus of attention for most coding services has been the inpatient record. Medicare's diagnosis-related groups (DRGs) demanded complete reporting of a patient's diagnoses and procedures, with special emphasis on the principal diagnosis and procedure, in order for a hospital to be paid appropriately. Now more than ever, the outpatient record has taken on new meaning. The demands of Medicare's ambulatory payment classification (APC) reimbursement system have illuminated the importance of complete documentation, coding, and billing for hospital outpatients.

Running on a parallel track with the APC system for outpatient reimbursement is Medicare's medical necessity requirements as defined in local coverage determinations (LCDs). Fiscal intermediaries have been producing LCDs to define Medicare coverage of outpatient services at a feverish rate. The LCDs include lists of diagnoses that define a medically reasonable and necessary diagnosis for the service. This has required a reexamination of the sparse information contained in many outpatient records so that documentation can be improved. The APC system looks at all the services rendered to an outpatient on a single day on a procedure-by-procedure basis. Thus, hospital coders must look at the documentation with a more critical eye.

Using Codes in the Clinical Database

Coded data produce the foundation for an organization's clinical database. Along with the abstracted information collected for each patient, such as physicians' names, dates of services, number of consultations, and special data collected for different patient types, the coded diagnoses and procedures describe what services were rendered. Various departments in a hospital use this information. For example, quality management departments use this information on a daily basis for clinical studies, process improvement of hospital services, and utilization review of services rendered. Endless questions can be asked about a hospital's patient population and services rendered by querying the clinical database, including:

- How many patients were admitted with pneumonia?
- How many patients had the principal diagnosis of respiratory failure?
- What was the most common outpatient surgical procedure for patients over age fifty?
- How many patients had a primary cesarean section?
- How many consultations did Doctor Jones have?
- What are the top ten diagnoses of hospital emergency room visits?

Using Codes for Decision Support

The clinical database becomes a richer information tool when it is combined with the financial information for each patient visit. The merging of clinical and financial data produces a database—commonly referred to as a decision support system—that is used for many business processes. For example, information can be gathered on the cost of hospital services compared to charges and to the actual reimbursement. Financial planners use these data for budgeting and forecasting. Individuals involved with managed care and other insurance contracts can use the clinical and financial information to negotiate payment contracts. The decision support system provides valuable information about the organization's business in both clinical and financial terms.

Managing Coding Services

To support an organization's information needs, clinical coded data must be timely, accurate, complete, and easily accessible. Accomplishing these goals requires effective management of coding services. This involves a coordinated effort between the coding manager and the medical staff, the financial departments, the registration or admitting departments, the information systems department, and the facility's administration.

Role of the Coding Manager in Various Facilities

In a large facility, a dedicated coding manager may direct a staff of a dozen or more coders and clerical support staff. The manager may not actually do coding but, instead, may facilitate communication among departments. He or she also provides support within the health information management (HIM) department that enables coders to perform their tasks with the necessary information for accurate coding. In a medium-size facility, the coding manager may be a supervisor who codes part of the day while maintaining the communication link with other departments. In a small facility with only one or two coders, the HIM department manager assumes the role of coding manager. This manager should keep in touch with coding-related issues and interdepartmental relationships.

Skills Required of Coding Managers

Coding managers need a unique balance of technical, communication, and process improvement skills to manage people, processes, and systems. These skills include the ability to:

- Appreciate the requirements of various coding systems for clear documentation and for adherence to coding guidelines and principles, especially when the manager does not have clinical coding skills

- Support the coding staff with effective recruitment, hiring, mentoring, and counseling

- Assume the role of teacher to keep staff members up to date on new coding issues and requirements

- Work effectively through strong interpersonal communication with people who have an impact on documentation and patient information outside the coding department

- Understand information systems and the transfer of patient care data between software applications by asking:

  —How do ICD-9-CM and CPT codes appear on the insurance claim?

  —What are the system's barriers to data transfer?

- See the big picture of healthcare data across the organization by appreciating the clinical needs of the organization as well as the financial or accounting requirements

Not all coding managers possess all of these skills. For example, one coding manager may have strong technical coding skills, but little understanding of management skills. Another coding manager may have strong management skills but may not understand the complexities of the coding systems and the documentation needed to support coding. The authors and publisher of *Effective Management of Coding Services* hope that coding managers will use the information and ideas presented here to improve their skill levels in all areas necessary to the coding process.

Introducing *Effective Management of Coding Services*

Effective Management of Coding Services, Third Edition, has been expanded to serve as a more detailed resource for coding managers across the continuum of healthcare settings. The book now includes chapters on classifications and terminologies, the uses of coded data in risk adjustment and payment systems, and coding in specialized care settings.

Part I. Scope and Organization of Clinical Coding Data

Part I, chapters 1 through 6, addresses the scope and organization of clinical coding data. Chapter 1 examines the role of the coding professional, identifies the primary resources of a successful HIM department, including qualified staff, and discusses the work process of coding, the importance of the physical setting, and the tools used in the coding function.

Chapter 2 takes a comprehensive look at recruitment, retention, recognition, and reward systems needed to staff a functional coding area. It also examines alternative staffing and work arrangements such as job sharing, telecommuting, and the use of external agencies to support the coding function.

Chapter 3 discusses the unique characteristics and considerations of coding in specialized care environments, such as physician offices, long-term care facilities, and home care and rehabilitation settings. It also addresses nonhospital issues.

Chapter 4 provides a historical perspective of the purposes and functions of coding in healthcare. It gives a general overview of the main coding classifications and terminologies used in today's healthcare environment and discusses current and future code set standards under the Health Insurance Portability and Accountability Act (HIPAA).

Chapter 5 discusses the role of coded data in risk-adjustment and payment systems and explains how coded data are used in the various prospective payment systems for hospital inpatient and outpatient, skilled nursing, home health, and inpatient rehabilitation settings.

Chapter 6 examines the role of the chargemaster in the overall coding process. The implications of the chargemaster, role of the chargemaster coordinator, quality data collection, reimbursement, and the organization of outpatient services are addressed.

Part II. Monitoring for Excellence of Service Delivery

Part II, chapters 7 through 10, examines strategies and techniques for monitoring the delivery of high-quality coding services. Chapter 7 considers performance management and process improvement and addresses the important issue of coding quality versus quantity. The chapter emphasizes the role of the coding manager in working with staff members to develop standards that address both quality and productivity.

Chapter 8 examines quality control issues by offering a plan for designing and implementing a data quality improvement program. The importance of auditing and monitoring the coding of inpatient and outpatient records is reviewed, as well as the use of coding consultants for independent quality review and coding assessment.

The important topic of compliance is addressed in chapter 9. The potential conflict between reimbursement optimization and ethical practices in coding is highlighted, with AHIMA's standards for ethical coding presented as part of a compliance program. The prevention of healthcare fraud and abuse is another focus of this chapter.

Chapter 10 examines reporting issues. This chapter can be used as a vehicle to define:

- The sources of data as they relate to the coding process

- The type of information necessary for creation of reports based on coded data

- How various users throughout the organization need and use clinical coded data

Part III. Financial Implications

Part III, chapters 11 and 12, considers the financial implications of coded data. Chapter 11 defines the links between coding services, the patient accounting department, and other departments within the healthcare organization. The movement away from "silo thinking" toward integrated teamwork is emphasized, with management of the revenue cycle viewed as an interdepartmental effort that emphasizes the good of the larger organization.

Chapter 12 examines the complex subject of case-mix management. Often misunderstood by financial managers, case mix is influenced by coding practices, but not completely driven by coded data. This chapter emphasizes that the coding manager must completely understand how case-mix numbers are determined, to both appreciate their role in the coding process and defend them when they might be inappropriately "blamed" for a case-mix decline.

Part IV. Future Considerations

Part IV, chapter 13, concludes the book. This final chapter examines the changing landscape of the professional coding community and looks ahead to what the future holds for the clinical coding process.

The goal of this book is to equip coding managers with a unique resource that focuses on the effective management of coding services. Whether they are prospective coding managers, new coding managers, or seasoned veterans—whether they have a professional health information background or have come to coding from another clinical healthcare area—this book provides coding managers with information essential to providing high-quality coding services. By taking advantage of the wealth of information supplied here, health information managers can advance their professional skills and contribute to an important organizational objective—the effective management of coding services.

Relevant terminology appears in boldface type in the text and is included in the glossary at the end of the book.

Note to educators: Ancillary materials are available to instructors in online format from the book's Web page in the AHIMA Bookstore or through the Assembly on Education (AOE) Community of Practice (CoP). Instructors who are AHIMA members can sign up for this private community by clicking on the help icon with the CoP home page and requesting additional information on becoming an AOE CoP member. An instructor who is not an AHIMA member or a member who is not an instructor may contact the publisher at publications@ahima.org. to request instructor resources. The instructor materials are not available to students enrolled in college or university programs.

Part I

Scope and Organization of Clinical Coding Data

Chapter 1

Structure and Organization of the Coding Function

Marion K. Gentul, RHIA, CCS
Nadinia A. Davis, MBA, CIA, CPA, RHIA, FAHIMA

Coding practice is the transformation of descriptions of diseases, injuries, conditions, and procedures from words to alphanumeric designations. The purpose of coding in healthcare settings is to use code sets, such as ICD-9-CM, ICD-10-CM, CPT, and Healthcare Current Procedural Coding System (HCPCS), or morphology codes, to classify patient encounters or episodes of care for historical and clinical reference. Additional code sets, such as Systematized Nomenclature of Medicine Clinical Terminology (SNOMED CT) and Logical Observation Identifiers, Names, and Codes (LOINC), link clinical documentation to the electronic health record to facilitate data analysis and interoperability of disparate computer systems. The actual code set used is determined by country, healthcare setting, provider practice, regulatory agency, or reimbursement system. (See chapter 4 for a discussion of coding and classification systems.)

Although the concept of coding is straightforward, the practice of coding is expanding and diversifying in many of today's healthcare environments. This expansion can be attributed to a number of factors, including:

- The increased use of coded data

- Shifts in coding procedures

- Changes in the physical layout of healthcare settings

- The impact of technology

- Major changes in the regulatory environment of healthcare

The coding of clinical data has been a responsibility of health information services since medical librarians established the profession in the early 1900s. For many years, coding has enabled healthcare facilities and associated agencies to tabulate, store, and retrieve disease-, injury-, and procedure-related data. However, coding has taken on increased significance with its linkage to reimbursement. Chapter 4 discusses the various coding services and their relationship to reimbursement. Coders must have a sophisticated understanding of both procedural and diagnostic coding as well as the ability to analyze and interpret patient health data. Further, as the healthcare industry moves to an electronic health record, the roles of coders can be expected to change. With changing roles, one can anticipate the need for different skill sets.

An effective health information service is essential to the success of any healthcare organization. The expertise of credentialed health information management (HIM) professionals is currently in high demand in hospitals and other healthcare institutions. This demand is fueled in part by the increasing emphasis on data quality, both within the organizations and from external forces such as regulatory agencies, accrediting bodies, and payers.

This chapter discusses the role of coding professionals at different levels and recent changes in the practice of coding.

Role of the Coding Professional

Coding professionals are persons who perform the coding function. Their abilities or skill sets can be measured in terms of education, experience, aptitude, quality, and productivity.

Knowledge of the Coding Function

The process of coding may vary among settings; however, the function of assigning codes does not change. Coders take clinical information—diagnostic terms and procedure descriptions—and assign a numeric code to each one according to a set of official guidelines designed to standardize coding. Coders take this clinical information from the physician's or primary caregiver's portion of the health record. The primary caregiver is responsible for providing coders with proper information. Regardless of the healthcare setting, information used to assign codes must be part of the legal health record, not part of an unofficial document such as a surgery log or registration list. In rare circumstances, exceptions to this rule may occur. However, an approved policy and procedure for these exceptions should be available to coders.

Coders must be able to assign codes to all codable information. Sometimes, however, the only information available consists of signs and symptoms. In such instances, coders must know where to look for pertinent clinical information for coding, how to ask the appropriate physician for more information, and how to identify information that is not pertinent.

There is no definitive timeline for learning and mastering coding. One reason for this is that the difficulty of coding between facilities varies significantly. For example, a coder at a community hospital may progress quickly to inpatient coding whereas a coder at a large teaching hospital may perform ambulatory surgery coding for years. Managers in individual facilities should ensure that coding personnel job descriptions accurately reflect the expectations of the facility regarding performance levels. Coder experience can be described in a number of ways. Three possible levels of distinction are entry-level, experienced, and expert.

Entry-Level Coders

Entry-level coders have little or no experience coding and may even have only superficial exposure to the healthcare setting in which they aspire to work. These individuals require significant training, after which they may be assigned limited responsibilities, such as coding only diagnoses in primary care clinics or coding ancillary testing encounters in hospitals or ambulatory care settings.

Many healthcare institutions provide critical on-the-job training for beginning coders. Other institutions rely on academic coding education programs to provide the first level of training. Individuals who have recently completed their coding coursework in a college or technical school program generally test at a beginning level, making them eligible for entry-level coding jobs.

Entry-level coders typically make a significant number of errors and code slowly. This is normal. All of their coding should be audited for accuracy and immediate feedback provided so that they can learn and improve.

Healthcare institutions that are unable to provide on-the-job training and/or close supervision for entry-level coders should seek out and hire experienced coders. It is frequently difficult for entry-level coders to find employment if they lack actual job experience. Job experience varies by institution, ranging anywhere from 6 months to several years. A shortage of qualified coders has been identified, yet many facilities are reluctant to hire new graduates of baccalaureate, associate degree, or coding programs. Smaller facilities and institutions struggling financially often cannot afford the "luxury" of hiring an entry-level coder who needs additional training and cannot quickly meet productivity standards. Thus, an entry-level coder may find it difficult to find employment without experience, but cannot gain employment experience if no one is willing or able to hire them in an entry-level position.

The American Health Information Management Association (AHIMA) has attempted to address this important issue in several ways. In 2005, AHIMA House of Delegates passed a resolution based on a Florida Health Information Management Association proposed resolution: "Bridging the Gap! Education to Employment" (Ellie 2005, AHIMA 2005). The intent of this resolution is "to enhance dialogue and actions to facilitate the employment of graduates from Commission on Accreditation for Health Informatics and Information Management Education (CAHIIM)-accredited HIM programs at the baccalaureate and associate degree levels, and AHIMA-approved coding programs at the predegree level" (appendix 1.1).

Experienced Coders

Once an individual has been coding for some time and has mastered the entry-level coding assignments, progressively more complex work may be assigned. Same-day surgeries and more complex ambulatory coding are logical steps. As the coder becomes more familiar with documentation and coding guidelines, inpatient coding tasks may be introduced—if that is the progression within the facility.

Experienced coders have probably been coding in their area of practice for at least a year. However, a move to another area of practice could put the coder at a lower level in the new area. For example, an experienced ambulatory surgery coder who moves to inpatient coding may be considered an entry-level inpatient coder. Facilities should make such distinctions clear and set specific performance guidelines for all available coding positions.

Experienced ICD-9-CM coders with several years of acute care hospital experience and with a demonstrated mastery skill level probably would be assigned responsibility for coding complex, acute care hospital cases. Such coders might be located physically in a healthcare facility's coding department, remote from the main HIM department, or might work at home if the technology is available to support electronic coding (e-coding) at a remote site. (A discussion of e-coding follows later in this chapter.)

Expert Coders

Expert coders have a demonstrated mastery skill level in their area of practice. They have many years of experience and have achieved a high level of productivity in terms of both accuracy and quantity of coding.

Because the variety of settings that require coding expertise is expanding, candidates for a coding position may be required to demonstrate a mastery skill level in several code sets. For example, a freestanding ambulatory care center or hospital outpatient department may require coding expertise in both ICD-9-CM and CPT coding systems. These facilities must use ICD-9-CM codes for diagnoses and CPT codes for procedures to report the services they provide to patients.

Expert coding professionals sometimes have strong preferences about the types of cases they want to code. Some coders prefer to maintain a high skill level in ICD-9-CM coding and to practice only in acute care hospitals. Although subspecializing may limit their practice options, it allows coders to become true experts in a particular area of coding.

Management of the Coding Function

Ongoing changes in healthcare delivery and reimbursement have brought about corresponding changes in the practice of clinical coding. The coding manager brings stability to this changing environment by structuring and organizing the coding function around certain basic resources. In addition, the coding manager is responsible for organizing the coding process so that documentation can be converted into meaningful data that meet the facility's various needs.

The main resources of a successful HIM department of any size or setting include:

- Qualified staff

- "Tools of the trade" and adequate information systems

- A well-designed physical environment

Qualified Staff

The primary resource in any coding area is qualified staff. Although credentials are not always part of the job description for a coding position, a credentialed coder is usually the most desirable candidate. The person who has earned and maintains a credential demonstrates measurable coding competency. (See chapter 2 for a discussion of credentials and competency.)

The title of **coder** denotes only that the person holding that position is assigned solely or primarily to the function of coding. The volume of work is such that a position has been created to support the coding function. The authors recommend that any extra roles and responsibilities enhance and enrich the coder's practice. Distracting tasks should be avoided whenever possible.

Many coders are "generalists" who are able to assign accurate codes to records across care delivery settings and service lines. Other coders are more specialized. The most common specialties are:

- Inpatient

- Service line

- Outpatient

- Coding/billing

Inpatient Coders

Inpatient coders, as the title implies, code inpatient medical records in an acute care hospital setting. They may be considered "generalists" in that they must be proficient in using ICD-9-CM codes to code all patient diagnoses and procedures that occur at their facility. They are able to communicate with physicians in all specialties. Inpatient coders have an in-depth knowledge of diagnosis-related groups (DRGs) and reimbursement implications, official coding rules, and state and government regulations.

Service-Line Coders

Service-line coders are proficient in all coding areas but excel in one particular service line, such as oncology or cardiology. They code inpatient and/or outpatient accounts for only one particular service line and thus can maintain a high level of coding accuracy. In addition, service-line coders are responsible for maintaining a dialogue with the clinical staff of their specialty regarding documentation issues and yearly coding and reimbursement changes. Service-line coders routinely ensure that appropriate clinical information is recorded in the health record. They often are considered educators to the degree that they communicate with clinical and finance staff regarding coding, documentation, and compliance matters.

Because service-line coders function in a subspecialty unit, they become part of the care management team. Coders who subspecialize are responsible for maintaining their level of expertise for both inpatient and outpatient coding guidelines and for all information regarding proper reporting of the unit's business for purposes of payment. They communicate routinely with patient fiscal services personnel, the coding manager or director, and the medical staff. Answering questions for physicians and nurses, who must continually review their documentation practices to ensure proper recording of patient care, is an important part of the service-line coder's job description. However, coding remains the most important function of this job, no matter how the nuances of the position may vary.

Outpatient Coders

Outpatient coders are responsible for assigning ICD-9-CM and CPT codes to ambulatory surgery or emergency department cases each day. The scope of their work remains in one of these settings and does not cross over into inpatient or physician office settings. In teaching hospitals, an outpatient coder may be responsible for coding **clinic cases** in which patients who are considered outpatients see physicians in a clinic within a teaching environment. The coding of clinic cases could be considered a subspecialty service line in an office-type setting.

Coders/Billers

Coders/billers work in ambulatory care and physician office settings. Generally, they are responsible for processing the **superbill,** or office form, that has been initiated by the physician and states the diagnoses and other information for each patient encounter. Coders/billers take the information about patient encounters and then process claims, or bills, for the patient's insurance company or for patients who self-pay or who choose to submit the claims themselves.

Tools of the Trade

Coding tools include codebooks, groupers, encoders and other software applications, official coding guidelines, dictionaries, texts, and other resource materials as well as Internet access.

Sources of Codes

The type of facility in which a coder works dictates the source of the diagnosis and procedure codes that are assigned. It is imperative that only current code sources be used. Regardless of the setting or the coding system used, an encounter that takes place in 2007 cannot be coded accurately with a 2001 codebook. The following sections contain brief explanations of the current code sources that are available and when they need to be updated. (See table 1.1 for a summary of code sources.) Under the Health Insurance Portability and Accountability Act (HIPAA) of 1996, the medical code set valid at the time healthcare is furnished must be used. The Web sites noted below should be checked frequently for any updates or revisions.

ICD-9-CM

The *International Classification of Diseases, 9th Edition, Clinical Modification* (ICD-9-CM) is currently used to code diagnoses in most settings, such as acute care, long-term care, rehabilitation, and ambulatory care. Volume III of ICD-9-CM is used for the coding of procedures in acute care and in other inpatient settings. Biannual changes in ICD-9-CM codes become effective for discharges after October 1 and April 1, respectively, coinciding with the beginning of the U.S. government's fiscal year and midyear. ICD-9-CM addenda and guidelines can be located online at http://www.cdc.gov/nchs/datawh/ftpserv/ftpicd9/ftpicd9.htm (CDC 2006a).

All coding materials related to ICD-9-CM must be updated biannually so that new and revised codes and descriptions can be assigned correctly on a timely basis. Coding materials can be ordered in advance from a chosen vendor or vendors for delivery and system installation as soon as they are available.

Printed codebooks are available in both updatable ring binder and bound versions. Layout, font size, color, and resources vary significantly among vendors, resulting in definite preferences among individual coders. Unless a significant price difference that materially affects the budget exists between books, coders should be allowed to choose the vendor and format of their choice. Budgets should allow for one book per coder, in addition to at least one book for general office reference.

Some coders prefer to own and maintain their own coding materials. This is an acceptable practice; however, coding managers must ensure that correct versions are always being used. For in-house coders, visual examination is sufficient. Offsite coders may need to sign a compliance statement periodically.

HCPCS

The *Healthcare Current Procedural Coding System* (HCPCS) is a two-tiered system of procedural codes used primarily for ambulatory care and physician services. A third tier, pertaining to codes developed by local payers, was eliminated as of December 31, 2003, in compliance with HIPAA standard procedure code requirements. HCPCS codes also are frequently attached

Table 1.1. Summary of code sources

Codes	Description	Uses	Updated	Maintained by
ICD-9-CM	Three volumes: Volumes 1 and 2: Diagnosis Tabular and Index Volume 3: Procedures	All diagnosis coding Procedure coding in inpatient settings	Semiannually Effective for discharges after October 1 and April 1	Cooperating Parties: CMS NCHS AHA AHIMA
CPT	Procedures and other services performed by or under the direction of physicians	Procedure coding in ambulatory settings; capturing charges in inpatient settings	Annually Effective for encounters after January 1	AMA
HCPCS	Procedures, services, supplies, and durable medical equipment	Procedure coding and capturing charge	Annually	CMS

to inpatient and outpatient charge description masters (CDMs) for convenience and to facilitate communication between providers and payers about services and supplies included in the CPT or HCPCS Level II system. (See chapter 6 for a detailed discussion of the CDM.)

Level I of CPT, developed and maintained by the American Medical Association (AMA), is the first level of the HCPCS coding system. CPT is a nomenclature designed to standardize communication between physicians and payers. It is used primarily for claims processing purposes for physician services and for reporting ambulatory care services. The primary focus of CPT is to describe to the payer the physician's care of the patient. When used for facility reporting, CPT reflects facility services rather than the physician's professional services.

The AMA updates CPT annually, with most codes effective January 1 each year. Although the Centers for Medicare and Medicaid Services (CMS) and other payers generally allow a 3-month grace period to implement new and revised CPT codes, facilities are nevertheless advised to obtain updated versions of the codes and to orient coding staff to them as soon as possible. Some CPT codes may be released with an effective date other than January 1.

Printed codebooks for CPT, like those for ICD-9-CM, can vary somewhat in their features and formats. Comments about coder preferences apply here as well. The budget should include a CPT codebook for every coder who is responsible for outpatient coding, and an additional book for general office reference. CPT errata and updates can be found at http://www.ama-assn.org/ama/pub/category/3884.html (AMA 1995-2006).

Level II codes are applicable to selected physician and nonphysician services, durable medical goods, drugs, and supplies. These codes, developed and maintained by CMS, the Blue Cross and Blue Shield Association (BCBSA), and the Health Insurance Association of America (HIAA), are updated as needed—currently, each quarter. The updates become effective when announced. Level II codes are used primarily for reporting purposes in ambulatory care for claims processing. Although many insurance plans recognize HCPCS Level II codes, the possibility exists that selected plans will reject these codes. HCPCS Level II updates can be found at http://www.cms.hhs.gov/medicare/hcpcs (CMS 2005a).

Groupers

In the acute care setting, two main types of Medicare grouping programs are used: DRGs for inpatient cases and ambulatory payment classifications (APCs) for outpatient cases. **Grouping** refers to a system of assigning patients to a classification scheme (DRG or APC) via a computer software program called a **grouper.** Normally, such a program is purchased from a vendor by a facility's information systems (IS) department.

In addition to Medicare, selected payers may adopt other grouping programs for non-Medicare inpatients. Other grouping programs may or may not use the same relative weights as the Medicare (CMS) grouper. The use of other grouping programs for non-Medicare patients varies from state to state. For example, New York and New Jersey use a DRG grouper distinct from the Medicare (CMS) grouper for non-Medicare cases.

DRGs and APCs: Similarities and Differences

The grouper systems for DRGs and APCs are both driven by coded data. Patient admissions or encounters are classified using grouping methodologies. Payments are weighted in both systems. The **weight** is the numeric assignment that is part of the formula by which a specific dollar amount, or reimbursement, is calculated for each DRG or APC. The principal difference between DRGs and APCs is that whereas one DRG is assigned for each inpatient admission, an outpatient encounter may be assigned one or more APCs. (See chapter 5 for additional discussion.)

Groupers and Diagnosis-Related Groups

DRGs are used for hospital inpatient reimbursement. In 1983, Congress amended the Social Security Act to include a national DRG-based hospital prospective payment system (PPS) for all Medicare acute care inpatients. CMS oversees this program. Acute care facilities are reimbursed for inpatient Medicare cases according to the DRG category to which each case is assigned by the CMS grouper.

Under a contract with CMS, 3M Health Information Systems has performed all annual updates or revisions to the Medicare DRG grouper. Each revision is called a grouper version. The revisions are necessary because biannual changes are made in ICD-9-CM and to the grouper itself. For example, version 23.0 was the grouper version effective from October 1, 2005, to September 30, 2006. Upcoming changes to the DRG grouper are published biannually in the *Federal Register* several months in advance of the effective date, so changes effective in October, for example, are typically published in final form the preceding August.

From a coding management standpoint, inpatient cases of patients discharged on October 1 must be grouped using the new grouper version. The HIM department should be in communication with the IS department to verify that the necessary software updates have been made by the time cases are to be entered into the facility's coding/abstracting system. Testing of some cases in which changes have been made may be necessary to verify that the updated software is functioning properly. Regarding systems updates, the coding manager may work closely with IS staff. At a minimum, the installation process and deadlines must be communicated. Additionally, the coding manager may "test" updates prior to the system going "live" in order to determine what, if any, changes should be communicated to the coding staff. For example, software changes or enhancements should be imparted to the coding staff to avoid data-entry errors and provide awareness of enhancements that may improve coding accuracy.

Even though grouper versions change yearly, historical data reflect the grouper version assigned at any given time. New DRGs have been added and others have been deleted over time. To ensure that year-to-year DRG comparisons are valid, the definitions manual of each grouper version may be used. Essentially, this manual is a printout of all data elements contained within each DRG.

Groupers and Ambulatory Payment Classifications

APCs are used in the outpatient prospective payment system (OPPS). Although facilities are reimbursed for each inpatient admission under DRGs, they are reimbursed for each patient encounter under APCs.

As with DRGs, CMS oversees APCs and OPPS. 3M Health Information Systems, under a contract with CMS, provides the APC grouper and updates. The initial final regulations for OPPS and APCs can be found in the *Federal Register* (OIG 2000). CMS has devoted a special section of its Web site to OPPS at http://www.cms.hhs.gov/providers/hopps/ (CMS 2006c). Coding managers should review this Web site periodically because it includes OPPS updates, corrections, frequently asked questions (FAQs), pricer logic, outpatient code editor (OCE) specifications and revisions, and program memoranda. The Web site also contains the Medicare OPPS training manual. Many excellent publications that focus on code selection and the impact of APC implementation on the HIM department are available from vendors.

Groupers and Other Prospective Payment Systems

The administration of other PPSs and the role of HIM personnel vary widely by type of facility. For example, in long-term care facilities, coded data are not the primary determinant of Medicare reimbursement. However, regardless of the HIM setting or the PPS under which it operates, groupers must be updated and tested by the effective dates. Likewise, personnel must be informed about any changes in the grouper and the impact those changes may have on coding practices and reimbursements to the facility.

Computer-Based Coding Sources

Printed coding materials are rapidly being supplemented with, or replaced by, computer-based coding sources. These sources include both simple code look-up software and comprehensive encoders.

Code Look-up Software

A **code look-up** is a computer file with all of the indexes and codes. Each record in the file may contain as few as two fields, one listing the code and the other listing the description. Because a coder still must search the index for the correct code and then verify it in the tabular section of the system, the code look-up is not an efficient application for routine coding. However, when used as accessory files to applications in which the code is already known, code look-ups can be used to fill in code description text. For example, when a coder enters a code into the hospital database, the computer accesses the look-up file in order to match the code with its description. This use of the look-up file allows code descriptions to be included in reports without the user having to type out the description manually. Moreover, look-up files may be useful for viewing historical data, particularly when old codes are no longer valid or their description has changed. A look-up file for the year in question would clarify the data.

Encoder Software

An encoder is a software program that enables the coder to assign codes based on using text typed into a look-up screen—analogous to the coder looking up a term in the index of the printed codebook. When the term is entered into the encoder look-up, the coder is given a selection of codes from which to choose. This corresponds to the coder referring to a code in the tabular section of the printed codebook. Encoders can also search on the code. This is useful for verifying a known code or looking up a particular description.

Encoding software products differ in the way they assist with the coding process. The primary application of encoding software is to assign diagnosis and procedure codes to hospital inpatient and ambulatory surgery records through computerization. Therefore, an encoder always contains ICD-9-CM codes and should contain HCPCS/CPT codes required for all types of reporting. To facilitate ambulatory surgery procedure coding, a software crosswalk may exist between the chosen ICD-9-CM code and the CPT codes. Because a one-to-one match does not always exist between the two code sets, the crosswalk may produce a selection of CPT codes from which the coder must choose.

Some types of encoders operate in the same way that codebooks do by merely supplanting the Volume 2 and Volume 3 indexes with a computer search and look-up. However, because the ICD-9-CM indexes also have embedded coding conventions and rules, a logic-based encoder may be designed to prompt the coder to answer certain questions before returning a response. For example:

> The keyword "hypertension" in the ICD-9-CM codebook leads to a table of possible codes, including certain comorbid conditions associated with hypertension. The encoder would return a question such as: Is the hypertension benign, malignant, or unspecified? The encoder may stop there and return the appropriate code from category 401. Some encoders may take the search further and ask for certain potentially related conditions, such as heart failure or renal failure, and whether the physician has specified a connection between the hypertension and these conditions. Upon coder input, the encoder would return the appropriate code.

Such encoder–coder interaction using software assistance leads some managers to believe that inexperienced or entry-level coders can function at a higher level than would ordinarily be indicated by their training and experience. Certainly, inexperienced coders may be able to look up codes quickly and prompts may remind them of nuances among codes, but unless the coders have been properly and thoroughly trained in coding guidelines, terminology, disease processes, and coding conventions, errors can occur during the encoder–coder interaction. Inexperienced coders may respond erroneously to encoder prompts and will not be assisted using encoders without a knowledge database. Thus, encoders do not replace coders with comprehensive coding education, experience, and analytical skills.

Use of encoder software offers a number of advantages. The following is an example:

A health record indicates that the patient has "arteriovenous (A-V) malformation of the intestines." The coder is not familiar with "A-V malformation." The codebook index does not specifically list this term in the alphabetic index. "Malformation" does not have a subterm for either "arterio" or "venous." Even creative searching leads only to congenital codes. Before proceeding to code this diagnosis, the coder obtains a medical dictionary to find out the definition of "A-V malformation." Unsuccessful in this pursuit, the coder turns to *Coding Clinic.* While searching *Coding Clinic,* the coder finds a reference that links A-V malformation to angiodysplasia and gives the correct code. Only then is the coder able to proceed with the code selection. This scenario occurs often enough that productivity can be dramatically affected for a coder encountering this type of problem for the first time.

In this scenario, an encoder with built-in resource references allows the coder to look up the definition within the computer program. In addition, most encoding software contains references the coder can access with just a keystroke or mouse click. Some references are: *Coding Clinic, CPT Assistant,* a CPT/ICD-9-CM Volume III crosswalk, a medical dictionary, a pharmacology reference, an anatomy and physiology reference, laboratory value resources, National Correct Coding Initiative (NCCI) edits, and reimbursement weights. The ability to access these references seamlessly within the encoding process makes encoding software a valuable tool. Even experienced, book-oriented coders can appreciate the convenience, accuracy, and productivity gains these resources can generate. In addition to these obvious procedural advantages, encoders contain validity edits and other edits to help coders decide whether certain codes are correct or whether reporting requirements have been met. For example, an encoder can prevent the code for uncomplicated childbirth (650) from being assigned accidentally to a male patient's hospitalization for benign prostatic hypertrophy (600.00).

Finally, an encoder almost always contains grouper capability. Some encoders may include only the federal (Medicare) grouper. However, in many states encoders provide multiple groupers that are specific to payer and time period. An encoder with this capability enables coders to compare selected cases between groupers by year or by version numbers. This is a useful tool for retrospective audits. Encoders and groupers also are used together to apply existing payer edits to a case and to show the impact on reimbursement prior to claims submission.

Some experienced coders find that using an encoder is slower than doing manual coding because they rely on their book-based notes and memory to code quickly. A significant disadvantage occurs when the encoder does not link to the hospital claims management/financial database. When the encoder is linked to the hospital database, codes can simply be entered, grouped, and examined as usual. Without this capability, the information must be entered twice—first to the encoder and then to the hospital indexing or claims management/financial database.

Yet another disadvantage to using encoders is that the software system must be updated at least quarterly to keep current with *Coding Clinic* and *CPT Assistant,* as well as ICD-9-CM and

CPT code updates and grouper updates. The coding of records discharged around scheduled code changes should be monitored carefully to ensure that the appropriate versions of code sets and groupers are being used. Coding managers should ensure that encoder vendors are obligated contractually to provide and install timely updates. In many facilities, the IS department oversees this process when a vendor is selected. The coding manager may want a copy of contractual obligations so that expectations are clearly defined and workflow can be planned.

Authoritative Coding References

Official coding guidelines and requirements, code changes, clarifications and interpretations of rules, edits, and other authoritative coding references come from the **Cooperating Parties for ICD-9-CM,** which is maintained and updated biannually by the Cooperating Parties. The Cooperating Parties are the American Hospital Association (AHA), CMS, AHIMA, and the National Committee on Vital and Health Statistics (NCVHS). The Coordination and Maintenance Committee of the Cooperating Parties meets in public forum semiannually to suggest, discuss, and recommend potential changes to ICD-9-CM codes. Detailed information on the recommendations and discussions can be found at http://www.cdc.gov/nchs/about/otheract/icd9/maint/maint.htm (CDC 2006b). AHIMA posts summaries of the proceedings at http://www.ahima.org/dc.

AHA/Coding Clinic

The AHA is responsible for issuing official advice via an editorial advisory board on behalf of the Cooperating Parties. Responses to coding questions posed by practitioners are published quarterly in *Coding Clinic for ICD-9-CM*. Individuals should send each coding question with as much clinical detail as possible. No patient or practitioner identifiers should remain on any of the documents submitted. At this time, questions may be sent to: American Hospital Association, ICD-9-CM Central Office, 1 N. Franklin Street, Chicago, IL 60606. It should be noted that a published response to a question requiring consideration by the ICD-9-CM Coordination and Maintenance Committee might not appear in *Coding Clinic* for many months, if at all.

Coding Clinic is the primary, authoritative reference for official coding guidelines pertaining to ICD-9-CM. It is available by subscription through the AHA by calling 1-800-261-6246. *Coding Clinic* is accessible in print, CD-ROM, and computerized formats. As previously mentioned, some encoders include *Coding Clinic* references with their packages.

CMS/Federal Register

Much of the authority for the universal application in the United States of rules pertaining to the use of the ICD-9-CM coding system comes from the federal government. CMS has adopted the ICD-9-CM codes and their associated rules as the official method of communicating inpatient diagnostic and procedural data between providers and Medicare/Medicaid agencies. Because CMS is a federal agency, coding and DRG changes are published in the *Federal Register.* Changes effective in October are published as proposed in May. Comments are accepted through July. Final changes appear in the *Federal Register* in August. Since 2005, changes take place biannually, effective October 1—the beginning of the federal fiscal year—and at midyear, April 1. However, while coding changes are possible twice a year, April 1 changes did not occur in either 2005 or 2006.

AMA/CPT Assistant

The AMA maintains the CPT nomenclature system and publishes *CPT Assistant,* a monthly publication that communicates CPT guidelines and changes and that addresses CPT coding questions.

CPT Assistant is available by subscription by calling 1-800-634-6922. A full listing of AMA products and services is available on the AMA Web site at https://catalog.ama-assn.org/Catalog/.

Other CPT Sources

HCPCS coding guidelines or conventions may be payer specific and found in payer manuals; however, the CMS Web site (http://www.cms.gov/) contains useful information concerning HCPCS codes. Most Medicare and Medicaid manuals are available on this Web site for downloading.

The NCCI is a set of edits to be applied to CPT codes for physician services and outpatient hospital claims. These edits were created by CMS in anticipation of the APC system and for use by intermediaries and carriers in Medicare Part B claims processing. *The NCCI Coding Policy Manual for Part B Medicare Carriers* can be purchased through the National Technical Information Service (NTIS) by calling 1-800-363-2068. The NTIS Web site can be accessed at http://www.ntis.gov/. The NCCI edits for hospital outpatients are included in the outpatient code editor (OCE).

Other "Drivers" of Coding

The official coding and reporting guidelines contain the authoritative coding rules that all coders must follow. However, third-party payers and some states also issue reporting guidelines and data collection requirements. These guidelines and requirements can create conflicts and present challenges for practitioners.

Third-Party Payer Requirements

In theory, third-party payers should conform to official coding guidelines and requirements for ICD-9-CM, as promulgated by the Cooperating Parties, or to the AMA's guidelines for use of CPT. For reimbursement by CMS, such confirmation is a requirement of HIPAA as part of the designated code sets. However, in practice, situations sometimes require that a facility or physician assign codes according to a third-party payer's reporting guidelines so that the facility is reimbursed appropriately for services. Occasions arise in which third-party payer guidelines appear to be—or are—in conflict with official coding guidelines.

Third-party payers do not necessarily provide their guidelines in writing. Often the only way a practitioner or coding manager can find out what is required is to review all claims **rejections** and directly contact the third-party payer or insurance plan administrator regarding a specific case. When contacting the payer, the coding manager should document the conversation. If there is still disagreement with the payer's guidelines, the coding manager should include a copy of the official coding guideline that supports the facility's position in the document. This document can be placed in the billing folder or in a comment field somewhere in the patient accounts section of the computer system. Before sending a copy of the document and attachments to the payer, the coding manager should discuss the situation with the patient accounts manager, practice manager, or whoever is most appropriate. In that way, the facility's administration is aware of the disagreement and the reason for any resultant delay in reimbursement.

Essentially, the goals are to code cases properly and still get paid; however, both goals may not always be possible to achieve. The coding manager, in conjunction with the patient accounts manager, should develop a written policy for handling situations in which a payer's coding instructions are in direct conflict with official coding guidelines.

Sometimes a facility determines that the more important goal is to be paid. The coding manager then should keep a record of those cases in which coding may have been compromised and what are believed to be the correct codes. In essence, the coding manager creates a separate database. This database may be necessary to track certain diagnoses or procedures in the future. Such a database also may serve as a reference should the third-party payer ever change its guidelines—the facility might be able to resubmit the cases and possibly recoup payment. Maintaining this separate database also demonstrates an effort by the facility to remain in compliance with official coding guidelines.

Another problematic issue in facilities is the debate over correct code assignment between coders and clinical personnel. With increasing emphasis on reimbursement, there is increasing oversight and a tendency for second-guessing the coder's decision, particularly in the matter of assigning a principal diagnosis. Although many clinicians and other quality-oriented personnel understand the treatment and documentation very well, they are not always thoroughly versed in coding guidelines. There is no simple resolution to such debates. As long as the coder can support the selected codes, based on authoritative coding guidelines, any controversies should be minimized. If the HIM department is experiencing a burdensome number of internal challenges to accurate, well-supported coded data, this may signal an opportunity to provide education to the other parties involved. In any event, policies and procedures should be in place to document and respond to such internal debates.

State-Specific Requirements

Some states have developed their own data collection requirements in addition to the minimum requirements set forth by CMS. For example, New Jersey requires the collection of "Z codes" to describe the physical location at which a traumatic injury occurred (at home, at work, in a public place, and so forth). Such data collection issues pose challenges to practitioners, who often must be extremely creative in devising an appropriate field in which to capture the data without having to recreate the entire patient database.

When finding "space" for the newly required data, practitioners should not compromise the depth of the diagnosis and procedure data being collected. Many older systems do not allow the capture of more than the maximum number of codes allowed (currently nine diagnosis and six procedure codes) on the standard Medicare billing form—the UB-92 (form CMS 1450). Currently, fields (form locators [FLs]) are available on the UB-92 for nine discharge diagnoses (one principal [FL67] and eight secondary [FL 68–75]), one admitting diagnosis (FL76), and six procedure codes (one principal [FL80] and five secondary [FL81]). Insertion of a code other than an appropriate diagnostic or procedure code into one of those fields can have a negative impact on the clinical database. Therefore, practitioners should make every effort to identify and effectively utilize another area of the database.

The National Uniform Billing Committee (NUBC) is in the process of updating the UB-92. The new form, UB-04, will retain the CMS 1450 designation. The new version will contain expanded diagnosis fields (18 as opposed to 9) and is designed to accommodate ICD-10 codes. Beginning March 1, 2007, healthcare providers (hospitals, skilled nursing facilities, hospice institutions, and other institutional claim filers) will begin transitioning from the UB-92 billing form to the UB-04. Effective May 23, 2007, all claims must be submitted using the UB-04 (CMS 2005b; NUBC 2005).

Facility-Based Coding Guidelines

The purpose of facility guidelines is to ensure accurate, uniform coding within the facility. Facility guidelines should supplement and support, but never contradict, official guidelines. Facility guidelines may be organized alphabetically, chronologically, or by topic or clinical service. Regardless of the method of organization, it is imperative that the guidelines begin with an index so that they can be referenced quickly and accurately.

All coding guidelines must be freely accessible to the coding staff and physicians to whom they apply. In situations where coders are not located in close proximity to one another, multiple copies of guidelines may be necessary or online copies may be placed on the encoding system or on the facility's intranet. Particular care must be taken to ensure that all copies of coding guidelines are complete and updated on a timely basis. Whenever a guideline is updated, all coders must be informed about the new procedure.

Clinical Guidelines

In addition to official guidelines, coding professionals benefit from guidance provided by physicians at an organizational level. Within the enterprise, selected practices may be standardized to assist in appropriate code selection for specified events.

It is inappropriate for coders to define clinical parameters for applying codes. Such a process would lead to inconsistency in coding and lack of comparability across data sources. *Coding Clinic* clearly states that in the absence of specific physician documentation to confirm code selection, a query must be made to the physician to validate code choices. However, because clinical practice for selected circumstances does not vary from physician to physician or patient to patient, clinical services within the enterprise may be called on to define or establish parameters that guide proper medical record documentation and resulting code selection. These guidelines must be clear, written, and universally applicable across the facility and must not contradict official coding guidelines.

Within a specific clinical service, defined protocols and care plans codify best practices in that service. For example, an insulin-dependent diabetes mellitus patient may be on a sliding scale insulin regimen to manage blood sugar effectively. The patient's blood sugar may be under control with this prescription. However, if the blood sugar for this patient is markedly high, even under this prescription, the condition may be considered "uncontrolled" for the purpose of code selection. A coding professional cannot decide from laboratory findings that the patient's diabetes is "out of control" and assign that code. However, if the hospital's endocrinology department has an established care plan that defines "two sequential blood sugars over 600 mg/dL" as uncontrolled, the protocol for coding would require the coder to query the physician to confirm the diagnosis so that the qualifier "uncontrolled" could be added to the resulting code set. Facility policy should describe how this additional information is incorporated in the medical record. Other common facility guidelines address postoperative blood loss anemia and hypokalemia. Best practice dictates that all conditions reported be reflected clearly in physician documentation in the medical record.

Operational Guidelines

In addition to clinical guidelines, certain operational guidelines are essential for uniform coding. For example, operational guidelines may address how and when to code blood transfusions, diagnostic radiology, and other procedures. Most inpatient facilities do not code routine chest x-rays using ICD-9-CM Volume III codes. Some inpatient facilities do not use ICD-9-CM Volume III to code any diagnostic radiology except CT scans and MRIs. Because these procedures rarely affect inpatient reimbursement, they are ignored for coding purposes in favor of invasive procedures.

Although there is space for 18 discharge diagnosis codes and six procedure codes on the UB-04, many systems allow more codes to be captured. Does the facility want the coder to continue adding codes in the system beyond UB maximum? Should the coder stop at other numbers, for example, 20 or 25, or continue coding ad infinitum? Consideration in reaching such a decision may rest on productivity concerns and the realistic use of coded data beyond the codes that appear on the UB-04 or those that are reported to outside entities.

Situations in which a system is limited to nine diagnoses and six procedures also must be considered. If significant or required diagnosis codes must be captured, how does the coder determine that? Should all diagnosis codes that are complication/comorbidity (CC) codes be given precedence over other codes for conditions relevant to the encounter? What if there are still more CC codes beyond the nine? Encoder/grouper software typically assists the coder by resequencing CC codes. However, that function is helpful only when the codes have already been entered into the computer. How does the coder determine which codes to capture? The answers to these decisions may lie in the type of service (medical or surgical) in which the patient is receiving treatment.

Another consideration is what data are truly useful to the facility. For example, a cancer institute may want all cancer cases reported, even though not all cancer codes are CCs. Certainly, however, a coder would not leave off a CC code if doing so would affect DRG assignment.

Leaving off a procedure code also could affect DRG assignment, so care must be taken to ensure that such a code does appear on the UB-04 claim form via the system. In cases of multiple surgeries, which often are entered chronologically, a procedure code beyond the system capabilities may be one that affects the DRG.

Because it is virtually impossible for a coder to mentally group these usually difficult and complicated cases, the coder will have to enter codes in a "test" mode and ensure that the correct codes are entered for the appropriate DRG prior to "finalizing" that account.

Supplementary Materials

A variety of additional materials exist that are helpful to the coding staff. Suggested minimum resources include the following:

- Official coding guidelines: For any resource, the quality of the source should be considered. Wherever possible, the original resource is preferable to a derivative. Official guidelines and related publications must be provided to all coding staff.

- Grouper guides: Although the computer routinely performs grouping, the coding department may find it useful to maintain a copy of the appropriate definitions manuals to resolve audit issues and to educate coders when questions arise as to grouping for a particular case.

- Terminology references: Because no coding source contains every possible variation of every term, a recent edition of a medical dictionary is necessary. Moreover, a good medical dictionary is useful when physicians refer to diseases using eponyms, which may not be found in the coding source. Because new terms arise constantly, a medical dictionary should be replaced about every 5 years. *Stedman's* and *Taber's* are both excellent medical dictionaries.

- Anatomy and physiology references: Although many coding sources now include basic anatomic diagrams, coders may encounter unfamiliar or detailed anatomy terms in health records. Unless the coding source specifically identifies the term, the coder may not be able to identify the correct anatomical site from the health record or the coding source. Therefore, an anatomy and physiology text can be useful. Again, this is not an annual expense. Replacement every 5 to 7 years is probably sufficient.

- Pathology references: Although not specifically a coding reference, a good pathophysiology book, such as the *Merck Manual,* can be helpful to a coder in framing a question to a physician.

- Pharmacology references: Part of the coder's analysis of any health record involves review of the physician's orders to determine what conditions are being treated. Coders quickly become familiar with the hospital's formulary; however, new drugs and generic drug names often make matching the drugs with the patient's conditions difficult. Therefore, a high-quality pharmacology reference is very useful. This reference book should be replaced at least biannually. Sometimes a facility's medical library or pharmacy department orders a new one every year. If so, the older reference book may be recycled into the HIM department.

- Diagnostic test reference: Another key analysis performed by the coder is the review of diagnostic testing. A reference that explains laboratory, radiology, and other diagnostic procedures can help with this process. A good reference will highlight the implications of results that are not within normal limits.

- Encoders often come with some or all of these reference materials, although often at additional cost. The HIM department should be involved in any decision making regarding such an additional purchase. The ease and reliability of accessing this material can improve productivity and coding accuracy and eliminate the purchase of hard-cover books, which can help to justify the costs.

Computer Access

As may be inferred from the preceding discussion, a computer is one of the key tools that should be on a coder's desk. Not only is the computer essential for encoding and grouping, but it also can facilitate coder activity, enrich the coder's job, optimize workflow, and encourage continuing education and research.

Clinical Data

Because more clinical data are captured and stored online, coders can access these data online and complete the coding process as soon as the information becomes available. Coders need not wait for paper copies to follow the record.

Patient History

As more data become available online, the coder's understanding of patients' clinical situations will be facilitated. All coding of patient encounters or discharges must be based on the documentation that pertains to particular visits or events. The coder cannot use prior documentation to "fill in the gaps" when current health records are incomplete. Nevertheless, access to prior records can help the coder frame a query to a physician or better understand existing documentation.

Administrative Data

Often coders are required to abstract specific data from the patient record in order to update the admission or discharge record online. Although the coder could perform this task, data-entry personnel could perform it more economically.

Internet Access

Internet access is a necessary tool for coding professionals because it provides research tools, resources, and the opportunity for continuing education from other sources. If coders do not have access to the Internet within the HIM department, access is often available in the medical staff library or other hospital locations. At a minimum, the coding manager should have Internet access. Coding staff may forward research questions to the coding manager.

With implementation of the AHIMA Communities of Practice (CoP), coders have the opportunity to reach other coders to discuss coding questions, procedural issues, best practices, coding guidelines, and other topics of interest. In addition, the AHIMA Web site provides Internet links, libraries of documentation, continuing education, and other useful research tools for coders.

However, the following negative aspects to Internet access have been identified:

- Unauthorized personal use of Internet access

- Excessive time spent posting unnecessary or non–job-related questions

- Potential inappropriate release of information

- Interruptions in service or system "downtime"

These issues must be addressed before access is provided to coders. Clear policies and procedures (appendix 1.2), effective supervision of personnel, and strong confidentiality statements (appendix 1.3) can limit the negative aspects of Internet access. Apart from the Internet, personnel should not have games or other non–work-related software, such as photo albums, on their personal computers.

Internal E-mail Access

Internal e-mail access can be very useful for communication among coders who work different shifts or at different locations for the same enterprise or system. User groups as well as informational files, policies, and procedures can be set up that can be accessed and updated or viewed by coder participants only.

Physical Environment

The location of the department or division responsible for coding and the location of its coders are important considerations in terms of access to information and productivity.

The location of the HIM department in a facility may not be negotiable. However, it can have a positive or a negative impact on the coding process because coders must have access to sources of information that are not always available within the department or in the health record. Sources of information include physicians, the Internet, and other departments. The types of information needed from these sources include:

- Clarification of documentation within the health record

- Research material, including disease processes and coding regulations

- Source documents (for example, pathology reports) that are not present in the health record at the time of coding but are needed for coding and are not available from the facilities system

Contact with Physicians

When the HIM department is located in a remote area, physicians may be unable or less inclined to visit and respond to coding questions. In such a situation, the coder must meet the physician on the patient unit or in some other, more convenient area.

Although physicians may be contacted by phone to clarify documentation, both documentation and coding are most accurate when physicians review the health records face-to-face with coders. At the time of the review and discussion, the physician should be asked to add or modify documentation in the record. Codes should be modified, changed, or deleted only after—or when—the physician documents in the medical record.

Contact with Other Departments

Because reports necessary for coding are often unavailable at the time the health record is being coded, they must be accessed online or obtained from the appropriate department. Such reports can include pathology reports, laboratory reports, and dictation. Retrieval of the reports can be handled easily by clerical personnel rather than by coders because discussion of the content of the reports is unnecessary. Collection procedures for these reports should be evaluated for cost-effectiveness.

Coding Staff Location within the HIM Department

Ideally, coders' work areas should be apart from the rest of the staff and away from high-traffic areas. In that way, coders can concentrate with a minimum of noise and distractions. Noise from copy machines, overhead pagers, telephones, moving files, radios, and other staff who must perform their functions while talking can be detrimental to productivity and coding accuracy.

Workstation Considerations

Coding workstations should be ergonomically correct and in compliance with the standards and requirements of the U.S. Department of Labor, Occupational Safety and Health Administration (OSHA). Additional information can be obtained from the OSHA Web site at http://www.osha-slc.gov/ergonomics-standard/index.html (OSHA n.d.).

Lighting Issues

Because the coding activity is based on reading, proper lighting is essential to prevent fatigue and eyestrain. Overhead ceiling lights are often inadequate for reading, so coders should have desk lamps that evenly distribute light in the work area. Bar lighting affixed to the bottom of cubicle shelves is one way to provide an even distribution of light. Moreover, an inexpensive glare shield positioned in front of the computer screen can minimize glare.

Space and Ergonomic Issues

Workspace requirements will vary depending on whether coding is performed from a paper record or scanned/electronic record. The workspace must be large enough to accommodate computers, books, keyboards, and open paper files of health records. Desks manufactured prior to the general use of computers in the workplace probably will be inadequate. Even in a "paperless" environment, coders currently are required to code from a paper record because of the hybrid nature of most facility's records.

Whenever possible, the coding manager should involve the coding staff in the process of selecting new workstations. Coders are able to provide input that only the persons who perform the tasks every day can give. Thus, the coding manager may avoid costly mistakes by obtaining staff input.

When designing or purchasing new workstations, coding managers should consider the following points with regard to space and ergonomics:

- Desk space is needed for one open health record, a stack of health records, a computer with monitor, a keyboard, and a mouse. Prior to any purchase, these items should be measured and arranged in the work configuration for each individual.

- If some or all of the coders are not currently using computers, the workstation plan should allow for the use of computers by all coding staff in the near future.

- Chairs are of critical importance for coders, who are required to sit most of the day. Although they are expensive, high-quality chairs with adjustable height, back, and tension configurations are a good investment. Chairs should have wheels and be able to swivel. Chairs with arms are probably unnecessary because arms would be in the way for most coding operations.

- Other considerations that can improve coder productivity and reduce downtime include the following:

  —A left-handed mouse for left-handed coders

  —Special access requirements

  —Products designed to prevent carpal tunnel syndrome

  —Overhead shelving with at least one shelf that can be reached from a sitting position

Shared Workstations

At times, coders share workstations. If possible, each individual should be assigned a drawer and a shelf to ensure the security of personal items and to provide a sense of individual space. In shared areas, coders should limit the number of personal items displayed. Coworkers who share space should leave the work area neat and clean for the next person. This is true whether the work area is shared among employees, outsource personnel, or reviewers.

Organization of the Workflow: Job Analysis

An advantage of remote or home-based coding is that workspace issues may be greatly minimized or even eliminated. Remote coders do not have to share workspace or work different shifts. Each job in the HIM department should be analyzed to ensure that appropriate personnel are performing the tasks and that the flow of work is optimized. Clearly, in a paper-based environment, staff members find the shifting of records from one side of the room to another to be time-consuming and enervating. Optimum workflow, therefore, depends not only on the efficient sequence of record-processing functions, but also on the physical location in which these functions are performed. Although a general discussion of HIM department workflow is outside the scope of this book, the following discussion includes the steps in the process that have an impact on coders, whether the coder is based in the HIM department or remotely, and whether or not the medical record is paper-based, or in a scanned or electronic format.

Availability of Clinical Data

Complete and accurate coding depends on the availability of clinical data in the health record. Those data provide a full report of the conditions treated and the services rendered to the patient and include the following:

- Physician documentation

- Physician communications, or query forms

- Laboratory data

- Pathology data

- Radiology reports

- Nursing documentation

- Social service notes

- Admission/discharge data

Physician Documentation

Because clinical coding represents the physician's diagnostic and procedural impressions and decisions, his or her documentation is critical in the coding process. Coders are expected to read the history and physical report, progress notes, orders, operative notes and reports, and the discharge summary. In addition, they should have available the physician's recording of diagnoses and procedures on the patient's registration record, or face sheet. In reality, the pressure to effect reimbursement pushes many coders to "read between the lines" of the health record, even in the absence or illegibility of some of the documentation. Most frequently missing are the face sheet notations and the discharge summary. When a coder is attempting to code an incomplete or a concurrent record, the facility needs to determine what elements must be present in order to complete the coding and "finalize" the record and account.

It is common practice that records missing pathology reports cannot be completed. But what if the specimen is a bullet or other nonorganic item? In some instances, a dictated operative report is missing, but an operative progress note is present. Is it up to the coder's judgment to complete coding or wait for the dictated report? What about a "final" diagnosis present or missing from a face sheet? Each facility must answer these questions and develop its own policies and procedures.

In addition, certain financial and other considerations must be discussed with patient accounts, the compliance officer, and medical staff leadership. For example:

- Will HIM delay billing for an account over $50,000 because of a blank face sheet when the final diagnosis is apparent in other documentation?

- When a record is coded in an incomplete state, will a potentially higher error rate be acceptable if codes would have been different had the record been more complete at the time of coding and an error is later cited upon audit?

- Will the medical staff support HIM in physician compliance with requirements regarding documentation and timely completion of records?

Physician Communications or Query Forms

When a coder is unsure of a diagnosis or procedure, or when ancillary documentation points to a condition not apparently documented by the physician, the coder should query the physician prior to making a final code assignment. Some facilities require that this query, or communication between coder and physician, whether oral or written, be documented formally by means of a query form.

When the query form has identified a documentation deficiency, the physician should go back and include the information in the health record. Late entries or corrections to the existing health record should be noted as such and include the actual date the late entry was made.

When the facility has determined that the physician query form is part of the medical record, the physician should sign off on the form, particularly when the person querying the physician has made the query verbally or over the phone. Otherwise, there is no true evidence that the verbal interaction occurred. The physician also could be present later and deny or revise what the query documented. The facility should have physician query guidelines that eliminate any appearance of coding without proper physician documentation in accordance with CMS regulations. (See chapter 9 for further discussion of compliance issues.)

When query forms are to be used for documentation quality improvement purposes, they may be retained in administrative files, organized by physician or service. Trends may be noted and followed up, with the goal of reducing the use of query forms for questions asked repeatedly.

Appendix 1.4 contains the AHIMA practice brief, "Developing a Physician Query Process," which provides a detailed discussion of current accepted standards for this area of HIM practice.

Laboratory Data

Coders need laboratory data to ensure that they have captured the patient's entire clinical experience. For example, the finding of "low hemoglobin" on a laboratory report may prompt the physician to order iron supplements. As a condition treated during the stay, this possible "anemia" is a codable event. However, in the absence of physician documentation or specific facility guidelines, the coder might not consider querying the physician regarding anemia as a diagnosis unless the laboratory report were available for review to prompt the query.

Pathology Data

Pathology reports are not always complete or available at the time of patient discharge. In some facilities, pathology specimens are sent to an outside pathology laboratory or another facility for diagnosis. Obtaining the final pathology report and coding from it is often critical to accurate coding, cancer reporting, and DRG assignment. Coders should never rely on other physician documentation in the record or code "rule-outs" without the final pathology report to confirm or provide an alternative diagnosis. In some instances, the attending physician should be required to amend a final diagnosis that conflicts with the pathology report, unless for some reason he or she disagrees with the pathologist. In such circumstances, the facility should have a guideline as to which or whose diagnosis to code.

Most facilities have a guideline stating that records are not coded without a pathology report. However, instances in which coding may be acceptable without a pathology report must be clearly defined. Such instances could include cases in which nonorganic objects, such as bullets, have been excised or removed.

Radiology Reports

Unlike pathology reports, radiology reports are usually available prior to discharge. Although radiology reports convey important information to physicians, they are less useful in alerting coders to potential codable events. However, radiology reports often clarify issues documented in the progress notes and help confirm ruled-out or nonspecific diagnoses that may not be clearly stated. For example, if a physician documents "fractured hip" throughout the record, yet the x-ray of the hip indicates "intertrochanteric fracture of the femur," then the fracture may be coded with greater specificity from the radiology report. Fractures also may be specified to a greater degree by the radiologist than by the physician.

Nursing Documentation

Coders may not use nursing documentation such as notes and graphics as the sole support for assigning diagnoses and/or procedures to a health record. However, nursing documentation is often a rich source of information that may assist the coder in querying the physician or in confirming illegible or vague physician documentation. In addition, nursing documentation confirms whether a medication has been administered and provides information that supports the coding decision. Bedside procedures are often well documented by nursing, compared to a relatively brief mention in the physician progress notes.

Social Service Notes

Social service notes may provide information concerning patient disposition/discharge status that cannot be found elsewhere in the record. For example, the physician may state "discharge to nursing home." If the coder or data-entry person is abstracting the actual name of the nursing home, the only place to find this information may be in the social service note. Often the patient transfer form is located with this note. Another important detail often found in social service notes is whether the patient will be receiving home care, such as a visiting nurse service. The transfer destination at discharge is extremely important because Medicare inpatient DRG reimbursement may be affected.

Admission/Discharge Data

Coders are often asked to "review" data that have been charted or entered into the hospital computer system by clerical or nursing staff at the time of admission and at the time of discharge. These data, which are often demographic data, are reviewed for errors that may affect coding. For example, if a patient's gender has been entered incorrectly (a female patient is listed as having prostate surgery), the system may not accept the correct gender-specific codes. Birth dates also may affect coding. For example, V30.00 would not be used as the principal diagnosis unless the newborn was born during that admission. If the coder were about to code a newborn record and saw that the admission and birth dates did not match, he or she would be alerted to review the record to see whether:

- The newborn had been born elsewhere and transferred into the facility.
- An error had been made in the recording of the admission date.
- An error had been made in the recording of the birth date.

Access to Prior Admissions

As discussed previously, the coding of each patient encounter must stand on its own documentation. However, access to documentation and coding of prior admissions may assist coders in identifying issues for a physician query. For example, a physician may document "cancer of the breast with metastasis." The coder needs to determine whether the patient has had surgery—therefore a "history" of cancer of the breast—and exactly where the cancer has metastasized. If the coder has access to documentation from a prior admission, the health record may contain information that can be presented to the physician and enable the physician to document consistently throughout all admissions. The physician must add the documentation to the record for each encounter or admission in order for the correct codes to be assigned.

Posted Charges

In some instances, the health record does not contain enough information to determine whether:

- A procedure was performed.

- A procedure that should have been reported with a code was missed.

- A procedure was coded but not performed.

For example, when coding the health record of a patient seen in the emergency department for a deep laceration, the coder would review the documentation to determine whether the laceration was sutured. If the physician has not documented the type of wound closure, the coder may be able to see if a suture tray was ordered by reviewing the charges posted for the account. Although the presence of an order and a bill for a suture tray suggests that the procedure was performed, it does not justify coding the procedure. The physician still must document the procedure to support assignment of the code. It may have been that the suture tray was ordered, but that the laceration was not sutured because the patient decided to leave against medical advice. In this case, the charge should be deleted. Coders should refer such cases back to the physician for clarification. For such referral, coders should follow the policy or process coordinated between the coding manager and the patient accounts manager or the practice manager.

Process Flow

The coding process can be broken down into the separate subtasks of data access, data assessment, data analysis, code assignment, and post-assignment processing, as well as auxiliary tasks.

Data Access

Coders must have access to pertinent documentation at the time codes are assigned. Data may be in the form of a paper record, an electronic record, or a combination of both. For example, laboratory test data are commonly computerized. Rather than search or wait for a paper laboratory report to catch up with a paper record, the coder may readily access the information via the facility's computer system. In the event of a transcription backlog, the coder should have permission to play back a dictated report and obtain the required information or to access the transcribed reports online.

Electronic Data Access for Offsite, Home-Based, or Remote Coders

Coders who work offsite—whether they are home-based, telecommuting, outsourced coders, or just working in another location within the facility—should have the same access to data as onsite coders. If this access cannot be achieved, offsite coding will be unsuccessful in terms of accuracy and quality of code assignment.

HIPAA security regulations state that "covered entities" (hospitals in this scenario) must ensure that electronic information pertaining to individuals remains secure. In planning for remote coding, the HIPAA "security rule delineates recommendations in three distinct categories (Keough 2004):

- Administrative procedures

- Physical safeguards

- Technical security services and mechanisms"

The coding manager's emphasis will be on administrative procedures, to include a home-based coding telecommuting policy and agreement, an electronic record policy and procedure, and a downtime procedure. He or she should work with IS and understand the physical safeguard requirements and implementation process. Technical services and mechanisms include system access, work distribution, and audit trails. Overall, it is essential that remote coding not compromise the confidentiality or security of patient records. (See appendix 1.5 for a sample home coder confidentiality policy.)

Policies and procedures should be established to ensure that remote coders have access to all pertinent documentation on a timely basis so that productivity does not suffer. Moreover, policies and procedures must be established to ensure that remote coders have the ability to obtain missing documentation in a timely manner. If, for example, incomplete records are transmitted for remote coding, it should be determined whether it is necessary to transmit the entire record or only parts of the record. For example, when the operative report is missing from the record, the coding manager should consider the following questions:

- Will the record still be transmitted?

- Will the record be held until the report is available?

- Will the operative progress note alone suffice?

In addition, the coding manager should ask the following questions:

- Can a clerical staff person make these determinations on a record-by-record basis?

- Does the staff member need to have a certain degree of coding knowledge to ascertain the "codability" of an incomplete record?

- Who will be held accountable if a record is coded incorrectly because a critical piece of the record was not transmitted?

Data Assessment

Coders must assess the completeness of the available documentation. Health records may be coded concurrently at any time during or after the patient's encounter or admission.

However, coding is performed most commonly postdischarge or postencounter. Even then, the health record is most often not finalized or complete. Official Coding Guidelines discourage the coding of incomplete records (CDC 2006a, 70). However, from a fiscal and practical perspective, coders cannot wait for every health record to be completely finalized prior to coding. They must consider that most regulatory bodies allow the physician 30 days to complete an inpatient hospital health record. Therefore, coders must possess the knowledge to determine which incomplete records can or cannot be coded and the facility must have policies in place to support coders in such a determination. For instance, coders should know whether it is acceptable to code a record that does not yet have a final diagnosis or discharge summary. When records are coded without this information, a method should be established to review the code assignments against the information when it becomes available.

Data Analysis

Coders review documentation to identify "codable" diagnoses and procedures. As previously mentioned, information may be noted in ancillary reports or nursing notes. These sources of data are not a substitute for physician documentation and should not be used for coding on their own.

Physicians may document conditions or diagnoses in the final diagnosis or discharge summary that existed previously ("history of") but are not currently being treated, do not affect the patient's care, or have no impact on the patient's length of stay. Coders must be able to identify and distinguish these conditions or diagnoses because they should not be coded.

Many procedures are performed, but not all are coded. For example, it is unlikely that an ICD-9-CM Volume III procedure code for a chest x-ray would be assigned for an inpatient admission. However, a CPT code assigned by the **chargemaster** would be used if the x-ray were the reason for an outpatient encounter. The determination of which procedures to code is often facility- or encounter-based. For inpatient admissions, all procedures affecting DRG assignment must be coded.

Code Assignment

Coders assign the appropriate codes from the appropriate code set—ICD-9-CM and/or CPT. As discussed previously, these code assignments may be made using the codebooks, the assistance of an encoder, or a combination of both.

Postassignment Processing

Coders abstract the data, including the diagnoses and procedure codes, and enter them into the computer or record them on the health record, or both. Many facilities have coders handwrite the codes and other abstracted data onto the health record face sheet in addition to entering the data into the computer. At first, this abstraction process may be considered redundant. Coders often need a worksheet, however, and use the face sheet for this purpose. Also, when a coding error has occurred, the handwritten codes can be compared to the codes entered into the system. In that way, it can be determined whether a true coding error was made or whether a data-entry or system interface error was made.

Some facilities use noncoding personnel to enter codes into the computer system. This approach frees coders from spending time entering data and thus enhances their productivity. However, a disadvantage to this approach is that errors entered unwittingly by noncoders, such as the transposition of code numbers, might not be caught. In addition, in the process of entering data, coders can note any edits, make any necessary changes, and confirm that the DRG assignment makes sense for each particular case. If noncoders are used to enter codes, a postentry audit process should be in place to ensure that the data are entered correctly.

Timing of the Coding Process

Hospital inpatient cases are most frequently coded retrospectively, or after the patient has been discharged and the entire health record has been routed to the HIM department. **Retrospective coding** is the model on which the previous discussion is based. In some hospitals, inpatient cases are coded concurrently, or while the patient is still in the hospital and receiving care. Under the **concurrent coding** model, coders may be located near the physician's "incomplete" area of the HIM department so they can query physicians during the patient's stay if documentation is vague, unclear, or incomplete. In concurrent coding, coders must travel to the medical and surgical units to review the case, begin a problem or diagnosis list from physician documentation, and assign ICD-9-CM codes while the patient is in-house. In this model, the cases may be reviewed and coded multiple times, an average of every other day. After the patient is discharged, health records are still routed to the coding department for completion, but the coders spend much less time postdischarge reviewing the records because they have already initiated the coding process. Concurrent coding is time-consuming compared to retrospective coding. Benefits are derived primarily from shortening the post-discharge processing time. The concurrent query process can improve documentation and also can shorten processing time.

Auxiliary Tasks

Coders may be required to perform a variety of tasks in addition to specific coding-related activities. Although task assignment is largely a function of staffing, workflow, and worksite, coders' daily noncoding activities should be limited to functions that enrich their work experience and utilize their training and abilities to the fullest.

Any task not directly related to coding should be evaluated to ensure that it moves the goals and objectives of the coding process forward. When a task is unrelated to coding, the coding manager should evaluate whether noncoding staff could perform it effectively. Coders should not routinely assemble or analyze health records, answer telephones, or handle general correspondence.

Assembly and Analysis

For the most efficient coding in a paper-based environment, the health record should be assembled and analyzed prior to coding. Assembly and routine quantitative analysis facilitate the reading of the health record and the coder's understanding of the data. In addition, abstracting of data, such as the identification of consultants and surgeons or of the dates of invasive procedures, helps the coder to follow the events described in the record and recognize whether critical data are missing.

When a coder receives an unassembled paper record, he or she might decide to assemble it to make it easier to read. For small records, such as those for ambulatory surgery, clinic visits, and normal newborns, this action may take seconds. However, for larger records, the minutes involved in assembly can seriously impair productivity. For appropriate utilization of resources, the coding manager should evaluate whether allowing overtime by other staff in the assembly and analysis area is less expensive than paying coders to assemble and analyze charts.

Reporting

Credentialed individuals such as registered health information technicians (RHITs) and registered health information administrators (RHIAs) have received training in statistical methods and can assist in reporting activities. Although coders understand clinical data, they are not always trained in statistical reporting methods. Depending on the facility's computerized support, coders can be trained to run routine reports and to create ad hoc reports. With some training in computerized spreadsheet programs, coders also can prepare other types of analyses.

Statistical and other types of reporting activities can be job enriching for some coders. Although not all coders will view these activities as such, others will welcome the opportunity to add to their job skills and achieve greater visibility within the facility.

Quality Analysis

As previously mentioned, the prescreening of identified record content can be effectively delegated to coders. Not only can this activity enrich the coder's job, but it also can be an effective use of facility resources. As always, the impact of other responsibilities on coding productivity is a concern. If quality analysis activities lead to outsourcing part of the coding function, the departments requesting these services may need to assist in funding them.

Postaudit Review

Many facilities require coders to preaudit records that payers and other auditors have requested for review. This activity is of limited benefit because the preaudit does not prevent the audit itself. The audit findings will be the same whether or not errors have been detected and corrected prior to the audit.

On the other hand, the postaudit review of problems is essential. If a payer audit or other audit results in the identification of possible errors, the records containing these errors should be reviewed. First, if the auditor is in error, the facility should resolve this type of finding immediately. Second, the nature of an actual error must be identified and the reason for it evaluated. Trends in errors found on audit often demonstrate the need for general or targeted retraining. One of the most common reasons for coding "errors" is missing or unavailable documentation at the time of coding. The coding manager should carefully evaluate the need to complete a health record versus the need to bill quickly, keeping in mind that errors found on audit can lead to payment reductions or denials.

Self-Auditing

The healthcare facility should not rely on payer audits to ensure coding quality or to identify problem areas; thus, routine quality control audits should be an integral part of every facility's coding function. When resources are limited, coders can audit themselves. However, self-auditing may be the least desirable form of review when motivating factors other than data quality are involved. If this type of auditing is performed, it can be done on a rotating basis, with the "auditor" role passing from one coder to the next on a specific schedule. This method works best when all coders are of equivalent experience.

Self-auditing also can be handled as a routine part of daily activities. Depending on the workload, 1 hour per day or per week can be devoted to reviewing selected records. Some or all of this audit activity can be handled on an overtime basis if the existing workload is heavy. The cost of overtime can be compared with the cost of hiring external quality auditors and consultants.

Finally, the coding supervisor should perform quality audits on a routine basis for performance evaluation. In some facilities, the coding supervisor's role is limited to audit activity and overload or fill-in coding but does not include routine coding.

Coders and External Audits

In any healthcare setting, coders may be given responsibility for responding to outside queries or external audits. If external auditors are scheduled to come into the facility to conduct an audit, the coding staff may be required to prepare or verify the health record **pull list,** which is the list of requested records to be pulled and provided to the auditors in either electronic or paper format. Moreover, coders may meet with the auditors after the audit is complete. For offsite coding audits, mail-in requests for copies of health records may be routed first to coders and then to the release-of-information department for processing.

More recently, state healthcare quality improvement organizations (QIOs), under contract with CMS, are conducting focused coding and documentation audits at the direction of CMS. As part of those audits, some review organizations are notifying hospitals that they must conduct internal audits and submit the findings to them. The audits may be routed to coders to initialize the audit process, particularly in rural settings.

QIOs are currently under contract with CMS to perform a Hospital Payment Monitoring Program (HPMP). Under HPMP, an auditing component targets specific DRGs and discharges that have been identified as at high risk for payment errors. The high-risk, hospital-specific data are identified in an electronic report called Program for Evaluating Payment Patterns

Electronic Report (PEPPER). The coding manager may be assigned to perform PEPPER audits or to work with the facility's internal auditing or quality improvement department. (More state-specific requirements and information about HPMP and PEPPER can be obtained from the state QIO.)

Expectations of Other Staff Members

Staff members in many departments of healthcare organizations rely on coded data to complete their work. The expectations of those departments for timely information must be factored into performance standards for coders.

Turnaround Time

Many facilities measure coding turnaround time by days past discharge. For example, a facility may use a threshold of "discharge plus 3 days" (3 days postdischarge) to describe its expectation of when health records should be coded. However, the currency of the coding is not as important as its accuracy. Allowing a reasonable period to assemble or scan all of the necessary documentation is usually better than forcing the coding of an inadequately documented medical record. As previously mentioned, some documentation is more critical to the coding process than other documentation. Although coding managers will wait for a pathology report before coding a breast biopsy, they might not delay billing for an orthopedic pin extraction. However, coding managers should be aware that there is a risk in forcing the coding of an incomplete health record.

Delayed Billing

The HIM department is responsible for coding, which in turn affects billing. Even if the patient's payer is not reimbursing the facility, based on a DRG, the payer still wants the chart to be coded. Failure to code can lead to failure to bill. For that reason, the HIM department should routinely receive a detailed list of all discharges for which no bill has yet been dropped. This list is often called the **discharged not final billed (DNFB)** list. Although delays in billing may be due to reasons other than coding, the DNFB list is an important tool in managing the coding process. The coding manager should examine the reasons health records have not been billed. Records that account for large amounts of unbilled dollars should be prioritized for timelier coding. This type of proactive management demonstrates the HIM department's commitment to facilitywide concerns. In addition, some facilities have an automatic **bill hold** on accounts to allow time for all charges to be entered. This bill hold time varies and may be up to 3 days. Thus, it is of no advantage to "guess" codes and risk errors if the bill will not drop anyway. The coding manager should find out from the patient accounts manager if there is a **bill hold period** and what that period is.

Medical Staff Office Support

Medical staff offices may request data pertaining to individual practitioners. Reports containing physician-specific data should not be provided without proper authorization as specified by medical staff rules and regulations. An example of routinely approved, reported data concerns physicians on cycle for reappointment to the staff, or "recredentialing." Often the purpose of such data is to review the types of cases the physician has had over a specified period. If the physician has performed a certain number of cases in a particular area, he or she may be "promoted" from one staff level to the next (for example, from associate physician to attending physician). Accurate coding is paramount to this process because it is the only method used to capture these kinds of data.

The medical staff office also may request data for a particular physician group or specialty. For example, the chair of the urology department wants the facility to open an impotence clinic and has asked the medical staff office to assist in some aspects of market analysis. Data concerning how many impotent patients were seen over the course of a year would be used as part of a market research and feasibility plan.

Conclusion

Coders are a valuable resource to their healthcare facilities. Although the competence of coders is reflected in coding quality, coding-specific credentials can evidence achievement prior to employment. To perform their function effectively, coders require high-quality continuing professional education. They also require specific tools that should be updated appropriately, including codebooks, reference texts, encoders, and groupers. The facility should support coders with access to official and facility-based coding guidelines, as well as to computers and the Internet. The physical environment affects coder productivity and should be evaluated for ergonomics and efficiency.

Coders require specific data to perform their functions effectively. Physician, laboratory, radiology, and pathology data are particularly important. The function of the coder is to assign accurate codes to the clinical data. To perform their job effectively, coders should not be assigned distracting tasks such as answering telephones.

In managing the coding function, turnaround time and billing are important considerations. Coders demonstrate professionalism and commitment by fulfilling customer expectations and responding to organizational requirements.

Coders must meet specific competency levels, as detailed in their job descriptions. Control and supervision of the coding function require appropriate supervisory oversight and continuous assessment.

References and Resources

American Health Information Management Association. 2005 (August). House Resolution: Increase Dialogue, Employment Opportunities. *AHIMA Advantage* 9(5).

American Health Information Management Association and Medical Transcription Industry Alliance. 1998 (January). Position statement: Confidential Health Information and the Internet. Available online from AHIMA Body of Knowledge.

American Health Information Management Association. 1997 (Jan. 2). Sample form: Employee/Student/Volunteer Nondisclosure Acknowledgment. Available online from AHIMA Body of Knowledge.

American Medical Association. 1995–2006. Code Information and Education. Available online from http://www.ama-assn.org/ama/pub/category/3884.html.

Centers for Disease Control and Prevention. 2006a (Aug. 02). International Classification of Diseases, Ninth Revision, Clinical Modification, Sixth Edition. Available online from http://www.cdc.gov/nchs/datawh/ftpserv/ftpicd9/ftpicd9.htm.

Centers for Disease Control and Prevention. 2006b (Aug. 23). ICD-9-CM Coordination and Maintenance Committee. Available online from http://www.cdc.gov/nchs/about/otheract/icd9/maint/maint.htm.

Centers for Medicare and Medicaid Services. 2006c (May 31). Hospital Outpatient PPS. Available online from http://www.cms.hhs.gov/HospitalOutpatientPPS//.

Centers for Medicare and Medicaid Services. 2005a (Dec. 15). HCPCS Background Information. Available online from http://www.cms.hhs.gov/medicare/hcpcs.

Centers for Medicare and Medicaid Services. 2005b (Dec. 14). Electronic Billing & EDI Transactions, Institutional paper claim form (CMS-1450). Available online from http://www.cms.hhs.gov/ElectronicBillingEDITrans/15_1450.asp.

Dougherty, M., and R.A. Scichilone (originally prepared by D. Fletcher). 2002 (July-Aug.). Practice brief: Establishing a Telecommuting or Home-based Employee Program. *Journal of American Health Information Management Association* 73(7): 72A–L.

Ellie, P.2005 (March 2). AHIMA House of Delegates Proposed Resolution (Florida), Bridging the Gap! Education to Employment.

Office of the Inspector General. 2000 (April 7). Medicare Program Prospective Payment System for Hospital Outpatient Services; Final Rule. 42 CFR Parts 409. *Federal Register* 65(68):18438–820.

Keough, T. 2004. Safe at home: remote coding meets HIPAA. *Journal of the American Health Information Management Association* 75(2): 42–46.

National Uniform Billing Committee. 2005 (April 19). UB-04 Proofs. Available online from http://www.nubc.org/public/whatsnew/UB-04Proofs.pdf.

Occupational Safety and Health Administration. n.d. Safety and Health Topics: Ergonomics. Available online from http://www.osha-slc.gov/SLTC/ergonomics/index.html.

Prophet, S. 2001 (Oct. 2). Practice brief: Developing a Physician Query Process. *Journal of the American Health Information Management Association* 72(9): 88I–M.

Appendix 1.1

AHIMA Resolution Based on "Bridging the Gap"

House Resolution:
Increase Dialogue, Employment Opportunities

In May, the House of Delegates passed a resolution sponsored by the Florida Health Information Management Association designed to bridge the gap between education and employment. This resolution intends to facilitate the employment of graduates from Commission on Accreditation for Health Informatics and Information Management Education-accredited HIM programs at the baccalaureate and associate degree levels and AHIMA-approved coding programs at the predegree level.

What the Resolution Means

Employment is a goal for students as they complete accredited and approved educational programs and begin their professional careers. Although many are successful at graduation, it seems that an ever-increasing number are being challenged to achieve the entry-level experience qualifications desired by employers. This seems especially true in the coding arena. As employers are pressed to have optimal productivity from every employee from the start date of employment, new graduates find it difficult to bridge the gap from education to employment.

AHIMA is addressing the clinical practice education issue with the creation of the e-HIM Virtual Learning Laboratory to facilitate ongoing skill development. This action is applauded, but it is not a full substitute for onsite clinical experiences. Another area of action is for organizations to create "preceptor" programs to smooth the transition from education to employment. Many facilities have these programs in place for new nursing graduates, why not HIM? It is desired that this document will generate the sharing of additional education to employment transition models that can be duplicated in other settings.

Preamble

Whereas, HIM students are the future of our profession;

Whereas, the goal of HIM students is to gain active employment in the HIM profession upon completion;

Whereas, initial employment appears increasingly challenging to qualify for;

Whereas, HIM employers appear to be requiring more skills and HIM experience before offering employment;

Whereas, HIM student/new graduate employment is necessary to continue to optimally recruit the next generation of HIM students;

Be it resolved, the HIM profession must heighten its awareness of this apparent phenomena to take corrective actions; and

Resolved, HIM accredited and approved educational programs will solicit feedback from advisory boards and others to determine the actual employment skills desired by employers; and

Resolved, HIM accredited and approved educational programs will, in cooperation with employers, attempt to provide optimal preparation to meet the skills expectations desired in the work force; and

Resolved, HIM employers must enhance their efforts to provide clinical education to HIM students from HIM accredited and approved educational programs to better prepare them for the work force; and

Resolved, HIM employers must further advance their efforts to employ recent HIM graduates from HIM accredited and approved educational programs by creating entry-level opportunities; and

Resolved, AHIMA will continue to support the development of the e-HIM Virtual Learning Laboratory to facilitate ongoing skill development for all members; and

Resolved, AHIMA BOD will continue to prioritize and be responsive to the development of new ideas and concepts addressing student education to employment transitional support; and

Resolved, AHIMA, component state associations, regional associations, and others are requested to promote the CAHIIM-accredited HIM programs at the baccalaureate and associate degree levels, and the AHIMA-approved coding programs at the predegree level in their respective areas via Web sites or other means to reduce confusion with unapproved options; and

Resolved, AHIMA, Foundation of Research and Education of AHIMA (FORE), educational programs, and/or members need to support formal research to statistically verify student employment at a base level and to evaluate the effectiveness of corrective actions toward improvement on an ongoing basis.

Resolved, all parties that have had experiences with "preceptor" transitional type programs are requested to share them in the CoPs. This will facilitate others evaluation of the feasibility of developing similar models that will facilitate bridging the gap from education to employment.

Approved May 17, 2005

Source: AHIMA 2005.

Appendix 1.2

Sample Procedure for Internet Use

Excerpt from AHIMA Position Statement *Confidential Health Information and the Internet*

Background

Recommendations

Health information applications on the Internet have the potential to bring great benefit to patient care but may also result in significant harm if they are improperly designed, monitored, or used. To protect the confidentiality and integrity of patient health information, the American Health Information Management Association (AHIMA) and the Medical Transcription Industry Alliance (MTIA) make the following recommendations:

- Applications on the Internet that contain patient-identifiable health information must be carefully designed to protect the confidentiality of the information.

- Appropriate security measures and available technologies should be employed to protect confidential health information from unauthorized access or alteration. These measures include encryption, secure transmission protocols, and firewalls.

- Text, voice, image, and other patient files transmitted or maintained on the Internet should be encrypted to protect their confidentiality. Whenever possible, patient-identifiable information should exist as a separate file rather than part of the transcribed text document.

- Photographs or other images that may identify a patient should be used in Internet applications only with the express written consent of the patient or his/her legal representative.

- When a transcriptionist completes a document, it should be transmitted back to the transcription service bureau with no files (text, voice, or image) remaining on the hard drive of the transcriptionist's computer. Temporary files containing patient-identifiable information should be deleted as soon as they are no longer needed. Files such as patient admission lists should be deleted automatically or returned to the originator when the transcriptionist logs off at the close of each business day. Any files stored outside the transcription service bureau should have the same level of physical and electronic security as files kept by the service bureau.

- Print functions should be limited. Off-site transcriptionists should not be allowed to print copies of reports.

- Audit trails should record all individuals who access, modify, or delete any report.

- If patients and caregivers will use electronic mail to communicate, such communications should be limited to nonconfidential information. If confidential information will be transmitted via electronic mail, that information should be encrypted to protect its confidentiality.

- If caregivers use electronic mail, bulletin boards, or online discussion groups to discuss a patient's case, no patient-identifiable information should be included. If electronic mail is used to discuss a case, that transmission should be encrypted.

- Client-side file caching by an Internet browser should be disabled. This prevents the localized save of patient data on the client machine.

- Transcription service bureaus should educate their employees and contractors about privacy and confidentiality issues, including use of electronic mail and online discussions ("chat rooms"). Written confidentiality agreements addressing these issues should be signed by each employee or contractor at the time of hire. Written acknowledgment should be signed on an annual basis thereafter to remind individuals of their ongoing responsibility for protecting the confidentiality of health information. Such agreements should be updated periodically to address issues raised by the use of new technologies.

- Organizations should develop, implement, and enforce policies and procedures to protect confidential information in Internet applications.

Source: AHIMA 1998.

Appendix 1.3

Sample Confidentiality Statement

Employee/Student/Volunteer Nondisclosure Agreement

[Name of healthcare facility] has a legal and ethical responsibility to safeguard the privacy of all patients and to protect the confidentiality of their health information. In the course of my employment/assignment at *[name of healthcare facility]*, I may come into possession of confidential patient information, even though I may not be directly involved in providing patient services.

I understand that such information must be maintained in the strictest confidence. As a condition of my employment/assignment, I hereby agree that, unless directed by my supervisor, I will not at any time during or after my employment/assignment with *[name of healthcare facility]* disclose any patient information to any person whatsoever or permit any person whatsoever to examine or make copies of any patient reports or other documents prepared by me, coming into my possession, or under my control, or use patient information, other than as necessary in the course of my employment/assignment.

When patient information must be discussed with other healthcare practitioners in the course of my work, I will use discretion to ensure that such conversations cannot be overheard by others who are not involved in the patient's care.

I understand that violation of this agreement may result in corrective action, up to and including discharge.

_____

Signature of Employee/Student/Volunteer

_____

Date

Note. This sample form was developed by AHIMA for discussion purposes only. It should not be used without review by your organization's legal counsel to ensure compliance with local and state laws.

_____

Source: AHIMA 1997.

Appendix 1.4

Practice Brief: Developing a Physician Query Process

Principles of Medical Record Documentation

Medical record documentation is used for a multitude of purposes, including:

- Serving as a means of communication between the physician and the other members of the healthcare team providing care to the patient

- Serving as a basis for evaluating the adequacy and appropriateness of patient care

- Providing data to support insurance claims

- Assisting in protecting the legal interests of patients, healthcare professionals, and healthcare facilities

- Providing clinical data for research and education

To support these various uses, it is imperative that medical record documentation be complete, accurate, and timely. Facilities are expected to comply with a number of standards regarding medical record completion and content promulgated by multiple regulatory agencies.

Joint Commission on Accreditation of Healthcare Organizations

The Joint Commission's 2000 Hospital Accreditation Standards state, "the medical record contains sufficient information to identify the patient, support the diagnosis, justify the treatment, document the course and results, and promote continuity among health care providers" (IM.7.2).[1] The Joint Commission Standards also state, "medical record data and information are managed in a timely manner" (IM.7.6).

Timely entries are essential if a medical record is to be useful in a patient's care. A complete medical record is also important when a patient is discharged, because information in the record may be needed for clinical, legal, or performance improvement purposes. The Joint Commission requires hospitals to have policy and procedures on the timely entry of all significant clinical information into the patient's medical record, and they do not consider a medical record complete until all final diagnoses and complications are recorded without the use of symbols or abbreviations.

Joint Commission standards also require medical records to be reviewed on an ongoing basis for completeness and timeliness of information, and action is taken to improve the quality and timeliness of documentation that affects patient care (IM.7.10). This review must address the presence, timeliness, legibility, and authentication of the final diagnoses and conclusions at termination of hospitalization.

Medicare

The Medicare Conditions of Participation require medical records to be accurately written, promptly completed, properly filed and retained, and accessible.[2] Records must document, as appropriate, complications, hospital-acquired infections, and unfavorable reactions to drugs and anesthesia. The conditions also stipulate that all records must document the final diagnosis with completion of medical records within 30 days following discharge.

Relationship Between Coding and Documentation

Complete and accurate diagnostic and procedural coded data must be available, in a timely manner, in order to:

- Improve the quality and effectiveness of patient care

- Ensure equitable healthcare reimbursement

- Expand the body of medical knowledge

- Make appropriate decisions regarding healthcare policies, delivery systems, funding, expansion, and education

- Monitor resource utilization

- Permit identification and resolution of medical errors

- Improve clinical decision making

- Facilitate tracking of fraud and abuse

- Permit valid clinical research, epidemiological studies, outcomes and statistical analyses, and provider profiling

- Provide comparative data to consumers regarding costs and outcomes, average charges, and outcomes by procedure

Physician documentation is the cornerstone of accurate coding. Therefore, assuring the accuracy of coded data is a shared responsibility between coding professionals and physicians. Accurate diagnostic and procedural coded data originate from collaboration between physicians, who have a clinical background, and coding professionals, who have an understanding of classification systems.

Expectations of Physicians

Physicians are expected to provide complete, accurate, timely, and legible documentation of pertinent facts and observations about an individual's health history, including past and present illnesses, tests, treatments, and outcomes. Medical record entries should be documented at the time service is provided. Medical record entries should be authenticated. If subsequent additions to documentation are needed, they should be identified as such and dated. (Often these expectations are included in the medical staff or house staff rules and regulations.) Medical record documentation should:

- Address the clinical significance of abnormal test results

- Support the intensity of patient evaluation and treatment and describe the thought processes and complexity of decision making

- Include all diagnostic and therapeutic procedures, treatments, and tests performed, in addition to their results

- Include any changes in the patient's condition, including psychosocial and physical symptoms

- Include all conditions that coexist at the time of admission, that subsequently develop, or that affect the treatment received and the length of stay. This encompasses all conditions that affect patient care in terms of requiring clinical evaluation, therapeutic treatment, diagnostic procedures, extended length of hospital stay, or increased nursing care and monitoring[3]

- Be updated as necessary to reflect all diagnoses relevant to the care or services provided

- Be consistent and discuss and reconcile any discrepancies (this reconciliation should be documented in the medical record)

- Be legible and written in ink, typewritten, or electronically signed, stored, and printed

Expectations of Coding Professionals

The AHIMA Code of Ethics sets forth ethical principles for the HIM profession. HIM professionals are responsible for maintaining and promoting ethical practices. This Code of Ethics states, in part: "Health information management professionals promote high standards for health information management practice, education, and research." Another standard in this code states, "Health information management professionals strive to provide accurate and timely information." Data accuracy and integrity are fundamental values of HIM that are advanced by:

- Employing practices that produce complete, accurate, and timely information to meet the health and related needs of individuals

- Following the guidelines set forth in the organization's compliance plan for reporting improper preparation, alteration, or suppression of information or data by others

- Not participating in any improper preparation, alteration, or suppression of health record information or other organization data

A conscientious goal for coding and maintaining a quality database is accurate clinical and statistical data. AHIMA's Standards of Ethical Coding were developed to guide coding professionals in this process. As stated in the standards, coding professionals are expected to support the importance of accurate, complete, and consistent coding practices for the production of quality healthcare data. These standards also indicate that coding professionals should only assign and report codes that are clearly and consistently supported by physician documentation in the medical record. It is the responsibility of coding professionals to assess physician documentation to assure that it supports the diagnosis and procedure codes reported on claims.

Dialogue between coding professionals and clinicians is encouraged, because it improves coding professionals' clinical knowledge and educates the physicians on documentation practice issues. AHIMA's Standards of Ethical Coding state that coding professionals are expected to consult physicians for clarification and additional documentation prior to code assignment when there is conflicting or ambiguous data in the health record. Coding professionals should also assist and educate physicians by advocating proper documentation practices, further specificity, and resequencing or inclusion of diagnoses or procedures when needed to more accurately reflect the acuity, severity, and the occurrence of events. It is recommended that coding be performed by credentialed HIM professionals.[4]

It is inappropriate for coding professionals to misrepresent the patient's clinical picture through incorrect coding or add diagnoses or procedures unsupported by the documentation to maximize reimbursement or meet insurance policy coverage requirements. Coding professionals should not change codes or the narratives of codes on the billing abstract so that meanings are misrepresented. Diagnoses or procedures should not be inappropriately included or excluded because payment or insurance policy coverage requirements will be affected. When individual payer policies conflict with official coding rules and guidelines, these policies should be obtained in writing whenever possible. Reasonable efforts should be made to educate the payer on proper coding practices in order to influence a change in the payer's policy.

Proper Use of Physician Queries

The process of querying physicians is an effective and, in today's healthcare environment, necessary mechanism for improving the quality of coding and medical record documentation and capturing complete clinical data. Query forms have become an accepted tool for communicating with physicians on documentation issues influencing proper code assignment. Query forms should be used in a judicious and appropriate manner. They must be used as a communication tool to improve the accuracy of code assignment and the quality of physician documentation, not to inappropriately maximize reimbursement. The query process should be guided by AHIMA's Standards of Ethical Coding and the official coding guidelines. An inappropriate query, such as a form that is poorly constructed or asks leading questions, or overuse of the query process can result in quality-of-care, legal, and ethical concerns.

The Query Process

The goal of the query process should be to improve physician documentation and coding professionals' understanding of the unique clinical situation, not to improve reimbursement. Each facility should establish a policy and procedure for obtaining physician clarification of documentation that affects code assignment. The process of querying physicians must be a patient-specific process, not a general process. Asking "blanket" questions is not appropriate. Policies regarding the circumstances when physicians will be queried should be designed to promote timely, complete, and accurate coding and documentation.

Physicians should not be asked to provide clarification of their medical record documentation without the opportunity to access the patient's medical record. Each facility also needs to determine if physicians will be queried concurrently (during the patient's hospitalization) or after discharge. Both methods are acceptable. Querying physicians concurrently allows the documentation deficiency to be corrected while the patient is still in-house and can positively influence patient care.

The policy and procedure should stipulate who is authorized to contact the physician for clarifications regarding a coding issue. Coding professionals should be allowed to contact physicians directly for clarification, rather than limiting this responsibility to supervisory personnel or a designated individual.

The facility may wish to use a designated physician liaison to resolve conflicts between physicians and coding professionals. The appropriate use of the physician liaison should be described in the facility's policy and procedures.

Query Format

Each facility should develop a standard format for the query form. No "sticky notes" or scratch paper should be allowed. Each facility should develop a standard design and format for physician queries to ensure clear, consistent, appropriate queries.

The query form should:

- Be clearly and concisely written

- Contain precise language

- Present the facts from the medical record and identify why clarification is needed

- Present the scenario and state a question that asks the physician to make a clinical interpretation of a given diagnosis or condition based on treatment, evaluation, monitoring, and/or services provided. Open-ended questions that allow the physician to document the specific diagnosis are preferable to multiple-choice questions or questions requiring only a "yes" or "no" response. Queries that appear to lead the physician to provide a particular response could lead to allegations of inappropriate upcoding.

- Be phrased such that the physician is allowed to specify the correct diagnosis. It should not indicate the financial impact of the response to the query. The form should not be designed so that all that is required is a physician signature.

- Include:

  —Patient name

  —Admission date

  —Medical record number

  —Name and contact information (phone number and e-mail address) of the coding professional

  —Specific question and rationale (that is, relevant documentation or clinical findings)

  —Place for physician to document his or her response

  —Place for the physician to sign and date his or her response

The query forms should not:

- "Lead" the physician

- Sound presumptive, directing, prodding, probing, or as though the physician is being led to make an assumption

- Ask questions that can be responded to in a "yes" or "no" fashion

- Indicate the financial impact of the response to the query

- Be designed so that all that is required is a physician signature

When Is a Query Appropriate?

Physicians should be queried whenever there is conflicting, ambiguous, or incomplete information in the medical record regarding any significant reportable condition or procedure. Querying the physician only when reimbursement is affected will skew national healthcare data and might lead to allegations of upcoding.

Every discrepancy or issue not addressed in the physician documentation should not necessarily result in the physician being queried. Each facility needs to develop policies and procedures regarding the clinical conditions and documentation situations warranting a request for physician clarification. For example, insignificant or irrelevant findings may not warrant querying the physician regarding the assignment of an additional diagnosis code. Also, if the maximum number of codes that can be entered in the hospital information system has already been assigned, the facility may decide that it is not necessary to query the physician regarding an additional code. Facilities need to balance the value of marginal data being collected against the administrative burden of obtaining the additional documentation.

Members of the medical staff in consultation with coding professionals should develop the specific clinical criteria for a valid query. The specific clinical documentation that must be present in the patient's record to generate a query should be described. For example, anemia, septicemia, and respiratory failure are conditions that often require physician clarification. The medical staff can assist the coding staff in determining when it would be appropriate to query a physician regarding the reporting of these conditions by describing the specific clinical indications in the medical record documentation that raise the possibility that the condition in question may be present.

When Is a Query Not Necessary?

Queries are not necessary if a physician involved in the care and treatment of the patient, including consulting physicians, has documented a diagnosis and there is no conflicting documentation from another physician. Medical record documentation from any physician involved in the care and treatment of the patient, including documentation by consulting physicians, is appropriate for the basis of code assignment. If documentation from different physicians conflicts, clarification should be sought from the attending physician, as he or she is ultimately responsible for the final diagnosis.

Queries are also not necessary when a physician has documented a final diagnosis and clinical indicators, such as test results, do not appear to support this diagnosis. Although coding professionals are expected to advocate complete and accurate physician documentation and to collaborate with physicians to realize this goal, they are not expected to challenge the physician's medical judgment in establishing the patient's diagnosis. However, because a discrepancy between clinical findings and a final diagnosis is a clinical issue, a facility may choose to establish a policy that the physician will be queried in these instances.

Documentation of Query Response

The physician's response to the query must be documented in the patient's medical record. Each facility must develop a policy regarding the specific process for incorporating this additional documentation in the medical record. For example, this policy might stipulate that the physician is required to add the additional information to the body of the medical record. As an alternative, a form, such as a medical record "progress note" form, might be attached to the query form and the attachment is then filed in the medical record. However, another alternative is to file the query form itself in the permanent medical record. Any documentation obtained postdischarge must be included in the discharge summary or identified as a late entry or addendum.

Any decision to file this form in the medical record should involve the advice of the facility's corporate compliance officer and legal counsel, because of potential compliance and legal risks related to incorporating the actual query form into the permanent medical record (such as its potential use as evidence of poor documentation in an audit, investigation, or malpractice suit, risks related to naming a nonclinician in the medical record, or quality of care concerns if the physician response on a query form is not clearly supported by the rest of the medical record documentation).

If the query form will serve as the only documentation of the physician's clarification, the use of open-ended questions are preferable to multiple-choice questions or the use of questions requiring only a "yes" or "no" answer. The query form would need to be approved by the medical staff/medical records committee before implementation of a policy allowing this form to be maintained in the medical record. Also keep in mind that the Joint Commission hospital accreditation standards stipulate that only authorized individuals may make entries in medical records (IM.7.1.1). Therefore, the facility needs to consider modifying the medical staff bylaws to specify coding professionals as individuals authorized to make medical record entries prior to allowing query forms to become a permanent part of the medical record.

Auditing, Monitoring, and Corrective Action

Ideally, complete and accurate physician documentation should occur at the time care is rendered. The need for a query form results from incomplete, conflicting, or ambiguous documentation, which is an indication of poor documentation. Therefore, query form usage should be the exception rather than the norm. If physicians are being queried frequently, facility management or an appropriate medical staff committee should investigate the reasons why.

A periodic review of the query practice should include a determination of what percentage of the query forms are eliciting negative and positive responses from the physicians. A high negative response rate may be an indication that the coding staff are not using the query process judiciously and are being overzealous.

A high positive response rate may indicate that there are widespread poor documentation habits that need to be addressed. It may also indicate that the absence of certain reports (for example, discharge summary, operative report) at the time of coding is forcing the coding staff to query the physicians to obtain the information they need for proper coding. If this is the case, the facility may wish to reconsider its policy regarding the availability of certain reports prior to coding. Waiting for these reports may make more sense in terms of turnaround time and productivity rather than finding it necessary to frequently query the physicians. The question of why final diagnoses are not available at the time of discharge may arise at the time of an audit, review by the peer review organization, or investigation.

The use of query forms should also be monitored for patterns, and any identified patterns should be used to educate physicians on improving their documentation at the point of care. If a pattern is identified, such as a particular physician or diagnosis, appropriate steps should be taken to correct the problem so the necessary documentation is present prior to coding in the future and the need to query this physician, or to query physicians regarding a particular diagnosis, is reduced. Corrective action might include targeted education for one physician or education for the entire medical staff on the proper documentation necessary for accurate code assignment.

Patterns of poor documentation that have not been addressed through education or other corrective action are signs of an ineffective compliance program. The Department of Health and Human Services Office of Inspector General has noted in its Compliance Program Guidance for Hospitals that "accurate coding depends upon the quality of completeness of the physician's documentation" and "active staff physician participation in educational programs focusing on coding and documentation should be emphasized by the hospital."[5]

The format of the queries should also be monitored on a regular basis to ensure that they are not inappropriately leading the physician to provide a particular response. Inappropriately written queries should be used to educate the coding staff on a properly written query. Patterns of inappropriately written queries should be referred to the corporate compliance officer.

Notes

1. Joint Commission on Accreditation of Healthcare Organizations. 2000. *Comprehensive Accreditation Manual for Hospitals: The Official Handbook.* Oakbrook Terrace, IL: Joint Commission.

2. Health Care Financing Administration, Department of Health and Human Services. 2000. "Conditions of Participation for Hospitals." *Code of Federal Regulations.* 42 CFR, Chapter IV, Part 482.

3. ICD-9-CM Official Guidelines for Coding and Reporting. Developed and approved by the American Hospital Association, American Health Information Management Association, Centers for Medicare and Medicaid Services, and the National Center for Health Statistics.

4. AHIMA is the professional organization responsible for issuing several credentials in health information management: Registered Health Information Administrator (RHIA), Registered Health Information Technician (RHIT), Certified Coding Specialist (CCS), and Certified Coding Specialist-Physician-based (CCS-P).

5. Office of Inspector General, Department of Health and Human Services. 1998. "Compliance Program Guidance for Hospitals." Washington, DC: Office of Inspector General.

References

AHIMA Code of Ethics, 1998.

AHIMA Standards of Ethical Coding, 1999.

AHIMA Coding Policy and Strategy Committee. "Practice Brief: Data Quality." *Journal of AHIMA* 67, no. 2 (1996).

Source: Prophet 2001.

Appendix 1.5

Sample Confidentiality Policy

Confidentiality and Nondisclosure Agreement

As an employee/contracted employee affiliated with the [name of organization], I understand that I must maintain the confidentiality of any and all data and information to which I have access in the course of carrying out my work. Organizational information that may include, but is not limited to, financial, patient identifiable, employee identifiable, intellectual property, financially nonpublic, contractual, of a competitively advantageous nature, and is from any souce or in any form (such as paper, magnetic or optical media, conversations, or film), may be considered confidential. The value and sensitivity of information is protected by law and by the strict policies of [name of organization]. The intent of these laws and policies is to ensure that confidential information will remain confidential through its use as a necessity to accomplish the organization's mission. Special consideration is expected for all information related to personally identifiable health information accessed in the course of your work.

As a condition to receiving electronic access and allowed access to a [system, network, or files] and/or being granted authorization to access any form of confidential information identified above, I agree to comply with the following terms and conditions:

1. My computer sign-on code is equivalent to my LEGAL SIGNATURE and I will not disclose this code to anyone or allow anyone to access the system using my sign-on code and/or password.

2. I am responsible and accountable for all entries made and all retrievals accessed under my sign-on code, even if such action was made by me or by another due to my intentional or negligent act or omission. Any data available to me will be treated as confidential information.

3. I will not attempt to learn or use another's sign-on code.

4. I will not access any online computer system using a sign-on code other than my own.

5. I will not access or request any information for which I have no responsibility.

6. If I have reason to believe that the confidentiality of my user sign-on code/password has been compromised, I will immediately notify [responsible party] by calling the helpdesk at [helpdesk phone number].

7. I will not disclose any confidential information unless required to do so in the official capacity of my employment or contract. I also understand that I have no right or ownership interest in any confidential information.

8. While signed on, I will not leave a secured computer application unattended.

9. I will comply with all policies and procedures and other rules of [name of organization] relating to confidentiality of information and access procedures.

10. I understand that my use of the [name of employer or organization] system may be periodically monitored to ensure compliance with this agreement.

11. I agree not to use the information in any way detrimental to the organization and will keep all such information confidential.

12. I will not disclose protected health information or other information that is considered proprietary.

Source: Dougherty and Scichilone 2002.

Chapter 2

Coding Staff Recruitment and Retention Issues

Nadinia A. Davis, MBA, CIA, CPA, RHIA, FAHIMA
Marion K. Gentul, RHIA, CCS

The goal of coding staff recruitment is to match the needs of the healthcare organization with the needs of the person performing coding functions. Inadequate supply of experienced coders may pressure some HIM department managers to hire candidates who are not fully qualified or adequately trained. Organizational demands to process accurate bills may make others reticent to hire and train entry-level coders. Experienced coders are likely to look for facilities that offer incentive plans or other attractive benefits, such as flexible work hours. Moreover, expert coders are often lured to jobs in the consulting field, where productivity is likely to be rewarded by compensation that is higher than it is in healthcare facilities.

This chapter presents basic guidelines that coding managers can use to assess their facilities' needs when recruiting applicants to fill a vacancy in the HIM department. It also discusses alternatives to filling vacancies with full-time employees.

Evaluating Candidate Qualifications

Matching the appropriate candidate to the open position challenges recruiters at all levels. Rethinking the requirements of the open position to take advantage of available candidates is sometimes necessary, particularly in a competitive market. Differences in coding environments make it difficult to distinguish between apparently similar candidates. One way to differentiate among candidates is through their credentials.

Coding Credentials

The two industry-recognized professional organizations that award coding credentials are the American Health Information Management Association (AHIMA) and the American Academy of Professional Coders (AAPC). Each of these organizations conducts credentialing examinations at various times throughout the year.

AHIMA offers the certified coding associate (CCA), certified coding specialist (CCS), and the certified coding specialist-physician based (CCS-P) credentials (AHIMA 2006a, AHIMA 2006b). The CCA examination tests the basic knowledge needed by new, inexperienced coders. The CCS examination emphasizes and tests the applicant's knowledge of hospital inpatient coding, specifically, the ICD-9-CM and associated coding rules and guidelines. The CCS-P examination also tests the applicant's knowledge of ICD-9-CM. However, the CCS-P examination emphasizes outpatient, ambulatory care, and physician practice-based coding, and it covers the HCPCS/CPT coding rules and nationally applicable reporting. Appendices 2.1–2.3 contain lists of competencies required for each of these AHIMA certifications.

AAPC offers two coding credentials. The certified professional coder (CPC) credential acknowledges competency for physician practice-based coding. The certified professional coder-hospital (CPC-H) credential recognizes competency for hospital-based coding. For individuals who have passed the required examinations but have not completed their work experience, AAPC provides interim designations: certified professional coder-apprentice (CPC-A), and certified professional coder-hospital apprentice (CPC-HA). AAPC also offers specialty credentials in evaluation and management, general surgery, and obstetrics and gynecology to members already certified as CPC, CPC-H, or CPC-A.

In general, hospital-based staff whose primary function is to perform inpatient coding should hold the CCS credential. Staff performing outpatient coding in hospital outpatient departments, ambulatory care settings, or physician practices may appropriately have the CCS-P or CPC credential. Many coders hold coding credentials from both AHIMA and AAPC. Coders also must meet continuing education requirements to retain their credentials. (A detailed discussion of continuing education appears later in this chapter.)

Some local colleges, trade schools, or Internet sites offer various sorts of "coding credentials" or "coding certificates." On an individual, case-by-case basis, a person possessing such a credential or certificate may meet the requirements for a coding position. However, it cannot be assumed that this person has achieved the same level of coding competence as one holding a credential from AHIMA or AAPC. Coding managers should encourage all staff members to work toward obtaining the credential or credentials most pertinent to their job functions. The best way to encourage is through cost reimbursement and/or compensation incentives.

In addition to coding credentials, AHIMA offers two general HIM credentials: the registered health information administrator (RHIA) and the registered health information technician (RHIT). These credentials are evidence of entry-level competence in general HIM practice and are useful in supporting job enhancement and enrichment opportunities for coding staff. (See table 2.1 for a summary of coding and HIM credentials.)

Membership in Professional Organizations

Professional coding organizations support coding initiatives and provide educational programs and services for coders. Without belonging to at least one professional association, coding professionals would find it difficult, if not impossible, to keep abreast of coding changes, reporting rules, and relevant legislation.

AHIMA, the national association of HIM professionals, is a diverse organization. Its members include coding staff personnel, as well as those who oversee coding functions and manage coding staff personnel. AHIMA offers coding resources, training, and continuing education, as well as the Society for Clinical Coding (SCC), a designated Community of Practice within the association. The membership of SCC includes coding professionals who work in settings throughout the healthcare continuum. AHIMA is also a member of the Cooperating Parties, which includes the American Hospital Association (AHA), the Centers for Medicare and Medicaid Services (CMS), and the National Center for Health Statistics (NCHS). The Cooperating Parties coordinate and maintain the ICD-9-CM coding system.

AAPC is a privately owned, professional coding organization. It offers both national and local continuing education opportunities, an informative bimonthly publication called *The Coding Edge,* and a strong network of local chapters.

Depending on the individual's job function and work setting, a coder might benefit from belonging to both AHIMA and AAPC. Staff members within the same healthcare facility who

Table 2.1. Summary of coding credentials and other HIM credentials

Credential	Title	Granting Organization	Requirements	Continuing Education
CCA	Certified coding associate	AHIMA	Passing national examination	10 hours per year
CCS	Certified coding specialist	AHIMA	Passing national examination	10 hours per year
CCS-P	Certified coding specialist—physician based	AHIMA	Passing national examination	10 hours per year
CPC	Certified professional coder	AAPC	Passing national examination, plus experience	18 hours per year
CPC-H	Certified professional coder—hospital	AAPC	Passing national examination, plus experience	18 hours per year (24 if both CPC credentials are held)
RHIT	Registered health information technician	AHIMA	Graduation from an accredited associate degree program and passing national examination	20 hours biannually
RHIA	Registered health information administrator	AHIMA	Graduation from an approved or accredited degree program and passing national examination	30 hours biannually

have memberships in different associations may share information with one another. Departments should budget funds for coding staff memberships in professional associations.

Experience

In recent years, the ability of many healthcare organizations to hire new coders has been hampered by industrywide economic pressures to reduce the number of coding positions and to keep salaries low in the face of declining inpatient occupancies. Meanwhile, the need for qualified coders in outpatient and other non–acute care settings has increased concomitantly with the focus on data quality and data integrity, corporate compliance, and the electronic health record. Because training a new coding professional can take a minimum of 6 months to 1 year, facilities have tended to drop training programs in favor of recruiting experienced coders.

In general, coders who have the appropriate credentials for their job functions, as well as at least 2 years of successful coding experience, are the most desirable candidates for coding positions. Unfortunately, even experienced coders may have difficulty adapting to different facility-specific guidelines and also must be trained and supervised. On the plus side, coders in new settings may provide their facilities with fresh alternatives and improvements to current practices. Coding experience and success in one setting may not always translate to success in another setting. A common misconception among noncoders is that "all coding is the same" or "a coder is a coder." This is not the case, because competency levels and documentation requirements differ from setting to setting.

For example, a coder with many years of experience at a local community hospital may not be proficient initially in a major teaching medical center. Similarly, inpatient coders who are moved to outpatient settings and outpatient coders who are moved to inpatient settings will need additional training because of differences in coding systems, documentation, and reimbursement reporting guidelines.

Continuing Education

Ongoing continuing education is vital to ensure accurate coding. Healthcare facilities should have specific policies and a formal process for continuing education for all coding staff positions. Appropriate continuing education is consistent with the National Correct Coding Initiative, the Joint Commission on the Accreditation of Healthcare Organizations' (JCAHO) criteria for staff competency, and compliance guidelines from the Department of Health and Human Services, Office of the Inspector General (DHHS OIG), which mentions the need for keeping coding staff up-to-date with regulatory requirements (CMS 2006, JCAHO 2002, DHHS OIG 1998).

Internal Continuing Education

Much continuing education can be accomplished without sending staff to costly outside seminars or workshops. The coding manager should consider the following suggestions for internal continuing education:

- Ask physicians from the medical staff to present short clinical topics pertinent to the patient population in a particular setting. Allow time for coders to ask questions of physicians within the different medical specialty areas. Consider pairing this presentation with a presentation of the associated coding issues.

- Have coders research pertinent clinical topics and present them to their colleagues. This activity can be done individually or in teams. Allow a specific amount of compensated time for staff to research the topics in the medical staff library, the local library, or on the Internet. The presentation should provide applicable coding assignments for the topics and include discussion of the impact on reimbursement, as appropriate.

- In hospital settings, allow coding staff to attend physicians' continuing education programs, "Tumor Board," or "Grand Rounds." Ask the medical staff office for a list of upcoming topics and obtain permission for coding staff members to attend.

- Consider using a "lunch-and-learn" format. Provide lunch to participants as a time-saver rather than using regular work hours for presentations. Busy staff and physicians will appreciate this accommodation. If the coding staff is large enough, consider forming coding teams and awarding token prizes, such as free food or movie tickets, for outstanding presentations. When creativity and fun are encouraged, the process can be motivating.

- Keep a log of topics presented by, and programs attended by, staff. Routine documentation presents a strong case to management and auditors that the HIM department and the facility are committed to data quality and accuracy and supports competence.

External Continuing Education

AHIMA and AAPC offer numerous external continuing education opportunities, often at local sites or by teleconference. Members of these organizations have the option of being automatically informed of upcoming events and topics. For example, the AHIMA e-Alerts advise members of upcoming events, continuing education opportunities, and other items of interest.

Many highly regarded training companies and consulting firms also offer pertinent education and training. Training companies and individual trainers often can customize presentations and materials specifically to meet an organization's needs. Codebook vendors or coding outsourcing firms are other sources of continuing education activities. To receive notice of these opportunities, coders should put their names on mailing lists and Internet notifications; for example: *hc*Pro at www.hcPro.com, CRN Institute at www.crn-institute.com and JustCoding.com. Coders should review notices of continuing education in professional journals and look for free seminars and web mailings from local insurance carriers and Medicare fiscal intermediaries. A current list of Medicare fiscal intermediaries is available on the CMS web site: http://www.cms.hhs.gov/center/provider.asp (CMS n.d.).

State hospital associations and AHA also offer educational opportunities. AHA periodically offers satellite presentations on clinical topics and coding changes.

Documentation of Continuing Education

When coders take part in any continuing education activities, their coding managers should document the credits awarded and the knowledge areas to which they apply, such as coding, computer technology, regulatory issues and privacy topics. (See table 2.2 for a sample continuing education log.) Coders should obtain a certificate of attendance for their personal files. In addition, employees attending in-house programs should receive a certificate of attendance or other documentation that can be used as evidence of continuing education for maintenance of credentials. Coding managers also should maintain a record of coders' attendance in the HIM department's file as evidence of coding education.

Table 2.2. Sample continuing education documentation log

NAME:_____			
Hire Date:_____			
Credential(s): _____			
Continuing Education Requirements: _____			

Date	Activity/Description (Attach program brochure)	Activity Sponsor	Hours Earned (Attach certificate of attendance)
cc: Human Resources			

Organizing the Coding Staff

The primary component of the coding staff is individuals with coding skills and experience. The number of coders, support staff, and supervisors of a coding area is completely dependent on the workload. Because no universally accepted criteria have been established for coding performance and because coders' responsibilities vary by facility and setting, no exact formula exists for determining how many coders are necessary.

Coding Skill Sets and Competencies

AHIMA has developed a specific set of work-based task competencies that credentialed coders should possess at both the hospital and physician-office levels. Those competencies are listed in appendices 2.1–2.3. In the absence of AHIMA credentials, employers must decide how coders will evidence competency. Employers may choose to make credentials a condition of employment. Alternatively, the hiring process may include a facility-based examination for all candidates.

As facilities move into an electronic environment, the need for coders to develop and maintain computer skills will grow. Some computer skill is already required in order to use the master patient index, an encoder, and to search for electronic reports. In using a truly electronic record, additional skills that may be required include report writing, data analysis, and online editing.

Job Descriptions

Job or position descriptions normally vary from one facility or organization to another, depending on the following factors:

- Size of the organization

- Services the facility offers

- Size and responsibilities of the coding staff

- Scope, setting, and oversight of the coding functions performed

Job descriptions should be reviewed annually and during an employee's annual performance review. Job descriptions should be updated whenever there are changes in responsibilities, oversight, or systems. They also should be updated when the organization has undergone a merger, acquisition, or reorganization. Facilities should ensure that job descriptions always reflect the most recent JCAHO requirements for job descriptions.

Job titles also vary from setting to setting. There is no "official" or preferred job title; however, the image conveyed by the title should be professional in tone.

The format of job descriptions also varies from organization to organization but, in general, should include:

- Job or position title.

- Department name: All coders within the organization may not be part of the HIM department even though they may have the same job or position title.

- Job or position title that the described position reports to, as it appears in the department's table of organization (TO) or organizational chart.

- Position summary: A brief statement or paragraph describing the major functions of the position as performed on a daily basis.

- Duties: A detailed explanation of the job functions that expands on the position summary. Duties should be listed in the order that the functions are performed, with the functions that are performed least frequently listed last. Many organizations include as the last duty, "other duties as assigned." If this phrase is not required by the facility or a union, it is best omitted. When "other duties" become apparent or are part of the coding function, they should be specified in the list of duties.

- Qualifications or requirements, including physical requirements such as lifting, sitting, reaching, computer skills, and specific knowledge of the organization's system. The requirements should specify whether a basic knowledge of the job is sufficient or whether the position requires special expertise in certain areas. For example, a coder must have expertise in coding, but not necessarily an extensive knowledge of the patient accounts function.

- Education, credentials, and experience should depend on the needs of the job as discussed previously in this chapter.

A sample job/position description is shown in appendix 2.4.

Control and Supervision

Each coding position also should be listed in the department's TO or organizational chart. Whenever a position is added or deleted or the job title changes, the TO should be updated. The TO shows how each position fits within the department and indicates lines of authority. In addition to the department's TO, the overall organizational TO demonstrates the authority and reporting lines and relationships among departments. Relationship and reporting lines within each department and among departments provide structure to the individual and can be used to foster cooperation within the organization.

Most traditional HIM departments have a director or manager who oversees the functions and duties of that department. If the HIM department has a small staff, the coding staff may report directly to the department manager or director. If the coding staff is large, coders may report to an assistant director, an assistant manager, a coding manager, or a coding supervisor. Regardless of title or other responsibilities, the person overseeing the coding function should have a strong coding background and the ability to act as a mentor and resource for new coders. He or she does not have to be the best coder in the department but must be able to facilitate the coding process and access all resources, professional and organizational, so that coders can function at maximum potential.

In a large organization or an integrated delivery system, coding positions may be delineated by the scope of services provided. Because of organizational complexity and the differences between inpatient and outpatient coding, separate job titles and positions may exist. For example, a coder who works in the long-term care division of an organization may have a different coding job title and job description than an acute care coder who works in the same facility. The difference in job descriptions reflects the variability in the scope of service, the setting, and the separate and distinct knowledge that each coder must have to perform the job.

Competency-Based Assessment

Job descriptions must contain measurable criteria for performance against which coders can be evaluated. Performance criteria include, but are not limited to:

- Number of charts coded
- Accuracy of coding as determined by a predefined audit process
- Maintenance of effective relationships with physicians and facility personnel

Coders should be evaluated at least quarterly, with appropriate training needs identified, facilitated, and reassessed over time. Only through this continuous process of evaluation can data quality and integrity be accurately measured and ensured.

Performing a Needs Assessment

When a vacancy occurs on the coding staff, the first thing the HIM department manager should do is to perform a **needs assessment.** This involves the following tasks:

- Performing a job analysis
- Assessing staff productivity requirements
- Analyzing the experience level of the coding staff
- Conducting a salary survey

Each of these tasks is a key element in helping the healthcare facility determine what coding positions are reasonable and necessary.

Performing a Job Analysis

The coding manager should not automatically try to fill a vacancy with a new coder who is just like the one who left. For example, filling a position vacated by a coder with 6 years of experience in the facility with a coder from outside the facility who also has 6 years of experience is not necessarily the best solution. The coding manager first should review his or her options. Questions to ask include:

- Should a new employee be hired and trained to fill the vacancy?
- Can the additional work be divided among current staff members?
- Can a current staff member be promoted to the position vacated?
- Should the department outsource the work?

During the vacating coder's time of service, the department may have hired, trained, and educated any number of coders, one of whom could be promoted to fill the open position. Obviously, when a current staff member is promoted to fill an open position, the vacancy simply shifts to another position. However, the position vacated by the promoted staff member may be easier to fill if it requires a lower skill level or less experience. Moreover, promotions within the department can boost staff morale, which is often needed when a staff member resigns.

During the time of a staff shortage, the coding manager should periodically review staff productivity and workload to assess their impact on morale and to avoid the loss of additional staff. Moreover, he or she can incorporate staff input when addressing pertinent issues, deciding whether to promote a staff member, or reorganizing work space and job responsibilities. When current staff must compensate for a vacancy, the coding manager should consider making whatever adjustments are necessary to balance the workload and to delegate some tasks temporarily to noncoding staff.

Finally, when the coding manager finds it necessary to hire a coder to fill a vacated position, he or she must justify that decision to the facility's administration. Thus, it is advisable to have benchmarking data and survey information completely up to date. In addition, the coding manager must know the costs for overtime or contract coding if the vacant position is not to be filled promptly. The longer a position is left unfilled, the likelier facility administration or owners are to decide that it is not really needed. Moreover, in times of layoffs, unfilled positions are often eliminated automatically.

Assessing Staff Productivity Requirements

The second part of the coding manager's needs assessment addresses staff productivity requirements. One approach is to review coder productivity (for both full- and part-time personnel) during regular hours and shifts. Such a review helps the coding manager determine whether productivity fluctuates at different times of the workday. For example, productivity is likely to be higher at night when fewer distractions or interruptions are present.

To compensate for productivity lost because of a change in personnel, the coding manager might be able to persuade some staff members to shift hours temporarily, perhaps by offering incentives such as a shift-differential increase in compensation. A shift-differential increase in pay may prove to be more cost-effective than overtime compensation.

Another approach to compensating for lost productivity is to arrange for coding staff to work when the HIM department is normally closed. This option requires notifying other departments and physicians as well as security staff that coders will be working after regular business hours.

Average discharges, productivity standards, and normal work hours all should be factored into the calculation of coding staff needs. Coders do not work every day. Vacations, sick days, holidays, downtime, continuing education, and noncoding responsibilities all must be considered. (See chapter 7 for a detailed discussion of productivity standards and the coding staff complement.)

In addition to assessing the productivity requirements of the HIM staff at his or her facility, the coding manager may want to conduct **benchmarking surveys** to determine the productivity requirements of local healthcare employers or those with a similar service mix. Some facilities may be willing to share this information directly. Local coding vendors also can be a useful source of information. Information items to be requested include hours worked, additional tasks performed, abstracting requirements, data-entry requirements, and vacation/sick days, in addition to the number of health records coded per time period. (See chapters 7 and 8 for a detailed discussion of benchmarking information.)

To have information available when recruitment becomes necessary, the coding manager should conduct benchmarking surveys on a routine basis. Routine benchmarking also helps the coding staff avoid complacency or the excessive assumption of unrelated tasks.

Analyzing the Level of Experience of Current Staff

The staff's level of experience is another critical factor to consider when deciding how to fill a vacancy. When the staff's level of experience is strong, hiring a trainee may be a possibility.

However, in the absence of experienced leadership or a staff resource person, a skeleton staff or a staff that is relatively inexperienced may be unable to support the hire of an untrained coder. One way to determine the experience level of the staff complement is to review each individual's current productivity and error rates and then compare them with previous productivity rates.

Conducting a Salary Survey

Understanding the economic marketplace is essential to any needs assessment. AHIMA is a good source of general salary information by region for AHIMA-credentialed coding staff. Local outsourcing coding vendors also are good sources of information, as are local colleges and universities with recent survey data for the region.

State hospital associations are another good source because they conduct salary surveys for all the main job categories generally found in hospitals. Hospital administrators and human resources (HR) departments frequently use this information. However, salaries can vary widely within a state and compensation is typically higher in metropolitan areas than in rural areas.

Salary surveys should be performed every 1 to 2 years. The HR department usually conducts them, but the HIM department may want to do job-specific surveys and then compare the results. One reason for this is that the two departments could have different hiring criteria. For example, the HIM department's main objective in hiring a coder is to find the best-qualified candidate whereas the HR department's main objective may be to lower the compensation level for the position. Indeed, some healthcare facilities offer their HR departments incentives to achieve savings in hiring practices. Thus, the coding manager must work with the HR department to ensure a balance in overall hiring goals and objectives.

Moreover, coding managers could use salary surveys done within their local marketplace to help them adjust compensation or environmental factors to better compete for coding employees. However, facilities competing for the same qualified candidates may not want to share information. When salary survey information is unavailable locally, coding managers will need to seek it from facilities with similar profiles that are located outside the immediate marketplace. In that way, competition for the same candidates is less likely.

Surveyors sometimes can increase their success by offering to share the results with everyone who participated in the survey. However, this usually will work only if the surveyors guarantee the participants' anonymity.

Recruiting and Hiring Coding Staff

When the HIM department makes the decision to fill a vacancy with a full-time staff member, it begins its effort to recruit candidates. This involves advertising the position and a sometimes-lengthy interviewing process. Although the traditional steps detailed below will probably need to be followed, it is also helpful to make known the need for and requirements of the position among colleagues. It is not unheard of to recruit at a professional association meeting, just as it is generally appropriate to take one's resume to such an event—just in case. Networking can be the most effective way to connect with the right individuals.

Choosing the Appropriate Advertising Vehicle

Many organizations limit their employment advertisements to local newspapers. However, to reach the maximum number of candidates, ads also may be placed in appropriate trade papers and magazines and on Web sites. If an expert coder is sought, it may be necessary to contact a professional recruiting firm in order to find the right individual. Although there is a fee involved in working with a recruiting firm, considerable savings may be obtained in terms of staff time reviewing multiple resumes and interviewing candidates. In a market where candidates are scarce, recruiting firms may present the best networking opportunity to identify candidates from other regions.

Determining the Content of the Ad

The HR department is generally responsible for writing and placing job advertisements. When job descriptions are updated annually, the HR department usually has the correct information on hand. However, sometimes inappropriate or outdated credentials have not been changed. An ad for an accredited record technician (ART), for instance, would reflect poorly on the department and the facility because this description of the credential was changed to RHIT in 2000. Thus, the coding manager should review ads for accuracy before they are placed.

In addition to checking for errors, the coding manager should read the ad for tone. HR departments use standard wording in recruiting advertisements. The coding manager should ensure that both the facility and the HIM department are described in a manner that makes them attractive to candidates and yet communicates a true picture of the working environment. Standard phrases such as "pleasant working conditions," "opportunity for advancement," and "full support for continuing education" are appropriate only when they are true.

Stating the Minimum Requirements

The ad also must specify the minimum requirements for the position. By itself, "high school education" is not an effective requirement for a coding position. Years of experience, if required, should be specified, in addition to all acceptable credentials. Depending on the duties of the coder, CCA, CCS, CCS-P, CPC, and CPC-H are the only credentials that pertain specifically to healthcare coding, although RHIT, RHIA, or credential "eligible" also are acceptable designations. "Eligible" generally refers to an individual who has completed all academic or other prerequisites but has not yet passed the required examination.

The issue of credentials can have an impact on employee morale. The coding manager must determine whether to hire a credentialed coder or one who is either not yet certified or preparing for certification. A staff composed entirely of credentialed coders may resent the hiring of an uncredentialed coder at a market salary. If obtaining an appropriate credential is a job requirement, the new employee may be hired on probation or paid a lower salary until he or she earns the credential. When a trainee is hired, any time limits imposed on obtaining the credential should be made in writing.

Finally, the ad should not state that the facility is willing to hire a trainee if it is looking for an experienced coder. Such a statement suggests that the position pays a trainee salary, which would discourage experienced coders from applying. On the other hand, if the facility is truly looking for a lower-salaried trainee, that should be specified.

Offering Sign-On Bonuses

Sometimes healthcare organizations offer sign-on bonuses to entice employees away from competing facilities. A **sign-on bonus** is a monetary incentive that is used to encourage a candidate to accept employment. However, any organization that offers a sign-on bonus should specify its criteria for qualifying for the bonus in a written contract. Having such criteria in writing discourages coders from "job hopping" from one sign-on bonus to another. Examples of such criteria include:

- The new coder must pass a probationary period.

- He or she must remain at the facility for a defined period of time, for example, one year following the probationary period.

- He or she must meet or exceed productivity standards at the milestone performance review(s).

Finally, when sign-on bonus criteria are not met, the contract might require the employee to reimburse the facility for the bonus amount. Alternatively, a portion of the "sign-on" bonus may be paid upon employment and the balance paid upon satisfaction of the stated criteria.

Selecting and Interviewing Candidates

Selecting and interviewing candidates involves a number of steps. These are explained in the following sections. As mentioned above, networking may produce a number of likely candidates. Be prepared to offer interviews to candidates who were obtained through networking. In some instances, you may want to interview such candidates even if they do not entirely meet your criteria, for the purpose of strengthening your network. Also, if a candidate is strongly recommended, he or she may have qualities and experiences that are not obvious from the resume.

Reviewing the Resume

The resume is typically the principal element on which organizations base their decision to interview job applicants. When reviewing resumes submitted for coding positions, the recruiter should look for:

- Level of experience—number of years, what type of coding, what type of facility

- Satisfaction of the minimum requirements—as derived from the needs assessment and stated in the advertisement

- Appropriateness of credentials—coding credentials versus general or unrelated credentials

- Gaps in employment—unexplained by educational experiences or other activities.

- Unrelated employment—supervisory skills that may transfer well from one industry to another and "second career" employees with excellent work habits learned in the previous career

- Length of service with previous employers—a long history of short employment unexplained by other activities, such as educational progress or spouse relocation

- Job responsibilities during coding employment that are unrelated to coding—including auditing, physician or coworker education, or cancer reporting

Any questions about the content of the resume should be noted. For example, gaps in employment are often due to relocation with a spouse or child-rearing issues. It is problematic whether some issues can be addressed in a job interview. One possible problematic reason for a gap in employment is a personality or productivity issue. It is not inappropriate to ask about gaps in employment and care should be taken to ensure that all gaps are explained.

It is also a "red flag" when an applicant does not have a reference from a recent prior employer. It is not unusual for an applicant to omit the current employer; however, failure to obtain a reference from a prior employer should be queried. Even if the previous supervisor has left the organization, it should be possible to contact that individual for a reference.

In addition to content, the recruiter should assess the resume and its cover letter for neatness, organization, spelling, grammar, and punctuation. The way applicants present themselves for employment is a possible indicator of how they will present themselves on the job. However, for many potentially excellent employees, English is a second, or sometimes a third, language. Thus, it may be difficult to determine whether grammar problems are the result of sloppiness or poor language proficiency. When grammar is the only problem with the documentation, it is best to err on the side of the applicant.

Sometimes, on paper, an applicant will appear to be overqualified for the position, as in the case of a consultant or a former department director. Such individuals should not be dismissed automatically. They may have personal reasons for seeking a position that is less stressful and/or that requires less overtime. Such applicants often have a good understanding of the "big picture" that enables them to model motivating behavior to others in the department.

Scheduling the Interview

Applicants who pass the resume review process become candidates for the position. Depending on the facility and the job being offered, the candidate will likely be interviewed by individuals in both the HR and HIM departments. If necessary, the interviews can be conducted over several days. Obviously, candidates who are currently working will be unable to schedule multiple interviews on different days during regular work hours. In such instances, interviews should be arranged to accommodate the candidates' schedules and, if possible, to include more than one interviewer at a time.

The facility attempting to attract and hire good candidates is, in effect, attempting to sell the open position and facility to the candidate. So, good first impressions are important to both parties. Respectful consideration should be shown to the candidate by allowing adequate time for the interview process. Rehearsing questions in advance is also helpful. If the coding manager is inexperienced in interviewing techniques, the HR department can provide assistance. When more than one candidate is being interviewed in a day, adequate time should be scheduled between interviews so that candidates do not meet and the interviewer can think about the interview. The interviewer should be punctual and not allow interruptions to intrude on the interview process.

Certain general questions should be asked of all candidates. (See table 2.3 for some classic interview questions and explanations of their purposes.) Type out the questions in advance and have a clean copy available for notes during each interview. Jot down notes during the interview. In the HIM profession, one can easily be in the position of interviewing an acquaintance. The coding manager should not skip any questions simply because he or she knows the candidate. When this is the case, someone from the HR department could join the interview to ask the questions. This strategy makes explanations easier when the candidate is not the best one for the position.

The interview process should include time for questions and replies, as well as time for taking a coding test, if required. It is essential that the candidate be informed in advance of the time frame both for the interview and the test. If the test needs to be scheduled at a different time than the interview, the candidate should be informed.

Table 2.3. Common interview questions and their purposes

Questions	Purposes
Describe your biggest accomplishment.	Can identify whether the individual is goal oriented or a team player. Is the biggest accomplishment being promoted or contributing to a major project?
	Illustrates the scope of the candidate's vision. Is the accomplishment related to a particular day's activities or to an organizationwide project?
	Focus on work- or school-related achievements. If the biggest achievement is personal, redirect the question.
What would you do if you were not a coder?	May lead to a discussion of the candidate's professional goals. Does he or she look for advancement to supervision and management? Is coding a step along the way of his or her chosen profession?
	Why the candidate is not doing this other activity may be important. Self-knowledge of lack of talent, for example, shows that the candidate has a realistic view of his or her skills and abilities.
	Some interviewers like to interpret unusual answers. "Broadway singer" might be interpreted as liking to be the center of attention and "baseball player" as a team player. However, this is dangerous territory and should be avoided.
Describe a problem you had and how you solved it.	Regardless of the origin of the problem, pay attention to how it was solved. Is this how you would want an employee to solve problems in your facility? Does the candidate's strategy fit into your corporate/department culture? If you are unsure, pose a problem that your coders have had and ask how the candidate would handle it.
All questions.	If you gain nothing else from the responses, you will gain an understanding of the degree of the candidate's verbal communication skills. Is he or she well prepared and articulate?

Analyzing the Interview

The best time to record impressions is immediately after the interview. Allow at least 15 minutes to think about the experience. Note the answers to specific questions. Be as objective as possible and extremely careful about notes written in the margins of the resume and on the question notes.

The purpose of a resume review and standard interview experience is to eliminate bias and subjectivity in hiring. Interviewers should not subvert that process by using discriminatory language in their interview notes. Now is a good time to think about follow-up questions for the particular candidate.

Testing for Coding Skills

The coding test may be standardized, with scenarios to which the coder assigns the appropriate codes. Examples of such tests may be taken from routinely published coding handbooks and texts. A local college or university may be able to assist in this process. The HIM department should review the test annually to ensure that it accurately reflects current codes and coding practices, as well as the actual work to be performed, as required by the Occupational Safety and Health Administration (OSHA 1998). To ensure compliance, it may be necessary to work with the facility/corporation's HR department to verify that the test is "fair" and accurately reflects the job skills required.

The test also may require the candidate to code health records. Although coding health records can take more time than a standardized test, it gives the coding manager a better idea of the candidate's level of productivity. If health records are used, they should be photocopied and redacted (patient identities obscured or removed). Health records used for this type of test should reflect common coding issues that arise in the facility. For example, if the facility has an active cardiac catheterization laboratory, and the coder would be expected to code these records, then such a health record should be included in the test.

The test results should be evaluated for accuracy, level of experience, and speed. However these elements are handled, all candidates must be treated equally in the scoring and analysis of the test.

Evaluating for Accuracy

Accuracy is the most important characteristic of the coder's work. An unfamiliar environment may impair the coding candidate's speed but should not affect his or her accuracy. The person evaluating the test should pay close attention to the types of errors made. These can indicate whether the coder merely needs training in a particular area (such as confusing a cardiac catheterization procedure) or whether he or she is sloppy or inattentive to detail (omitting a fifth digit on an ICD-9-CM code). If necessary, a test debriefing that queries the candidate about incorrect responses can be scheduled. This debriefing is part of the interview process and should be treated as such. The way the candidate handles critique of the coding can be indicative of the way he or she will handle supervision and audit results in the future.

Evaluating for Level of Experience

Test results should be evaluated to determine the applicant's stated level of coding experience. For example, a coder who has never seen an arteriovenous (A/V) fistula procedure for renal dialysis may not code it accurately but should at least be close. A coder with years of experience who states that renal procedures were routine at a previous position should be able to code the procedure correctly, without hesitation.

Evaluating for Speed

The least important factor in the coding test is speed. An experienced coder would certainly be expected to complete the test more quickly than a trainee. However, an unfamiliar format and environment can have a negative effect on productivity.

Making the Offer

Depending on facility policy, either the HIM department manager or someone in the HR department makes the actual offer of employment. If the coding manager is so designated, the two departments must resolve a number of specific issues, including:

- How long the offer will be in effect
- What leeway the coding manager will have in negotiating salary
- What specific issues or benefits the HR department will handle
- How to schedule preemployment requirements, such as physical examinations and facility orientations
- What the appropriate start date will be

The offer of employment should always be made in writing. Most currently employed individuals will not resign a position without a written offer in hand. After the prospective employee has accepted the offer, it is appropriate to e-mail or fax confirmation of the acceptance.

After the position has been filled, the courteous and common business practice is to inform the other candidates. This notification also should be done in writing as soon as possible.

Taking the New Employee through the Orientation Process

Many, if not most, healthcare facilities have a regularly scheduled 1- or 2-day orientation program for all new employees, regardless of job function. The purpose of the orientation program is to introduce new employees to:

- The organization as a whole
- The department in which he or she will work
- The specific job responsibilities

Orientation to the Organization

Depending on facility policy, new employees may be required to attend an orientation to the overall organization before attending the department-specific orientation. Therefore, their start date is not necessarily the date they actually begin to produce work. As a practical matter, coding managers should assume that the new employee's first week is devoted primarily to orientation.

Orientation to the overall organization might include discussion of:

- JCAHO requirements
- OSHA requirements
- Issues related to the Health Insurance Portability and Accountability Act (HIPAA)
- State requirements
- Employee benefits
- Expectations of conduct

When possible, orientation topics should be presented in order of importance. For example, the facility's confidentiality policies should be presented before the location of the cafeteria is discussed. Typically, the HR department conducts the orientation to the organization, with support from other departments. For instance, the coding manager may be asked to present the topic of confidentiality to new employees. Certainly one purpose of this process is to impart the tone and culture of the organization. However, the orientation also gives new employees the opportunity to ask questions they may have thought of since accepting employment. It is important that new employees receive accurate answers to their questions. Orientation, therefore, should be conducted by experienced individuals who can provide answers themselves or query others effectively to obtain prompt answers.

Orientation to the Department

The new employee's workstation should be ready upon his or her arrival. Orientation to the department should begin after he or she has settled in. Introductions should be the first order of business and can be made during an informal tour of the department.

The coding manager or designee overseeing the orientation to the department should have a checklist of items to be discussed and information to be disseminated. (See table 2.4 for a sample orientation checklist.) The facility may use a generic form with space included for departmental specifics. Current JCAHO standards can be used to ensure that the checklist includes all the requirements of continued employment, such as verification that the employee has read and understood the organizational mission statement and confidentiality policy.

The policy and procedure manual and the HIM department's TO also should be reviewed and discussed. Sections that do not necessarily pertain to the employee's immediate job function may be included to provide an overall picture of the department's functions and responsibilities. The department also may have the new staff member rotate through all or most of the job functions. Actually seeing the functions in action helps to clarify the department's role within the healthcare facility.

Table 2.4. Sample orientation checklist

Departmental Orientation	Trainer Initials	Employee Initials	Date
General:			
Workstation location			
Policies regarding workstation appearance			
Work hours			
Sign-in procedures			
Sick day procedures			
Vacation day procedures			
Introduction to staff			
Departmental grievance procedures			
Functional:			
Job description			
Performance measurement			
Work distribution			
Computer training			
Telephone training			
Daily tasks			
Weekly tasks			
Other periodic tasks			
Physician query procedures			
Problem chart procedures			
Missing information procedures			
Coding guidelines			
Coding resources			
Coding question procedures			
Subsequent work flow			
Departmental work flow			

The new employee should sign off on the checklist to indicate that the orientation process has been completed. The checklist then should be signed and dated by the HIM manager or a supervisor. It may be kept in the HR department or in the employee's file within the HIM department. In addition, a confidentiality statement should be signed with the signature witnessed and dated. The confidentiality statement then should be reviewed annually or according to organizational policy. Any employee-specific confidential information, such as computer passwords, must be kept in a secure location.

Orientation to the Functions of the Job

The next part of the new employee's orientation is to address the specific functions of the job. To be fully functional in, and comfortable with, the new position, the new coder first must be instructed on the department's operations. For example:

- How is work distributed?
- What tasks are to be performed in addition to coding?
- What happens to the health record after it is coded?

These and other functional orientation questions are listed in table 2.4 (p. 65). One important reason for formalizing this review is to document that it occurred. This ensures that a lack of knowledge of job functions cannot be used as an excuse for incomplete work.

Orientation to the functions of the job also should:

- Review the regulatory requirements that affect the position
- Determine the need for training
- Clarify the standards used to measure the employee's progress
- Explain the probationary period
- Discuss the job productivity expectations

Regulatory Requirements

Healthcare facilities and their employees must meet numerous regulatory and accreditation standards. The coding manager should review the facility's corporate compliance, coding compliance, and performance improvement programs with the new coder.

Often the arrival of a new employee gives the HIM department the opportunity to involve the entire coding staff in a formal review of the facility's regulatory and compliance programs.

Need for Training

A new employee's need for training can be based on the areas of weakness identified from the coding test taken during the interviewing process. The coding manager should schedule education and training in these areas before the coder begins the actual work of coding.

The coding manager should discuss all identified coding errors with new employees. Occasionally, the reviewer is wrong. Unless the error is clear, new employees should be given the opportunity to defend their coding with authoritative references. This process enables them to develop a collaborative relationship with the coding supervisor and with coworkers that will have long-term benefits.

Standards of Measurement

One goal of the functional orientation is to ensure that the new coder understands the standards that will be used to measure his or her job performance. For example:

- How often is performance reviewed?

- Who performs the review?

- How will errors be handled?

All employees should be given routine, collaborative, and educational feedback. This feedback is particularly important for new coders, who find it unproductive and stressful to wonder for weeks or months how well they are doing.

Probationary Period

An employee hired to fill an open position generally serves a period of probation. The intent of the **probationary period** is to give the employee the opportunity to demonstrate his or her ability to perform the duties of the position.

Most states specify the duration of the probationary period, which typically is 3 months. The probationary period is the last opportunity the employer has to rectify a hiring error with minimal effort. Probationary periods typically can be extended at weekly or monthly intervals for any length of time, although usually no more than 6 months.

If the new employee's work during the probationary period is unsatisfactory, the coding manager should identify the specific areas that need improvement and then discuss possible remedies with the probationary coder. Ideally, the new employee will demonstrate steady progress throughout this period. When he or she has progressed, even though not meeting every expectation, the coding manager must decide whether to extend the probationary period or remove the coder from probationary status.

During the probationary period, healthcare facilities often compensate an employee at less than full pay and withhold certain benefits, such as health insurance. The purpose of the probationary period is to ensure that the potential coder is qualified for the position, not to "buy time" to interview other candidates. The coding manager should not "string along" an individual for an extended period of time without making a decision. Organizations that engage in such unfair and unethical hiring practices will soon become known in the coding community and begin to experience hiring difficulties.

Terminating an employee after he or she has been taken off probation can be difficult and stressful. Thus, to avoid difficulties, the coding manager should be aware of all written policies, legalities, and union agreements regarding probationary periods and the hiring and firing of staff.

Productivity Expectations

The productivity expectations of the position should be clearly stated. An employee's failure to meet productivity standards can be grounds for dismissal. The coding manager who treats productivity expectations lightly is likely to end up with unproductive employees.

As indicated earlier, two indicators of a coder's skill are the types of errors he or she makes and the speed at which he or she can work. For example, coders who achieve 100 percent accuracy in assigning principal diagnoses and DRG groupings but occasionally miss an additional diagnosis are more accurate than those who make mistakes selecting principal diagnoses and DRGs but correctly code everything else. All coding is important, but correct coding of principal diagnoses and DRGs produces the most benefits and the least need for recoding after quality audits.

However, it is clear that the coder who completes only one health record per day with 100 percent accuracy is not productive. The speed at which a coder can work depends on a number of factors, including the quality of the documentation in the health record and the extent of his or her responsibilities. Coders can code more health records in a day when they do not also have to abstract and enter data. On the other hand, coders who enter their own data have the opportunity to review the results and correct errors at the time of entry.

Impact of Noncoding Activities

Noncoding activities negatively affect accuracy and speed. It is very important to view departmental functions as a whole. Some employees seem to attract unrelated projects, either because of their helpful personality traits or the desire for job enrichment or because they wish to demonstrate supervisory capabilities. Therefore, supervisory personnel should monitor employee activities to ensure that work distribution and workflow are appropriate.

Choosing Alternatives to Full-Time Staffing

The past 20 years have seen the emergence of a number of viable alternatives to the hiring of full-time, permanent employees. These include **job sharing,** telecommuting, and outsourcing.

Job Sharing

Employee morale and productivity often suffer when staff have to share the workload left by an unfilled position. Job sharing refers to the situation in which two or more individuals share the tasks of one job or of one full-time equivalent (FTE) position. Typically, the employees occupy one work space and are rarely in the office at the same time.

Advantages of Job Sharing

Job sharing is a good alternative when the position calls for a full-time coder, but the pool of qualified candidates consists exclusively of part-time workers. Moreover, cost savings can occur if no benefits are paid in a job-sharing arrangement.

The major advantage to job sharing is that the work can still be done even though the position has not been filled. Often a job-sharing position can be retained as a full-time position rather than converted to two part-time positions.

Disadvantages of Job Sharing

Job sharing also has disadvantages. For example:

- The resignation of one of the individuals sharing the job can create replacement problems.

- Performance evaluation may be problematic depending on how the job is shared (which is often left up to the employees). Although actual coding tasks can be reviewed, non-coding activities such as customer relations and collaboration with other departments may be difficult to assess. For example, one person sharing the job may leave a telephone message and the other may take the return call and complete the task. Moreover, if a performance problem occurs, the supervisor may be unable to determine where it originated.

- Because the employees sharing the job must work as a team to complete the job function, the coding manager may need to spend extra time monitoring their working relationship and to pay close attention to any reported issues of miscommunication or evidence of incomplete tasks.

Using Current Staff in Job Sharing

When job sharing is not feasible, other staff may be cross-trained to assume the clerical tasks of the coding position. One part-time employee could then perform coding tasks.

Overtime hours and pay may be an attractive incentive for staff to participate in job sharing in the short term, particularly during holidays and/or summer vacation time. However, employees may question the fairness of the compensation when required to do additional work over the long term.

Telecommuting

Telecommuting is an arrangement in which an employee works from home and communicates with the office via electronic means. It allows employees to be hired who are not in routine commuting distance from the facility.

Technically, many **contract coders** are types of telecommuters. They work for a coding service vendor but perform services at the healthcare facility. They submit time sheets and expense reports to the vendor and receive instructions and assignments electronically from the vendor. Indeed, many contract coders have never set foot in their actual employer's office. For the purpose of this discussion, however, a telecommuting coder is one who works at home using electronic data provided by the facility.

Some employees combine working at home and in the office. This is most common when they live within commuting distance from the office. However, a growing number of employers are willing to work with and periodically fund the transportation of employees from distant sites.

Telecommuting attracts individuals who prefer either to work at home or not to relocate. Without question, a healthcare facility's ability and willingness to allow telecommuting increases the pool of potential candidates. In addition, the use of telecommuters can decrease the physical work space allocated to a position.

Work-at-home coders must have consistently high professional standards to counteract negative stereotypes, such as the perception that patient records are visible at a coder's kitchen table while the neighbors are sitting around drinking coffee. Sometimes telecommuters are perceived by in-house staff as doing less work, being elitist, and placing a burden on the facility. One drawback of telecommuting is that the bonding among employees that facilitates collaboration may be lacking. Thus, coding managers should orient new telecommuters on-site and encourage networking among the coding staff via e-mail. Thanks to videoconferencing, telecommuters can participate in staff meetings and informal discussions as readily as if they were on-site.

Advantages of Telecommuting

Telecommuting may increase productivity because of the focus on the coding task and the limitation of noncoding activities. Telecommuting also increases the pool of potential employees. The cost of installing hardward, software, and communications lines may offset the cost of hiring contract coders. Facilitation of telecommuting is one of the rationales for scanning records.

Disadvantages of Telecommuting

Telecommuting is often justified on the basis of increased productivity. However, increased productivity is not always obtained. Sometimes, the distractions inherent at home are an encumbrance. For example, coders who think that working at home is a substitute for obtaining alternative child care are often surprised to discover how little can be done with a small child in the house. Telecommuters should be self-starters with good productivity in the office-based environment. While working from home may effectively boost the productivity of that worker, it will do little for an employee who spends half the day on personal phone calls. Finally, a coder who is highly productive in a paper-based environment may be impaired in an online environment, because of the physical limitations of a scanned record.

Telecommuting is a viable alternative only when all technical, confidentiality, and access issues can be resolved. The fact that communication with telecommuters is largely electronic makes supervision of their work challenging. Moreover, technical support can be difficult, particularly if the employee is located outside the normal commuting range. Ensuring the confidentiality of data is a primary concern.

Outsourcing

Outsourcing of the coding function from consulting firms can be a long- or short-term alternative when a shortage of qualified candidates makes hiring difficult or when the HIM department has insufficient resources to train in-house staff. Consulting firms tend to attract talented coders with high productivity levels.

As a long-term alternative, a healthcare facility can cover its coding function by using a combination of in-house employees and contract coders. This strategy is typically used in a job market with a shortage of qualified coders.

Advantages of Outsourcing

The outsourcing of coding tasks offers several advantages, including:

- Contract coders who perform unsatisfactorily are more easily replaced than in-house coders who perform unsatisfactorily.

- Contract coders may be more experienced and productive than full-time in-house coders.

- The facility can use contract coders to fill temporary needs caused by vacations and illness.

- Contract coders may be willing to work outside regular business hours.

Disadvantages of Outsourcing

The disadvantages to outsourcing include:

- Coding managers or department supervisors have little control over contract coders beyond monitoring the quality of their work.

- Nothing prevents contract coders from leaving the facility when their productivity requirement has been met for the day or when a better job placement comes along.

- Generally, contract coders are not assigned noncoding tasks and cannot be expected to "pitch in" when an in-house employee is absent. The contract coder may have gone into consulting partly to get away from that type of burden, which also helps to explain contract coders' generally high levels of productivity.

- In-house coders sometimes resent what they perceive to be the elitist attitude of contract coders. The coding manager should not minimize or ignore the potential impact of this issue on regular coding employees.

Using Coding Vendors

The decision to use coding vendors involves finding potential candidates, writing requests for proposals (RFPs), evaluating the proposals submitted, and contracting with the selected vendor. Several levels of vendors provide coding services, including independent consultants, coding contractors with multiple employees, and multiservice contractors for whom coding is just one part of the business. There are advantages and disadvantages associated with each type of vendor.

Independent Consultants

Independent consultants perform coding services either as solely independent contractors or to supplement their regular employment. Because of low overhead, they tend to be relatively inexpensive compared with coding companies. Independent consultants often have a wealth of knowledge and can provide excellent advice on processing procedures, productivity issues, and physician relations. Sometimes they can become engaged in departmental affairs, even to the point of attending staff meetings and office parties. The Internal Revenue Service (IRS) has very clear guidelines about what constitutes an independent contractor (2006). (See appendix 2.5.) Any independent consultant contract should include a standard independent contractor clause. An independent contractor who has only one organization as a client for a significant period of time looks like an employee to the IRS and probably should be put on the organization's payroll.

Multiservice Contractors

Some **multiservice contractors** are small, local companies that provide coding services as well as coding-related services, such as DRG audits. Despite their name or apparent corporate status, some of these companies are actually sole proprietorships or independent contractors who subcontract to other independent contractors or other coding companies. For example, the staff of "Fast Coding, Inc." may consist entirely of Mary Coder. When Mary obtains a contract that requires additional staffing, she calls her friend Bob, who used to work for another consulting company and is now an independent contractor. Thus, coding managers may encounter contract coders who have been in their department under different organizational umbrellas at different times. Although there is nothing inherently wrong with this situation, some increased risk may be attached, because the burden of responsibility in the event of error may be unclear. In order to eliminate this risk, the contract between the facility and the contractor must clearly specify who will be doing the work and what remedies are available in the event of error. Careful construction of the RFP and detailed reading of the contractor's response to the RFP should identify any problematic issues.

Contractors with Multiple Employees

Some coding contractors are large enough to hire trainees. These coding companies have the resources to maintain stable training schedules and are in a better position to hire trainees than healthcare facilities might be. Coding managers should know, however, whether the contract coder is a trainee, how long he or she has been or will be in training, and what, if any, burden this will place on the HIM department. Coding quality is the coding manager's top priority and, as such, should be the key issue in contracting.

Another issue with large contractors is that coding is sometimes a very small part of their business. Although they do have coders on staff, they may recruit additional coders as contracts require (similar to smaller companies). Pay particular attention on the RFP to who is actually going to do the work. The opposite may also be true. Large contractors may have a very large staff, which affords the facility a high degree of assurance that coding coverage will be stable and consistent.

Writing a Request for Proposal

A **request for proposal (RFP)** is the means used by facilities to solicit information in writing from vendors about specific services and their costs. The RFP should be simple and clear and should specify a predetermined format for responses, particularly for pricing and productivity. Some vendors charge by the health record, others by the hour. To compare rates, the RFP can require all the vendors to standardize their pricing and to give a per-record rate based on their hourly rate and on standard productivity requirements.

The following issues should be addressed in every RFP for coding services:

- Coding quality

- Price

- Volume productivity

- Noncoding tasks

Coding Quality

Because the facility is contracting with a vendor as opposed to hiring an employee, it should determine how the vendor plans to assure the quality of the services it is providing. Answers to the following questions can help the coding manager determine whether the vendor's quality program is in line with the HIM department's coding compliance concerns:

- Does the vendor have a quality assurance (QA) plan, in-service training program, and/ or some other continuing education plan?

- Will the vendor audit the quality of its work?

- How does the vendor determine coding quality?

- Will the vendor accept a penalty clause if coding quality falls below a certain level?

- Will the vendor respond to quality challenges by insurers and/or regulators?

Price

Obviously, the price of services is important. However, coding managers should avoid simply hiring the vendor who offers the cheapest price without examining the proposal for add-ons. For example, $10 per health record may look less expensive than $11 per health record, but when the $10 proposal includes a surcharge for any length of stay (LOS) of more than 6 days and the facility's average LOS is 5 days, the actual fees may regularly exceed $11 per health record. Thus, the price and any variations mentioned must be fully considered in evaluating which vendor's pricing is best.

Volume Productivity

Although the vendor's volume productivity requirements are generally nonnegotiable, the coding manager should definitely examine the vendor's employee policies regarding productivity. For example, if the HIM department has 100 health records available to code and the contract coder's productivity requirement is 50 health records per day, will the coding manager have the opportunity to give the contract coder additional work? Or will the coder leave when the requirement is fulfilled? A contract provision that allows the coding manager to request, for example, three to five health records in addition to standard productivity specifications may enable the HIM department to complete a full discharge day of work or to code an extra record with high unbilled charges. If the facility wants a coder to be available for a full work day, regardless of productivity, this must be stated in the contract. Additionally, the facility must take into consideration the contractor's productivity expectations in relation to its own. If the contractor only expects 25 records per day and the facility expects 30, that expectation gap must be resolved or a different contractor hired.

Noncoding Tasks

The HIM department should not assume that a contract coder will perform noncoding tasks such as filing loose sheets, entering data, calling other departments for reports, contacting physicians, or answering the telephone. Although these tasks are often included in the normal operating procedures for employee coders, contract coders are not required to perform them unless the contract so specifies. Thus, if the contract coder is expected to perform noncoding tasks, the HIM department should specify them, along with detailed procedures, in the RFP so that they can be factored into the overall price of the service. Expect a large price differential for nonroutine coding tasks, becaue of impaired productivity. For example, if 50 charts per day becomes closer to 40 when abstracting and data entry are added, the facility can expect a 25% increase in the per-record price of services.

Evaluating Vendor Responses

Before responding to an RFP, a vendor may request a meeting to discuss the requirements of the job and the case mix. In this way, the vendor can observe the state of the HIM department's records at the time of coding and become acquainted with all the quirks of the department's processing. Many outsourcing contracts end disastrously when this kind of information is not requested or conveyed up front. Indeed, coding managers should be wary of a vendor whose quote for coding services falls well below the quotes of the other bidders. Such a vendor probably has not taken into consideration the case mix, the difficulty of the health records, or the unique processing requirements, or noncoding tasks, of the system.

An objective review of the proposals is essential for making a sound hiring decision. The review should be based on specific criteria that are defined in advance, including:

- Qualities—Does the contractor have business practices that are consistent with those needed by the facility?

- Characteristics—Is the contractor a good fit for the facility?

- Skills—Check the staff roster for the skill sets that are needed

- Experience—Ensure that there is evidence that the contractor has experience in the appropriate type of coding

- Price—Read the proposal to ensure that the prices are calculated in a comparable manner

When a vendor does not respond as requested, the coding manager must decide whether to ask for clarification or to eliminate the vendor from consideration. Generally speaking, it is safe to assume that a vendor whose RFP response does not conform to requirements will be similarly negligent in dealing with processing requests.

The coding manager should rank his or her priorities and weight the responses in a decision matrix. (See table 2.5.) This method of analysis helps to focus on the vendors who most closely meet the organization's needs. Each vendor's weighted score is the sum of the criterion scores times the criterion's rank. In table 2.5, for example, the total score for vendor 1 is 24: $[(3 \times 3) + (5 \times 2) + (5 \times 1) = 24]$.

The rankings of priorities can be more complex. For example, if quality assurance is significantly more important to the facility than cost, its weight (rank) might be 4 instead of 3. To ensure an objective evaluation, the HIM department should develop criteria priorities and measures for scoring in advance of reviewing the RFPs.

Avoiding Common Pitfalls

Both in-house employees and outsource personnel sometimes have conflicting perceptions about issues such as customer service, staffing, productivity, and work flow that can negatively affect the HIM department's relationship with its vendor. If the vendor's contract does not address these issues, the parties should consider an addendum.

Customer Service Issues

The customer service relationship between the HIM department and the coding vendor is very important. The contract should address how problems in this area will be resolved and by whom. For example:

- Will vendor personnel be required to interact with noncoding personnel and physicians?

- How will the contract coder's physician queries be handled?

- How will coder errors be handled?

This last question is particularly important. Even though the vendor may have a quality assurance plan, the healthcare facility is ultimately responsible for ensuring the quality of its

Table 2.5.   Sample decision matrix for vendor selection

Rank	Criteria	Vendor 1	Score	Vendor 2	Score	Vendor 3	Score
3	Quality assurance	Limited	3	Full Program	5	Full Program	5
2	Continuous coverage guaranteed	Yes	5	Yes	5	No	1
1	Cost per chart	$7	5	$13	1	$10	3
	Weighted score		24		26		20

Scores range from 1 to 5, with 5 being the highest and 1 the lowest.

coding. Thus, the work of contract coders should be included in the HIM department's routine quality audits. However, the department should follow its protocols at all times. Like employee coders, contract coders must be afforded the opportunity to review and defend their work.

Staffing Issues

The vendor's contract may call for the coding of a certain number of health records during a period of time but not address how to achieve that productivity level. If the vendor sends a different contract coder every week, the work flow in the HIM department is disrupted. Even new contract coders must be oriented and their work reviewed. Therefore, if "revolving door" staffing is problematic for the HIM department, it should be prohibited in the contract.

Productivity Issues

As mentioned previously, the productivity quantity standards for employee staff and consultant staff may differ significantly. For example, it is not unusual for employees to code 25 to 30 inpatient records per day, compared to a contract coder's rate of more than 50 inpatient records per day.

Productivity standards for consultant staff should be stated in the contract. When no quality issues exist, it is absolutely inappropriate for the coding manager to ask the contract coder to slow down to match the employee rate. Rather, the coding manager should explain the differences in the requirements and point out to the regular staff that they may be performing noncoding duties that contribute to those differences. Indeed, the coding manager may find it more difficult to explain the differences in productivity rates to his or her administrative superiors who are unfamiliar with departmental processing issues. The coding manager must be prepared to defend the department's internal productivity requirements or to reevaluate them as needed.

Without question, consultant coders are an expensive line item in the HIM department's budget. Some departments attempt to justify the cost by having the consultant code the most difficult records. If this is the plan, the coding manager should explain it up front so that the vendor can determine an appropriate price. If the coding manager agrees to a normal case mix and does not provide it, the HIM department can expect to lose the consultant or to face a significant rate hike as soon as the contract permits.

Work Flow Issues

Problematic work flow issues include loose paperwork, available paperwork, and analysis. Optimally, the contract coder should be provided with an agreed-on number of records that have been preassembled and analyzed (although production delays may occasionally present challenges). If the production cycle places coding before analysis, this should be specified up front to bring the price quotes in line with reality and to prevent problems down the road.

Technology Issues

If the coding services are being provided on a telecommuting basis, the RFP process and subsequent contract must specifically address how the technology will be provided, what penalties, if any, will apply in the event of technological failure, and how technology problems will be addressed.

Amending the Proposal

The vendor's response to the RFP is a proposal, not a legal contract. Thus, the coding manager should not hesitate to require the amendment of any item in the vendor's response that does not meet the HIM department's requirements. However, it should be noted that amendments to the proposed terms will likely result in a change in the quoted price for services.

During the contract negotiation or amendment process, some of the previously discussed issues may come to light. For example, the RFP may have asked for a proposal to code 100 health records per week but not have specified the hours the department would be open to the consultant, with the result that the vendor quoted a price based on regular business hours. During the amendment process, the vendor discovers that the facility is willing to allow the consultant to work evening and Saturday hours. Such clarification may provide more choices in terms of the consultants who are available to fulfill the contract.

Finalizing the Contract

If the coding manager does not have the authority to sign the vendor contract, it may have to pass through administrative, purchasing, and legal reviews. When this is the case, parties from those areas should be involved in the final selection and negotiation process in order to avoid delays in executing the contract. (See table 2.6 for a summary of key vendor contract issues.)

The coding manager would be wise to have the facility's corporate counsel review the contract in its preliminary stages so that any legal concerns can be addressed in the negotiation stage. Involving legal counsel at the negotiation stage ensures that the final contract will

Table 2.6. Key vendor contract issues

Issue	Questions	Comments
Productivity	What are the productivity measures and requirements?	Understanding the "available work" requirements (How many records need to be ready to code?)
	How will they be enforced?	Important for keeping current with the coding function
	Are there any "minimum available work" requirements?	Understanding the vendor's policies and procedures if work is unavailable
Quality control	How will coding quality be measured and reported?	Not only what the vendor's standards are, but also how to go about resolving differences
	How will necessary quality interventions be conducted?	How to handle identified errors and other quality issues
Employee relations	Who will actually do the coding?	Understanding the relationship between the vendor and the workers that it provides
	How will unsatisfactory workers be handled?	How easy will it be to replace an unsatisfactory worker?
	Is coverage guaranteed when a scheduled worker is not available?	Exploring depth of the vendor's coding staff
Department interaction	Exactly what tasks are the consultant coders expected to perform?	Ensuring that the vendor is aware of all information
	Who will provide training for those tasks?	Fully discussing whether trainee coders will be used
Cost variances	How is payment for services rendered calculated?	Ensuring the validation of invoices
	What, if any, variances in payment are expected, and how are they calculated?	Length-of-stay variances, case-mix variances
Confidentiality	What confidentiality policies and procedures are in place?	Particularly in reference to distance coding, how is compliance assured?
	Who will sign the facility's confidentiality agreement?	HIPAA privacy regulations will require a formal agreement

be reviewed and executed in a timely manner. Legal review also ensures the protection of both the coding manager and the healthcare facility.

Designing Retention Strategies

Like organizations in other industries, healthcare facilities often use financial and other incentives to maintain staff loyalty in a competitive marketplace. HIM departments might use various strategies such as bonuses, job enrichment, promotions, and training to ensure the retention of coding staff.

Bonuses

Most healthcare facilities offer annual wage increases, merit increases, or both. However, when these incentives prove inadequate, the coding manager may find it necessary to offer bonuses.

Service Bonus

A **service bonus** is a monetary reward given to long-term staff in recognition of their skills and commitment to the facility. Working with the HR department, the coding manager should determine whether other departments in the facility, such as critical care nursing or physical therapy, have service bonuses in place. If so, he or she should review the process used by these departments to determine service bonuses. However, if no written policy and procedure is in place for service bonuses, the coding manager should work with the HR department to draft a generic policy that would apply equally to all positions in the facility. Documentation to support service bonuses should include the costs of recruitment, training, and vacancy coverage. Service bonuses may be awarded on a yearly basis and designed to be more financially attractive than the sign-on bonuses mentioned earlier. No criteria other than successful passing of the yearly performance review may be needed to receive a service bonus.

The cost of low morale is difficult to assess. Unproductive hours, absenteeism, and feelings of underappreciation, however, are legitimate factors to consider when the facility's goals include the retention of qualified staff. Service bonuses acknowledge and reward long-term staff through employer recognition of their skills and commitment.

Productivity Bonus

Healthcare organizations also sometimes use **productivity bonuses** to reward exceptional performance or to motivate improvements in performance. For example, productivity bonuses might be considered for:

- Coders who consistently perform above and beyond established productivity standards: These are the employees that the facility most wishes to retain, but the most likely to be offered financial rewards by competitors.

- Coders who, for various reasons, slow down or stop coding when they have met the usual quantity standard: These individuals might be inspired to maintain high performance if financial rewards for increased productivity were in place.

- Coders who consistently produce more than others in the department: These individuals may eventually become resentful if they perceive that they are being compensated the same as less-productive staff.

Before offering productivity bonuses, however, the coding manager must determine whether current productivity standards are realistic and a fair exchange for present compensation. Bonuses should be offered only when the normal standards are far exceeded. If the standards are properly designed, this should not occur on a daily basis.

For example, when the quantity standard is 25 health records coded daily, coders will qualify for a bonus only when they exceed 30 or 35 health records with acceptable accuracy. If coders consistently code 30 to 35 records per day, the quantity standard has probably been set too low. However, raising the quantity standard after the productivity bonus program is in place could make the facility appear insincere in its intent to reward productivity—the reward will seem perpetually out of reach and lose its meaning as an incentive. Conversely, if the bonus is too easy to get, staff may wonder why it is not simply included in their usual wages or may come to believe their usual wages are inadequate.

In addition to volume productivity, it is important to maintain coding accuracy. Records must be distributed in such a way that each coder is given a similar mix of easy-to-difficult cases. Coders should never be rewarded for quantity in the absence of meeting quality standards.

Staff Recognition

Appreciation for a job well done can be shown in many low-cost ways that can enhance staff's professional pride, team building, and loyalty to the facility. HIM Week is an excellent time to "show off" staff to the rest of the facility. Materials for HIM Week can be downloaded from the AHIMA Web site. Small items such as pens or t-shirts can be purchased for staff as small tokens of appreciation. A recognition luncheon can be provided.

Job Enrichment

Money is not the only motivator that retains employees. Location, environment, and self-actualization can be equally important. Thus, an important part of the coder's annual review is to determine whether he or she has any personal or professional goals that the organization can help to satisfy. For example, the coder may want to become involved with quality audits. Rather than ignore this goal and risk losing the employee, the coding manager could assign new duties that will satisfy the coder's desires and interests. Table 2.7 offers a list of possible job-enrichment activities.

It is not always possible to achieve job enrichment for every employee. In addition, the desires of individual coders must be balanced with the needs of the department. In any event, whenever a coder is asked to perform additional tasks, the HIM department must provide appropriate training.

Table 2.7. Possible job-enrichment activities

Quality assurance activities	• Qualitative analysis screening • Coding audit activities
Interdepartmental reporting	• Routine medical staff activity reporting • Analysis of procedure index versus ancillary department activity
Staff development	• Continuing education
Physician interaction/liaison	• Physician query process coordination • Physician education

Promotion

It is impossible to promote every employee who wants to be promoted. Likewise, not every employee who wants to supervise has the temperament, talent, or training to be a supervisor. Moreover, not every promotion leads to supervisory responsibilities. Several levels of coding staff can be defined. The following job titles represent potentially nonsupervisory positions with progressively more responsibility:

- Trainee
- Outpatient coder
- Inpatient coder
- Coding specialist
- Lead coder
- Coding supervisor/head coder
- Clinical data analyst

Table 2.8 describes the responsibilities of employees in these positions.

Table 2.8. Progressive coding position descriptions

Level	Title	Responsibilities
1	Coder trainee	Abstracting, data entry, filing loose sheets, coding of a limited case mix with 100% review
2	Outpatient coder	Abstracting, data entry, filing loose sheets, coding of emergency and clinic records; 100% review until accuracy productivity benchmarks are met
3	Inpatient coder	Abstracting, data entry, filing loose sheets, coding of inpatient and ambulatory surgery records; 100% review until accuracy productivity benchmarks are met
4	Coding specialist	Abstracting, data entry, filing loose sheets, coding of a wide variety of records; performs coding accuracy reviews under the direction of the coding supervisor and researches coding questions
5	Lead coder	Abstracting, data entry, filing loose sheets, coding of a wide variety of records; performs coding accuracy reviews under the direction of the coding supervisor; researches coding questions, compiles and prepares productivity reports, compiles and prepares ad hoc reports based on diagnosis, DRG, physician, and/or service
6	Coding supervisor	Performs coding accuracy reviews, researches coding questions, compiles and prepares productivity reports, compiles and prepares ad hoc reports based on diagnosis, DRG, physician, and/or service; consults with clinical staff regarding coding guidelines, maintains coding policies and procedures, supervises coding staff, prepares staff evaluations under the direction of the department manager
7	Clinical data analyst	Performs a wide variety of activities for which coding is the foundation skill. In some facilities, this is an expert coder. In other facilities, candidates might need additional education and credentials and the position could involve extensive training, statistical analysis, high level of communication skills, and management experience

One problem with this approach is that employees and the HR department both may assume that the highest-level coder in the progression should be next in line for promotion to coding supervisor. However, many coders do not want the responsibilities of the supervisory role. The coding manager must ensure that the appropriate person is being groomed for the supervisory position. Only by talking to employees on a regular basis can the coding manager determine their needs and professional goals.

Continuing Education

Credentialed coders require continuing education to maintain their credentials. Regardless of the specific credential, maintenance of coding skills should be a job requirement. Thus, the job description should reflect the mandatory nature of continuing education and describe the measures required to satisfy it.

Beyond the maintenance of credentials, some coders regard continuing education opportunities as a route toward career advancement. It is the HIM department's responsibility to provide support to such coders. Coding managers should have input into the process of continuing education to ensure that coders are both maintaining and developing their professional skills.

Conclusion

To ensure effective recruitment of coding staff, managers must know the needs of the facility and understand the needs of coders. Performing a needs assessment through job analysis, productivity review, analysis of staff complement, and salary survey helps the manager improve his or her recruiting efforts.

Effective advertising focuses on the appropriate medium and ensures that the recruitment language is correct and clear. Interviewing should be consistent among applicants, with attention paid to resume specifics and courtesy to the applicants. If testing is to take place, it must reflect the actual work the applicant would be expected to do.

Orientation to the facility, the department, and the specific job responsibilities should be standardized and documented. Training must continue through the probationary period with clearly defined productivity expectations. Employee retention may be improved with the effective use of productivity bonuses.

Alternatives to full-time staff include part-time staff and job sharing. Telecommuting and outsourcing are alternatives when the existing applicant pool is inadequate. The effective coding manager will carefully address productivity, work flow, and cost issues when recruiting staff for traditional and alternative coding positions.

References and Resources

American Health Information Management Association. 2006a (March). AHIMA Candidate Handbook: Certified Coding Associate (CCA). Available online from http://www.ahima.org/certification/documents/2006/06-CCAhandbook.pdf.

American Health Information Management Association. 2006b. AHIMA Candidate Handbook: Certified Coding Specialist (CCS) and Certified Coding Specialist—Physician-based (CCS-P). Available online from http://www.ahima.org/certification/documents/2006/06-CCS-CCSPhndbk.pdf.

Centers for Medicare and Medicaid Services. 2006 (April 20). National Correct Coding Initiatives. Available online from http://www.cms.hhs.gov/NationalCorrectCodInitEd/.

Centers for Medicare and Medicaid Services. n.d. All fee-for-service providers. Available online from http://www.cms.hhs.gov/center/provider.asp.

Department of Health and Human Services, Office of Inspector General. OIG Compliance Program Guidance for Hospitals. 1998 (Feb. 23). *Federal Register* 63(35): 8989 Available online from http://oig.hhs.gov/fraud/complianceguidance.html#1.

Internal Revenue Service. 2006 (June 27). Topic 762—Independent Contractor vs. Employee. Available online from http://www.irs.gov/taxtopics/tc762.html.

Joint Commission Guide to Staff Education. 2002 (Dec. 1). Joint Commission Guide to Staff Education. Oak Brook, IL: JCAHO.

Occupational Safety and Health Administration. 1998 (Rev. July 1, 2002). Uniform Guidelines on Employee Selection Procedures, *29CFR1607.5* 29(4): 204–205. Washington, DC: U.S. Government Printing Office. Available online from http://a257.g.akamaitech.net/7/257/2422/14mar20010800/edocket.access.gpo.gov/cfr_2002/julqtr/29cfr1607.5.htm.

Appendix 2.1

CCA Competency Statements

Domain 1: Health Records and Data Content

1. Collect and maintain health data
2. Analyze health records to ensure that documentation supports the patient's diagnosis and procedures and reflects progress, clinical findings, and discharge status
3. Request patient-specific documentation from other sources (such as ancillary departments, or the physician's office)
4. Apply clinical vocabularies and terminologies used in the organization's health information systems

Domain 2: Health Information Requirements and Standards

1. Evaluate the accuracy and completeness of the patient record as defined by organizational policy and external regulations and standards
2. Monitor compliance with organization-wide health record documentation guidelines
3. Report compliance findings according to organizational policy.
4. Assist in preparing the organization for accreditation, licensing and/or certification surveys

Domain 3: Clinical Classification Systems

1. Use electronic applications to support clinical classification and coding (such as encoders)
2. Assign secondary diagnosis procedure codes using ICD-9-CM official coding guidelines
   a. Assign principal diagnosis (Inpatient) or first listed diagnosis (Outpatient)
   b. Assign secondary diagnosis(es), including complications and comorbidities (CC)
   c. Assign principal and secondary procedure(s)
3. Assign procedure codes using CPT coding guidelines
4. Assign appropriate HCPCS codes
5. Identify discrepancies between coded data and supporting documentation
6. Consult reference materials to facilitate code assignment

Domain 4: Reimbursement Methodologies 7 2 0 9

1. Validate the data collected for appropriate reimbursement
   a. Validate Diagnosis-Related Groups (DRGs)
   b. Validate Ambulatory Payment Classifications (APCs)
2. Comply with the National Correct Coding Initiative
3. Verify the National and Local Coverage Determinations (NCD/LCD) for medical necessity

Domain 5: Information and Communication Technologies 4 1 0 5

1. Use personal computer to ensure data collection, storage, analysis, and reporting of information
2. Use common software applications (such as word processing, spreadsheets, or e-mail) in the execution of work processes
3. Use specialized software in the completion of HIM processes

Domain 6: Privacy, Confidentiality, Legal, and Ethical Issues 3 7 3 13

1. Apply policies and procedures for access and disclosure of personal health information
2. Release patient-specific data to authorized individuals
3. Apply ethical standards of practice
4. Recognize and report privacy issues/problems
5. Protect data integrity and validity using software or hardware technology

---

Source: AHIMA 2006a.

Appendix 2.2

Certified Coding Specialist (CCS)

The CCS examination consists of two parts:

Multiple Choice—Part I consists of 60 four-option multiple-choice items (50 "scored" items, and 10 "pretest" items). Pretest items are unscored items that are included in the examination to assess the item's performance prior to using it for operational use in a future examination. The pretest items are scrambled randomly throughout the examination and do not count toward the candidate's score.

Medical Record Coding—Part II requires candidates to code 13 medical records, which contain seven outpatient records (four ambulatory surgery, one emergency department, and two records from Cardiac Cath/Interventional Radiology/Pain Management) and six inpatient records. Inpatient diagnoses and procedures are to be coded with ICD-9-CM volumes 1–3; ambulatory care diagnoses are to be coded with ICD-9-CM volumes 1 and 2; and ambulatory care procedures with CPT.

I. HEALTH INFORMATION DOCUMENTATION

1. Interpret health record documentation using knowledge of anatomy, physiology, clinical disease processes, pharmacology, and medical terminology to identify codeable diagnoses and/or procedures.
2. Determine when additional clinical information is needed to assign the diagnosis and/or procedure code(s).
3. Consult with physicians and other healthcare providers to obtain further clinical information to assist with code assignment.
4. Consult reference materials to facilitate code assignment.
5. Identify patient encounter type to assign codes (such as inpatient versus outpatient).
6. Identify the etiology and manifestation(s) of clinical conditions.

II. DIAGNOSTIC CODING GUIDELINES

1. Select the diagnoses that require coding according to current coding and reporting requirements for inpatient services.
2. Select the diagnoses that require coding according to current coding and reporting requirements for hospital-based outpatient services.
3. Interpret conventions, formats, instructional notations, tables, and definitions of the classification system to select diagnoses, conditions, problems, or other reasons for th encounter that require coding.
4. Sequence diagnoses and other reasons for encounter according to notations and conventions of the classification system and standard data set definitions [such as Uniform Hospital Discharge Data Set (UHDDS)].
5. Determine if signs, symptoms, or manifestations require separate code assignments.
6. Determine if the diagnostic statement provided by the healthcare provider does not allow for more specific code assignment (such as fourth or fifth digit).

7. Recognize when the classification system does not provide a precise code for the condition documented (such as residual categories and/or nonclassified syndromes).

8. Assign supplementary code(s) to indicate reasons for the healthcare encounter other than illness or injury.

9. Assign supplementary code(s) to indicate factors other than illness or injury that influence the patient's health status.

10. Assign supplementary code(s) to indicate the external cause of an injury, adverse effect, or poisoning.

III. PROCEDURAL CODING GUIDELINES

1. Select the procedures that require coding according to current coding and reporting requirements for inpatient services.

2. Select the procedures that require coding according to current coding and reporting requirements for hospital-based outpatient services.

3. Interpret conventions, formats, instructional notations, and definitions of the classification system and/or nomenclature to select procedures/services that require coding.

4. Sequence procedures according to notations and conventions of the classification system/nomenclature and standard data set definitions (such as UHDDS).

5. Determine if more than one code is necessary to fully describe the procedure/ service performed.

6. Determine if the procedural statement provided by the healthcare provider does not allow for a more specific code assignment.

7. Recognize when the classification system/nomenclature does not provide a precise code for the procedure/service.

IV. REGULATORY GUIDELINES AND REPORTING REQUIREMENTS FOR INPATIENT HOSPITALIZATIONS

1. Select the principal diagnosis, principal procedure, complications and comorbidities, and other significant procedures that require coding according to UHDDS definitions and official coding guidelines.

2. Evaluate the effect of code selection on Diagnosis-Related Group (DRG) assignment.

3. Verify DRG assignment based on Prospective Payment System (PPS) definitions.

V. REGULATORY GUIDELINES AND REPORTING REQUIREMENTS FOR HOSPITAL-BASED OUTPATIENT SERVICES

1. Apply guidelines for bundling and unbundling of codes.

2. Apply outpatient PPS reporting requirements:
   a. Modifiers
   b. CPT versus HCPCS II
   c. Medical necessity (for example, linking diagnosis to procedure/service)
   d. Evaluation and Management (E/M) code assignment

3. Select the reason for encounter, pertinent secondary conditions, primary procedure, and other significant procedures that require coding.

4. Verify ambulatory payment classification (APC) assignment based on outpatient prospective payment system (OPPS) definitions.

VI. DATA QUALITY

1. Assess the quality of coding from an array of data (such as reports).
2. Educate physicians and staff regarding reimbursement methodologies and documentation rules and regulations related to coding.
3. Participate in the development of institutional coding policies to ensure compliance with official coding rules and guidelines.
4. Analyze health record documentation for quality and completeness of coding (such as inclusion or exclusion of codes).
5. Review health record documentation to substantiate claims processing and appeals (such as codes, discharge disposition, patient type, charge codes).
6. Analyze edits from the Correct Coding Initiative (CCI) and Outpatient Code Editor (OCE).

VII. DATA MANAGEMENT

1. Manage accounts (such as unbilled, denied, suspended).
2. Recognize UB-92/UB-04 data elements.
3. Identify Charge Description Master (CDM) issues (such as revenue codes, units of service, CPT/HCPCS, text descriptions, modifiers).
4. Identify accounts subject to the 72-hour rule.
5. Identify hospital-based outpatient accounts subject to the "to/from" dates of service edits.
6. Identify cases needed for health record reviews (such as committee, clinical pertinence, research).
7. Analyze case-mix index data.

Appendix 2.3

Certified Coding Specialist—
Physician-Based (CCS-P)

The CCS-P examination consists of two parts:

Multiple Choice—Part I consists of 60 four-option multiple-choice items (50 "scored" items, and 10 "pretest" items). Pretest items are unscored items that are included in the examination to assess the item's performance prior to using it for operational use in a future examination. The pretest items are scrambled randomly throughout the examination and do not count toward the candidate's score.

Medical Record Coding—Part II requires candidates to code 13 medical records, which contain seven outpatient records (four ambulatory surgery, one emergency department, and two records from Cardiac Cath/Interventional Radiology/Pain Management) and six inpatient records. Inpatient diagnoses and procedures are to be coded with ICD-9-CM volumes 1–3; ambulatory care diagnoses are to be coded with ICD-9-CM volumes 1 and 2; and ambulatory care procedures with CPT.

I. HEALTH INFORMATION DOCUMENTATION

1. Interpret health record documentation to identify diagnoses and conditions for code assignment.
2. Interpret health record documentation to identify procedures or services for code assignment.
3. Determine if sufficient clinical information is available to assign one or more diagnosis codes.
4. Determine if sufficient clinical information is available to assign one or more procedure or service codes.
5. Consult with physicians or other healthcare providers when additional information is needed for coding and/or to clarify conflicting or ambiguous information.
6. Consult reference materials to facilitate code assignment.
7. Identify the etiology and manifestation(s) of clinical conditions.

II. CODING

1. Assign ICD-9-CM code by applying "Diagnostic Coding and Reporting Guidelines for Outpatient Services (Hospital-Based and Physician Office)."
2. Interpret ICD-9-CM conventions, formats, instructional notations, tables, and definitions to select diagnoses, conditions, problems, or other reasons for the encounter that require coding.
3. Interpret CPT and HCPCS II guidelines, format, and instructional notes to select services, procedures, and supplies that require coding.
4. Assign CPT code(s) for procedures and/or services rendered during the encounter.
5. Assign codes to identify Evaluation and Management (E/M) services.
6. Recognize if an unlisted code must be assigned.

7. Exclude from coding those procedures that are component parts of another reported procedure code.
8. Code for the professional vs. technical component when applicable.
9. Assign HCPCS II codes.
10. Append modifiers to procedure or service codes when applicable.

III. REIMBURSEMENT METHODS AND REGULATORY GUIDELINES

1. Apply global surgical package concept to surgical procedures.
2. Apply bundling and unbundling guidelines (such as National Correct Coding Initiative [NCCI]).
3. Interpret health record documentation to identify diagnoses and conditions for code assignment.
4. Apply reimbursement methods for billing or reporting (such as OIG, CMS (HCFA), *Federal Register*).
5. Link diagnosis code to the associated procedure code for billing or reporting.
6. Evaluate payer remittance or payment (such as EOB, EOMB) reports for reimbursement and/or denials.
7. Interpret Local Medical Review Policies (LMRP) or payer policies to determine coverage.
8. Process claim denials and/or appeals.

IV. DATA QUALITY

1. Validate assigned diagnosis and procedure codes supported by health record documentation.
2. Validate assigned E/M codes based on health record documentation using the E/M guidelines.
3. Assess the quality of coding and billing using routinely generated reports.
4. Verify that the data on the claim form correctly reflect the services provided.
5. Verify that the data on the claim form correctly reflect the conditions managed or treated during the encounter.
6. Validate the accuracy of the required data elements on the claim form.
7. Conduct coding and billing audits for compliance and trending.
8. Determine educational needs for physicians and staff on reimbursement and documentation rules and regulations related to coding.
9. Participate in the development of coding and billing policies and procedures for reporting professional services.
10. Evaluate payer remittance or payment (such as EOB, EOMB) reports for data quality.

Appendix 2.4

Sample Job Description

Job Title:

Certified coding specialist

Job Description:

- Reviews patient records and assigns accurate codes for each diagnosis and procedure

- Applies knowledge of medical terminology, disease processes, and pharmacology

- Demonstrates tested data quality and integrity skills

Education:

A minimum of a high school degree,* plus successful obtainment and maintenance of the AHIMA credential—certified coding specialist (CCS)

Qualifications:

Two years of coding and abstracting experience in ICD-9-CM, DRGs, and CPT, including modifiers and APCs

Job Skills:

- Thorough knowledge of the related prospective payment systems (PPSs)

- Broad knowledge of pharmacology indications for drug usage and related adverse reactions

- Knowledge of ancillary testing (laboratory, x-ray, electrocardiogram)

- Knowledge of anatomy, physiology, and medical terminology

- Understanding of coding practices and guidelines

- Experience with personal computer and mainframe applications and with encoding systems

- Auditing skills for coding quality and compliance

- Strong process management skills

---

*Many HIM professionals with advanced degrees have taken the CCS in order to demonstrate coding knowledge.

Appendix 2.5

Determining Whether an Individual Is an Employee or an Independent Contractor

Topic 762—Independent Contractor versus Employee

To determine whether a worker is an independent contractor or an employee under common law, you must examine the relationship between the worker and the business. All evidence of control and independence in this relationship should be considered. The facts that provide this evidence fall into three categories—Behavioral Control, Financial Control, and Type of Relationship.

Behavioral Control covers facts that show whether the business has a right to direct or control how the work is done through instructions, training, or other means.

Financial Control covers facts that show whether the business has a right to direct or control the financial and business aspects of the worker's job. This includes:

- The extent to which the worker has unreimbursed business expenses,

- The extent of the worker's investment in the facilities used in performing services,

- The extent to which the worker makes his or her services available to the relevant market,

- How the business pays the worker, and

- The extent to which the worker can realize a profit or incur a loss.

Type of Relationship covers facts that show how the parties perceive their relationship. This includes:

- Written contracts describing the relationship the parties intended to create,

- The extent to which the worker is available to perform services for other, similar businesses,

- Whether the business provides the worker with employee-type benefits, such as insurance, a pension plan, vacation pay, or sick pay,

- The permanency of the relationship, and

- The extent to which services performed by the worker are a key aspect of the regular business of the company.

For more information, refer to Publication 15-A (PDF), *Employer's Supplemental Tax Guide* or Publication 1779 (PDF), *Independent Contractor or Employee*. If you want the IRS to determine whether a specific individual is an independent contractor or an employee, file Form SS-8 (PDF), *Determination of Worker Status for Purposes of Federal Employment Taxes and Income Tax Withholding.*

Source: IRS 2006.

Chapter 3

Coding in Specialized Care Settings

Lynn Kuehn, MS, RHIA, CCS-P, FAHIMA

Where do credentialed clinical coders work? Although not specifically addressing coders, a 2002 AHIMA member survey identified the current employers of AHIMA members (AHIMA 2002; Wing et al. 2003). The survey reported that 30 percent of credentialed AHIMA members gave their primary job title as coder/clinical data specialist or clinical data analyst. Perhaps this survey could be descriptive of the work sites of clinical coders as well. More than 61 percent of AHIMA members were employed by hospitals with inpatient and outpatient services. The remaining 39 percent of respondents identified nearly 40 different settings, none with more than 8 percent of respondents. Among the more frequently reported settings that could possibly hire clinical coders were physician offices (7.2 percent), skilled nursing facilities (4.0 percent), mental health facilities (1.4 percent), home health agencies (1.3 percent), rehabilitation hospitals (1.2 percent), correction facilities (0.2 percent), and hospices (0.2 percent).

Coding practice varies from setting to setting based on clinical factors, reimbursement issues, services provided, uses of coded information, time factors, staff availability, technology, and coding classification system(s) used. The type of coding performed is consistent: ICD-9-CM codes for diagnoses or reasons for visits, ICD-9-CM for hospital inpatient procedures and CPT/HCPCS codes for the outpatient/ambulatory visits, procedures, therapies, and tests. Billing is typically performed using the CMS-1500 format for professional fee billing in the nonhospital setting. However, the CMS-1450 or Uniform Bill 92 (UB-92) is used for some nonhospital organizations, such as home health agencies and hospices. Changes are being made to both the CMS-1500 and the UB-92, now to be the UB-04, during 2006 and 2007 (CMS 2006 and NUBC 2005). See chapter 4 for more information on the UB-04.

This chapter describes the practice of coding in a variety of different settings other than general acute care hospitals. Each setting is defined and discussed in terms of its individual coding needs.

Coding Practice in Various Nonacute Care Settings

Each of the settings discussed below presents its own unique challenges. Many of these settings may not be the best place for the new coder to start a career without a strong support system, such as that offered by an experienced coder/mentor in the same setting. Experience counts in these special settings because reporting rules, reimbursement requirements, and clinical conditions vary widely.

Ambulatory Care

Ambulatory care settings are locations where patients are seen by a physician or other healthcare provider as outpatients on an episodic basis. The patients may have appointments or may be provided service on a "walk-in" basis. In ambulatory care settings, coders are often located close to actual areas of patient care so that they can interact regularly with the healthcare providers. They serve not only as coders, but also as documentation specialists and health record completion managers. Coders in ambulatory care settings are likely to code a higher volume of cases per day because of the limited amount of information they must review in each case. Sometimes ambulatory care coders are assigned responsibility for communicating with insurance companies and prior-authorization firms that represent the patient's benefits plan.

For ambulatory surgery, urgent care, and other ambulatory care services, coders follow a method of coding practice similar to that used for inpatients in hospitals. They receive copies of health records in their work areas, review each record, and assign both ICD-9-CM diagnosis codes and CPT/HCPCS procedure codes to each account.

When portions of health records are stored on-line, coders may be required to access those portions on a computer screen and incorporate the information into their code assignment process. Coders then print out a final code summary and attach it to the hard copy of the health record, thus signing off on the case.

When the entire ambulatory care record is on-line, coders use a split-screen program to view the health record on one side of their computer screen and the encoder on the other side. They then follow the same basic process of assigning codes and finalizing the account. Accounts that coders deem incomplete are flagged in the computer system via the abstract or billing screen to be held until a complete health record has been compiled.

Physician Offices and Clinics

Physician offices and clinics can vary widely in terms of setting. A physician office may consist of one or two physicians in practice together or may be a large multispecialty group practice with anywhere from a dozen to several hundred physicians. Physicians may own such practices as a professional corporation or may be salaried members of a hospital-owned or other investor-owned corporation. Within an academic medical center, a medical faculty foundation may exist that provides physician office or clinic services tied to the university hospital. Moreover, different medical and surgical specialties offer outpatient services in a physician practice–type setting.

The term *clinic* once referred to a location where free care was provided. Today, however, the term may refer to many different forms of ambulatory care settings, ranging from the privately owned physician practice to the academic outpatient healthcare center. Perhaps closer to the older clinic concept are physician offices designated as community health centers that serve uninsured or underinsured geographic areas. Many of these clinics are grant funded, with restricted budgets that may not permit the hiring of a credentialed clinical coder. The providers are likely to code the diagnoses and procedures themselves. The difference at a community health center is not in how codes are assigned but, rather, in how the patient care visit is billed. Some services are billed based on the visit, and other services may be factored into the center's yearly cost report to its funding sources.

Although physician office and group practices are hiring a growing number of credentialed clinical coders, many are hiring only one, thus limiting his or her resources within the practice. In the past, many physician practices did not value the expertise of the coding professional; buying current books or sending staff to seminars or educational sessions was viewed as cost prohibitive. However, this view is changing. Physician practices are not only finding that accurate coding improves their insurance claims submission process, but that the coder's review of the documentation to verify the level of service assignment for the CPT code is a valuable compliance factor.

Coders in physician office and clinic settings, especially in the smaller practices, are likely to have multiple responsibilities, including coding, billing, collections, fee schedule or encounter form management. The coder in this setting has a much closer, hands-on relationship with the reimbursement side of healthcare than in a hospital setting and must be more of a reimbursement expert. Although ICD-9-CM coding is important to describe *why* the patient is receiving services, the accuracy of CPT coding in a physician office and clinic setting is more essential to describe what services were provided. The coder must recognize the difference between inpatient and outpatient coding in terms of the ICD-9-CM coding guidelines. Regarding CPT coding, the coder must be very familiar with CPT principles and how and when to use CPT/HCPCS modifiers accurately. Coders must understand the structure and format of CPT in order to understand what is a "comprehensive" service and what is a "component" part of the total service. Using Medicare's National Correct Coding (NCCI or CCI) edits is an essential activity of the coder.

Coders who also serve as billers must be familiar with the physician's personal fee schedule, the Medicare Fee Schedule Database, and contracted PPO fee schedules, as well as the NCCI edits. The fee schedules, like the NCCI edits, may dictate when certain CPT codes are used or when they are used in combination. Coders working for surgeons must understand the concept of global surgical periods and know when a patient can be billed for a service and when the service is included in the surgical package (such as preoperative visits, the surgery itself, and normal follow-up office visits). Few encoders, or computerized coding software products, are used in physician offices, so the coder in this setting must know how to use the indices in all the coding books effectively.

Other billing issues that are important to the coder/biller in the physician setting are:

1. linking of a diagnosis to a procedure on the CMS-1500 form to establish medical necessity

2. proper application of the professional and technical modifiers for component procedures such as radiology examinations

3. billing supplies using HCPCS to a separate Durable Medical Equipment payer rather than the regular Medicare carrier.

Coders in physician office and clinic settings may have their own office or share space with the medical billing staff. Alternatively, coders in these settings may be placed in the registration and discharge area of the clinic or office because the coding function is tied to the actual process of generating a demand bill—one that patients can take with them. This may amount to coding the information the physician checks off on a superbill or encounter form that lists the many visit or procedure options and diagnoses. However, more practices are moving the coding function away from the front desk. The medical visit level and any procedures/diagnoses taken from the encounter form are more likely to be verified against the health record prior to being entered into the billing system to finalize the CMS-1500 claim form. After the patient's claim has been submitted, the coder may be involved with insurance tracking of the claim. He or she may be required to supply more information to the payer in terms of documentation or explanation of coded information supplied. After the claim is paid, the coder may be involved in comparing what was billed with what was paid. In consultation with the physician(s), the coder may work with an insurance payer to justify payment for denied services.

Physicians look to coding professionals for details on reimbursement-related issues, such as proper application of the Medicare Resource-Based Relative Value Scale (RBRVS) as the basis for the Medicare Fee Schedule and how payments are calculated. Medicare has set the unit of service for physician reimbursement as the "procedure," coded with a single CPT or HCPCS code. Many of the CPT and HCPCS codes are assigned a relative value weight or relative value unit (RVU). Others are paid at a flat rate by fee schedule, such as laboratory tests, drugs and supplies.

The RVUs measure the differences between procedures based on the physician work involved, practice costs, and the malpractice expense associated with the particular procedure. These units are then weighted with a geographic multiplier (geographic practice code index or GPCI) and finally are multiplied by a conversion factor to determine the approved amount for Medicare. The conversion factor is set annually by Congress and is published in the *Federal Register* each December, along with the RVUs for each procedure and the GPCI for each Medicare carrier and locality.

Many physician practices use the same RVUs and a higher conversion factor to determine or manage their own fees. Some payers have adopted the RBRVS with a different, usually higher, conversion factor as their standard fee schedule for payment.

The formula for calculating a Medicare-approved amount using RBRVS is:

$$[(W(RVU) \times G(W))) + (P(RVU) \times G(P)) + (M(RVU) \times G(M))] \times CF = Approved\ Amount$$

W(RVU) = Work RVU
R(RVU) = Practice expense RVU
M(RVU) = Malpractice RVU
G(W)   = Work geographic practice cost index (GPCI)
G(P)   = Practice expense GPCI
G(M)   = Malpractice GPCI
CF   = Conversion Factor

Physicians also look to coding professionals for documentation requirements associated with the evaluation and management codes found in CPT. The CMS and the American Medical Association (AMA) have published two sets of guidelines known as the 1995 Documentation Guidelines for Evaluation and Management Services and the 1997 Documentation Guidelines for Evaluation and Management Services. Both sets are valid for use by all physicians and can be found on both the CMS and AMA web sites. The 1995 set is a basic set of guidelines that is favored by most primary care physicians. The 1997 set has detailed criteria for examination documentation and is preferred by many specialists (Kuehn 2006, 40–72 and 279–280).

In a practice where coding and billing are recognized as two different skill sets, coders and billers work as a team to share their respective expertise in order to correctly identify the reasons the patient was seen and the services provided that justify reimbursement to the healthcare provider.

Ambulatory Surgery Centers

An **ambulatory surgery or surgical center** (ASC) is a distinct entity that operates exclusively for the purpose of providing surgical services to patients who do not require hospitalization. Medicare and other third-party payers have identified a set of procedures that are safe to perform in a nonhospital setting such as an ASC. Generally, covered procedures do not exceed 90 minutes to perform and do not require more than 4 hours of recovery time. Patients are able to return home with minimal at-home assistance from healthcare providers. Medicare does not allow an ASC to keep patients overnight at the center, but other payers may allow overnight stays in order to give the patient more time to recover and be monitored postsurgically.

The first ASC opened in 1970. Today, more than seven million surgeries are performed each year in the more than 3,300 surgery centers across the United States. ASCs that receive Medicare payments must meet the program's certification criteria and receive payments only for those procedures that have been approved by Medicare. More than 2,400 ASC procedures have been granted that approval. In 2002, most procedures performed in ASCs were in either ophthalmology or gastroenterology. At particular ASCs, surgeries may be performed in a variety of specialties or services dedicated to one specialty, such as eye care. More than 50 percent of ASCs specialize in a single specialty, and 49 percent provide services in multiple specialties. (See the Federated Ambulatory Surgery Association Web site at www.fasa.org.)

Coding in an ASC is similar to acute care hospital coding. Visits are coded after the procedure is performed and the record completed. However, like the coder in the physician practice, the coder in the ASC is closer to the billing or reimbursement aspects of the healthcare setting. Coders at an ASC may not wear as many "hats" as in the physician practice setting but may have more responsibilities in managing a health information management (HIM) department in terms of record completion and coordination of the HIM activities.

ICD-9-CM coding is important to describe the patient's diagnosis or reason for surgery. Unlike coding in a physician practice to reflect the professional fee, coding in an ASC reflects the facility fee, which is reported by the CPT code for the procedure performed. The CPT code includes the facility, nursing, preoperative and postoperative care, supplies, and drugs. Medicare and other third-party payers group all CPT/HCPCS codes into one of nine payer fee groups. Other payers pay for each CPT code. Multiple CPT codes means multiple payments, 100 percent for the highest-valued CPT code and 50 percent for additional procedures. The coder in the ASC setting must use the Medicare NCCI edits and CPT/HCPCS modifiers to ensure correct reporting of comprehensive procedures and to prevent unbundling of services.

Radiology Services

A rather new employer of credentialed clinical coders is the freestanding radiology or imaging center or an independent group of radiologists who practice at a local hospital. The radiology coder assigns the CPT codes for radiology procedures, including the complex CPT codes for interventional radiology procedures that require a minimum of two CPT codes from the surgery and radiology chapters of the CPT book. In addition, the radiology coder must provide an ICD-9-CM diagnosis code(s) for the reason and/or outcome of the radiology examination. Usually the coder has limited access to the patient's hospital or outpatient record and is dependent on complete documentation by the radiologist who writes the report. The radiology coder also must consider the NCCI or CCI guidelines for CPT codes that may or may not be used together.

Moreover, the radiology coder may be involved in medical necessity and coverage issues. By becoming an expert in these coverage policies and local coverage decisions (LCDs), he or she can assist the radiologist in correcting, describing, and billing the services provided to meet medical necessity requirements. Specialty coding credentials are available for the radiology coder, such as a radiology certified coder (RCC) credential offered by the Radiology Coding Certification Board (www.rccb.org).

Correctional Institutions

Prison systems have to maintain a comprehensive healthcare delivery system for inmates. With such a system comes the need for an HIM department that includes coding and recording of all healthcare activity. Most prisons have only an infirmary or ambulatory care setting; others have "inpatient" units and chronic disease facilities. The aging population in prisons has brought new services into correctional healthcare. Some prisons are expanding their healthcare services to meet the needs of the prison population internally, thus reducing the number of transfers to external healthcare providers. Although coders who work in prison settings are generally classified as ambulatory care coders, coding positions in prisons may carry unique responsibilities and challenges.

The coding of the inmate's healthcare service is done primarily for statistical purposes. Billing an insurance company or third-party payer is usually not done because the state or federal government (depending on the type of facility) pays for everything.

The types of services and reasons for the healthcare services for an inmate can prove challenging for the coder because of the unique situation. Many inmates have both medical and psychological conditions, including drug dependencies. Correctional healthcare providers must address drug-related problems, suicide attempts, infectious diseases, exposure to infectious and other diseases, and mild to moderate trauma as the result of fights and altercations, in addition to many chronic illnesses. Administratively, the inmate must be examined whenever he or she requests as well as when procedures dictate. Inmates are examined after use of force by a correctional officer and for other administrative purposes, such as clearance for certain activities or privileges. A condition that might be considered minor in another setting (for example, a runny nose or a sore throat) is often the reason for the visit to "sick call" and must be coded. In some instances, inmates may try to fake an illness to avoid another situation in the prison. Thus, documentation is crucial in the correctional healthcare setting not just to assist in coding, but also to stand as evidence of what did or did not occur during the visit because disputes between inmates and the facility over healthcare issues are common.

Coders in correctional healthcare often are challenged to fit the ICD-9-CM coding system into a setting that is not the same as most healthcare environments. Many generic or unspecified codes are used as well as many V codes for administrative services when the inmate is not sick, and many E codes are used to describe what happened to the inmate, such as a recreational or work injury, assault, and so on. Coders are not pressed by reimbursement requirements but, rather, the record and coding are subject to other types of legal scrutiny within the correctional healthcare setting.

Home Health Services

The term **home health services** refers to the items and services furnished to an individual under the care of a physician by a home health agency or by others in an arrangement with such agency and under a plan established and periodically reviewed by a physician. Such items and services are provided on a visiting basis in a place of residence used as the individual's home.

Home health services can include:

- Part-time or intermittent nursing care provided by, or under the supervision of, a registered professional nurse (part-time is less than 8 hours each day and 28 or fewer hours each week; intermittent may be less than 8 hours each day for of 21 days or less)

- Physical or occupational therapy or speech-language pathology services

- Medical social services under the direction of a physician

- Home health aide

Patients who receive home health services are likely to have been recently discharged from an acute care hospital or a skilled nursing facility and require ongoing care. Patients may also be referred by their primary physician without a previous hospitalization.

Coders in home health agencies must understand the concept of coding for Medicare reimbursement. Under the home health prospective payment system (HH PPS), a case-mix-adjusted payment for up to 60 days of care is made using one of 80 **home health resource groups** (HHRGs). Health insurance prospective payment system (HIPPS) rate codes represent specific sets of patient characteristics or case-mix groups on which payment determinations are made. On the Medicare claims, the HHRGs are represented as HIPPS codes. HIPPS codes are determined based on assessments made using the Outcome and Assessment Information Set (OASIS). Grouper software uses specific data elements from the OASIS data set to assign beneficiaries to an HIPPS code. The grouper outputs the HIPPS code, which must be entered on the claim.

The coder assigns ICD-9-CM diagnosis codes for the following three possible data elements on the OASIS data set:

- M0230: To determine the primary or first-listed diagnosis for M0230, the coder must determine what patient condition is most related to the current home health plan of care. The diagnosis may or may not be related to a patient's recent hospital stay but must relate to the services rendered by the home health agency. If more than one diagnosis is treated concurrently, the diagnosis that represents the most acute condition and requires the most intensive services should be entered first. Skilled services (skilled nursing, physical, occupational, and speech therapy) are used in judging the relevancy of a diagnosis to the plan of care and to data element M0230. If a patient is admitted for surgical aftercare, the relevant medical diagnosis is coded only it if still exists. If the medical diagnosis no longer exists (for example, surgery eliminated the disease or the acute phase has ended), a V code, such as surgical aftercare, is generally appropriate for use as the primary diagnosis. Effective October 1, 2003, if a provider reports a V code in M0230 in place of a case-mix diagnosis, the provider has the option of reporting the case-mix diagnosis in data element M0245. The coder must select the code(s) that would have been reported as the primary diagnosis under the original OASIS-B[1] (8/2000) instructions, which did not allow V codes. A case-mix diagnosis is defined as a primary diagnosis that assigns patients with selected conditions to an orthopedic, diabetes, neurological, or burns/trauma diagnosis for Medicare PPS case mix assignment. Case-mix diagnoses may involve manifestation coding.

- M0240: Data element M0240 collects **secondary diagnoses,** which, in home health, are defined as "all conditions that coexisted at the time the plan of care was established, or which developed subsequently, or affect the treatment or care of the patient." M0240 should include not only conditions actively addressed in the plan of care, but also any comorbid conditions affecting the patient's responsiveness to treatment and rehabilitative progress, even if they are not the focus of the home health treatment. Home health codes avoid listing diagnoses that are of historical interest and have no impact on the patient's progress or outcome.

- M0245: M0245 payment diagnosis is an optional OASIS item that home health agency coders may use when a V code is listed in M0230, primary diagnosis, according to ICD-9-CM coding guidelines. In order to determine the payment, a code other than a V code must be entered in M0245 as the Medicare PPS payment diagnosis. Diagnoses that can be entered into M0245 include: no surgical codes, list the underlying diagnosis; and no V or

E codes, list the relevant medical diagnosis. If the patient's primary home care diagnosis is coded as a combination of an etiology code and a manifestation code, the etiology code should be listed in M0245 (a) and the manifestation code should be entered in M0245 (b). A M0245 code is not required if a V code has been reported in place of a diagnosis that is not a case-mix diagnosis.

(Note: Coding is also performed on M0190 [Hospital Inpatient Diagnosis] which is not part of the HHRG payment).

The home health coder must work closely with the OASIS coordinator and the home care nurses to obtain all the patient information required for coding. Home health is a branch of medicine dominated by nurses. According to state practice acts, nurses cannot diagnose patients; therefore, physicians are legally responsible for the plan of care. The intake department should collect information from the referral source and the clinician should verify any information in question with the physician.

The coder rarely has an opportunity to obtain more information from the patient's attending physician. This is also one branch of medicine where experience as an inpatient or other healthcare setting coder may be a handicap. Home health coding is unique in its relationship to the OASIS data set elements. The concept of coding for "why the patient is receiving services" and the definitions of the OASIS data elements M0230, M0240, and M0245 can be a challenge for the clinical coder coming to work in a home health agency.

The following Web sites offer information on home health prospective payment, coding, and OASIS:

- www.medicare.govHHCompare/home
- www.cms.hhs.gov/OASIS
- www.cms.hhs.gov/HomeHealthQualityInits
- www.oasisanswers.com

Hospice Programs

A **hospice program** is a public agency or private organization primarily engaged in providing the care and services to an individual considered to be "terminally ill" (with a life expectancy of 6 months or less). Hospice services are provided in the individual's home, on an outpatient basis, in a long-term care facility, and on a short-term inpatient basis. Hospice services also may be provided in an inpatient residence. Services are designed to address the physical and emotional pain through palliative treatment when a cure for an individual's illness is no longer an option. The patient and the family accept that no further treatment for the condition will be attempted. Comfort measures and palliative care are the focus of attention in hospice care.

Hospice services are provided by an interdisciplinary team composed of at least one physician, one registered nurse, one social worker, and a pastoral or other counselor. Hospice care covered by Medicare is chosen for specified amounts of time known as "election periods." Initially, the physician may certify a patient for hospice care coverage for two initial 90-day election periods, followed by an unlimited number of 60-day election periods. Payment is made for each day of the election period based on one of four per diem rates set by Medicare, commensurate with the level of care. Covered services include medical and nursing care usually for pain management; medical equipment such as wheelchairs and beds; pharmaceutical therapy for pain relief and symptom control; home health aide and homemaker services; social work services; physical, occupational, and speech therapy; diet counseling; bereavement and other counseling services; and case management. Volunteers also play a unique role in hospice care and hospices must document the cost savings achieved through the use of volunteers.

Coding for hospice services is similar to coding for home health. On admission, the coder must identify and code the diagnosis that qualifies the patient to meet the hospice certification of "life expectancy of 6 months or less." Procedures are not coded. During the hospice stay, the diagnosis may change and would be updated upon recertification or at the time of the patient's discharge or expiration. Secondary diagnoses also are coded because patients often have multiple medical conditions.

Long-Term Care/Skilled Nursing Facilities and Intermediate Care Facilities

Long-term care facilities provide a variety of services to aged and disabled individuals. This section focuses on **skilled nursing facilities** (SNFs) and **intermediate care facilities** (ICFs). A SNF is primarily engaged in providing skilled nursing care and related services to residents who require medical or nursing care or may provide rehabilitation services for injured, disabled, or ill residents. SNFs provide this type of service to a resident for a specific period of time while he or she recovers from a recent illness or injury and has the ability to benefit from rehabilitation services. A patient may transition from a SNF to an ICF or be admitted directly to an ICF for long-term care services. ICF residents do not receive skilled nursing services but, rather, general nursing services to support activities of daily living when they are no longer able to care for themselves.

In long-term care facilities, a **Minimum Data Set** (MDS), a standardized patient assessment tool developed by Medicare, is used to collect coded diagnostic information on nursing facility residents (Gottschalk 2000, 1–14). MDS information is reported to a federal data repository. Nursing facilities also may report coded diagnostic information in individual resident records and in aggregate disease indexes in the facility.

Reporting diagnosis codes for reimbursement is required in nursing facilities. ICD-9-CM diagnosis and procedures codes are reported on the UB-92/UB-04 claim form to all third-party payers. In terms of the Medicare PPS for long-term care, the diagnosis codes generally do not determine payment directly. However, accuracy of the codes can affect Medicare audit results. Errors in the diagnoses reported on Medicare billing claim forms can result in rejections of claims and delays in payments.

Coding guidelines for long-term care have been developed and approved by the Cooperating Parties in conjunction with the Editorial Advisory Board of *Coding Clinic* to standardize the process of data collection for long-term care and to assist coders in coding and reporting such cases (AHA 1999). The diagnostic listing in long-term care is dynamic, depends on many factors, and has a longer time frame than is the case for an acute care stay. ICD-9-CM codes are assigned on admission, concurrently as diagnoses arise or the MDS is updated, and at the time of the resident's discharge, transfer, or expiration. Other diagnoses present that affect the resident's continued care also should be coded. The Uniform Hospital Discharge Data Set (UHDDS) definition of principal diagnosis does not apply to the long-term care facility. The listing of the diagnoses may vary depending on the circumstances of the resident's admission or continued stay in the facility.

The diagnosis that is chiefly responsible for the resident's admission to, or continued residence in, the nursing facility is the first-listed diagnosis. The first-listed diagnosis on admission may be coded with a V code for rehabilitation or for surgical or fracture aftercare, for example, or it may be coded to reflect a medical condition. If the coder is assigning diagnosis codes during the resident's stay, the first-listed diagnosis would be the condition chiefly responsible for the continued stay in the facility and referred to as the "primary" diagnosis.

Coders in long-term care facilities are continually updating codes and changing information based on the resident's changing status (for example, from skilled care to intermediate care) or as the resident's medical conditions change. Residents may be admitted to the SNF for one reason but end up staying in the facility for a different reason after the skilled services are completed. The coder must keep in mind the reason for the resident's continued stay as well as what diagnoses need to be reported on the MDS and for payment purposes.

Coding Practice in Acute Care Specialty Hospitals

Acute care hospitals that specialize in certain populations such as children and those with long-term acute care needs have coding issues that are unique to their populations. This section introduces the coding practice issues in children's hospitals and long-term acute care hospitals. Although other specialty hospitals—such as orthopedic hospitals or heart hospitals—exist, coding practice issues tend to be similar to those in acute care with a concentration on diseases or injuries in their specialty area. The two types of acute care specialty hospitals discussed here have coding and reimbursement issues that set them apart.

Children's Hospitals

Children's hospitals serve as regional centers for child health, with the most technologically advanced facilities and top specialists focused 100 percent on the unique needs of children. They draw patients from rural to metropolitan areas for a full range of care from routine cases to emergency and complex inpatient care.

Freestanding children's hospitals represent just one percent of all hospitals, but for all children hospitalized in the United States, children's hospitals account for 39 percent of admissions and 49 percent of inpatient days. On average, children's hospitals devote 60 percent of their care to children under 6 years, nearly 25 percent of their care to newborns, and 26 percent of their beds to intensive care units (compared to only 9 percent in general hospitals). Moreover, combined with the country's major teaching hospitals, in which many children's hospitals and pediatric departments are located, children's hospitals provide most highly specialized care for the nation's children with complex and rare conditions.

Freestanding children's hospitals alone treat:

- 52 percent of all children needing heart or lung transplants

- 42 percent of all children with cancer requiring inpatient care

- 45 percent of all children hospitalized for cystic fibrosis

- 40 percent of the five most costly and complex conditions

Children's hospitals and major teaching hospitals together treat:

- 98 percent of all children needing heart or lung transplants

- 88 percent of all children with cancer requiring inpatient care

- 76 percent of children hospitalized for cystic fibrosis

- 83 percent of the five most costly and complex conditions

Children's hospitals can belong to two organizations, and many are members of both. The largest association is the National Association of Children's Hospitals and Related Institutions (NACHRI), a not-for-profit group of 194 children's hospitals and large pediatric units of medical centers in the United States, Australia, Canada, Italy, Mexico and Puerto Rico (http://www.childrenshospitals.net). Another association is the Child Health Corporation of America (CHCA), a business alliance owned by approximately 40 freestanding children's hospitals in the United States (http://www.chca.com).

The coder working in a freestanding children's hospital is most likely located in the facility's HIM department. His or her record-processing and coding functions are similar to other acute care inpatient settings. Coders in children's hospitals become experts in coding newborn conditions, maternal conditions that affect the newborn or child, congenital anomalies, and reconstructive surgery. The coder may be confronted with very complex medical records with many conditions and procedures requiring ICD-9-CM codes. In this setting, the coder needs an especially good line of communication with the physicians because of the many complex conditions being described in the records. Pediatricians may occasionally cite "syndromes" that may not be included in the ICD-9-CM codebooks. In these cases, the coder must assign multiple codes to describe the various conditions that exist in the so-called syndrome. Coders in pediatric specialty hospitals must be more familiar with the congenital and acquired perinatal conditions than their counterparts in the general acute care hospital. To help promote consistency of coding in this complex coding environment, CHCA uses a roundtable format for the coders within their member hospitals. They develop and circulate guidelines for use in their hospitals and advocate about pediatric coding issues with AHA *Coding Clinic for ICD-9-CM*.

Children's hospitals are exempt from Medicare's inpatient acute care prospective payment system, but many children's hospitals still categorize patients by the Medicare DRG system to provide comparative data for internal use. Some children's hospitals are paid by state Medicaid plans using All-Patient DRGs (AP-DRGs), a system that contains diagnosis groups for patients of all ages. Both NACHRI and CHCA collect data from member hospitals and provide comparative data back to the hospitals based on the severity of illness indicated in the All Patient Refined DRG (APR-DRG) system. This system has diagnosis groups for patients of all ages and also subdivides each group into four levels of severity of illness. Therefore, it is possible that coders in children's hospitals need to be aware of how all three of these DRG systems work and the differences between the systems.

Long-Term Acute Care Hospitals

In general, **long-term care hospitals** (LTCHs) are defined as hospitals that have an average Medicare inpatient length of stay (LOS) of more than 25 days. LTCHs typically provide extended medical and rehabilitative care for patients with clinically complex conditions and who may suffer from multiple acute or chronic conditions. Services typically include comprehensive rehabilitation, respiratory therapy, head trauma treatment, and pain management. The following Web sites offer information on prospective payment for LTCHs:

- www.medicare.gov

- www.cms.hhs.gov/MLNMattersArticles/downloads/MM3335.pdf

- ms.hhs.gov/providers/longterm/

LTCHs should not be confused with long-term care nursing facilities such as SNFs and ICFs because their services and patients are very different. The LTCH PPS, which now sets payments for more than 300 long-term acute care hospitals, was designed to ensure appropriate payment for services to the medically complex patients treated in these facilities, while providing incentives to hospitals to provide more efficient care to Medicare beneficiaries. The PPS for LTCHs classifies patients into distinct diagnostic groups based on clinical characteristics and expected resource needs. The patient classification system groupings are called LTC-DRGs, which are based on the existing CMS DRGs used under the hospital inpatient PPS that have been weighted to reflect the resources required to treat the medically complex patients in LTCHs.

Coding and reporting for long-term care hospitals have received more attention with a recent article in *Coding Clinic for ICD-9-CM* (AHA 2003, 102–3). The Official Guidelines for Coding and Reporting for ICD-9-CM were updated for coding in LTCHs. The definitions of principal and other diagnoses from the guidelines are the same as those used in acute care hospitals.

The nature of LTCHs requires coders to be closely connected to the clinical care team and the physicians. Many coders attend team conferences on patients in order to clarify issues related to the patients' continued-stay conditions and procedures performed. The coder needs to be directly involved from preadmission screening through discharge to capture all the clinical information and to meet LOS guidelines. Many V codes are acceptable for admitting diagnoses to describe aftercare or status post conditions. Concurrent coding is a major issue because patients' conditions can change and new problems can arise over the course of weeks or months.

Health records in LTCHs are voluminous and can take 60 to 90 minutes to review. Discerning the principal diagnosis can be difficult because patients are often extremely ill with numerous serious conditions. Because LTCH patients have multiple complex medical problems, the most important secondary diagnoses should be reported within the top nine diagnoses to appear correctly on the UB-92/UB-04 claim form. Coders also must be wary of the PPS interrupted-stay rules and decide when two separate LTCH stays are coded as one or are combined. Depending on where the patient is transferred and what occurs in the other setting, coding for the LTCH can change. Implementation of the new PPS rule for LTCHs can challenge even the most experienced coders.

Coding Practices for Other Special Care Types

The disease and injury characteristics of behavioral health and physical medicine and rehabilitation put them in a healthcare class by themselves. Although totally different from each other, care for these conditions can be provided in similar ways—across almost all settings from inpatient to outpatient to home care. The unique coding practices of each are discussed here.

Behavioral Healthcare

Behavioral healthcare settings include hospitals, hospital units, ambulatory care centers, physician offices and clinics, as well as other private and public-sponsored healthcare settings. In behavioral healthcare settings, physicians, psychologists, and other healthcare professionals work together as a team to ensure effective treatment for all persons with mental disorders, including mental retardation and substance-related disorders. Recognized mental illnesses are described and categorized in *Diagnostic and Statistical Manual of Mental Disorders, Fourth Edition, Text Revision (DSM-IV-TR)* (APA 2000).

Behavioral healthcare institutions frequently set up designated work areas for coders similar to those in acute care hospitals. In these settings, coders use the health record to assign codes, to follow the reporting process, and possibly to complete a **clinical abstract** for each patient.

Coders in behavioral healthcare settings, both inpatient and outpatient, function much as those in hospitals and ambulatory care centers. Depending on the setting, some providers use DSM-IV-TR for data collection for internal purposes but must use ICD-9-CM for billing. Thus, the coder in the behavioral healthcare setting must have knowledge of the crosswalk between the two systems.

Behavioral health clinicians describe a patient's psychological and medical conditions with DSM-IV-TR using an AXIS I, II, III, IV and V outline. A coder often must code from documentation in a psychiatric evaluation and discharge summary using the physician's DSM-IV-TR terminology but must use ICD-9-CM inpatient rules and codes. One of the greatest challenges is coding the AXIS III or medical diagnoses presented in this format. The medical conditions may not be listed concisely by the psychiatrist, and the coder may not have the detail necessary to accurately describe the condition with an ICD-9-CM diagnosis code.

Medicare implemented a prospective payment system for inpatient psychiatric facilities (IPFs) in 2005. A complete analysis of the final rule is available from AHIMA (2004), and the full final rule can be found in the *Federal Register* (CMS 2004).

This system provides a per diem base rate for claims with a psychiatric principal diagnosis, found in chapter 5 of ICD-9-CM. The system uses the regular Medicare DRGs but provides an adjustment factor for 15 DRGs that relate to the psychiatric principal diagnoses. This adjustment factor provides reimbursement based on statistically significant cost differences for care within an IPF. The system also provides an additional adjustment factor for cases with comorbidities in 17 categories thought to require comparatively more costly treatment, for example, coagulation factor deficit, renal failure, or infectious diseases. Therefore, it is vital that coders code each secondary diagnosis that was evaluated or managed while the patient was in the IPF, not just the psychiatric principal diagnosis. A facility-level adjustment will also be provided for IPFs that maintain a qualifying emergency department to help account for those additional costs. IPFs can expect annual updates to the provisions of the PPS for their facilities.

Physical Medicine and Rehabilitation

Physical medicine and rehabilitation (PM&R) services may be provided on an inpatient or outpatient basis. These services may be provided in a dedicated freestanding rehabilitation hospital or as a dedicated unit within an acute care hospital. Medicare reimburses both settings on a prospective payment basis. Coding for rehabilitation services is similar to that for acute care, long-term care, and home care coding, yet is unique in its own requirements.

The coding for outpatient PM&R is not difficult because it is no different than coding for any outpatient therapy service in an acute hospital setting. The ordering physician must provide the diagnosis or reason for the therapy on the prescription or referral form. This information is converted to an ICD-9-CM diagnosis code. The coder must take note of all the therapies provided (for example, physical therapy and speech therapy) and provide a specific diagnosis code for each service if different medical conditions are being treated. The CPT procedure codes for physical, occupational, and speech therapy services are usually included in the chargemaster and not assigned individually by the coder.

Coding for inpatient PM&R services is performed for two reasons: (1) to complete the Inpatient Rehabilitation Facility Patient Assessment Form [IRF PAI]; and (2) for billing using the UB-92/UB-04 form. Codes assigned for the IRF PAI do not follow acute care hospital coding guidelines. Rather, the IRF PAI instructional manual describes how information must be collected. A code for the impairment group is not an ICD-9-CM code but, rather, a code unique to the IRF PAI. A code for the etiology, which is the acute condition that caused the impairment, and the date that it occurred also are reported. This code would not be reported on the medical record coding for the UB-92/UB-04. Additionally, codes for comorbid conditions, complications, and the reason for an interrupted stay or death are reported. Assignment of these additional diagnosis codes follows standard coding guidelines with a few exceptions. A complication documented on the day of discharge or the day prior to discharge is not reported on the IRF PAI but is reported on the UB-92/UB-04. Comorbid conditions included in the code for the impairment group or the etiology are not reported as comorbid conditions.

Coders also code for submitting diagnosis and procedure codes on the UB-92/UB-04. *Coding Clinic for ICD-9-CM* advises that the reason for admission (the principal diagnosis) should be a V57.xx code, Admission for rehabilitation (AHA 2002, 18–19). Physicians never document this as the principal diagnosis, so the coder must know to report the principal diagnosis as a V57 category code. The next diagnosis should be the actual reason for admission, but there is no unanimous agreement as to what this condition should be, for example, the impairment, the late effect, or some other diagnosis. If the coder is using a DRG grouper rather than the CMS grouper, codes are not resequenced correctly and the coder can find a code reported that is a CC for DRGs but has little to do with the reason the patient was admitted to the rehabilitation unit. Complicating this situation is the fact that other insurance/third-party payers do not follow the coding guidelines and want various codes reported as the principal diagnosis, such as:

- Admit for rehabilitation services V57.xx

- A code for the impairment, such as paralysis

- The acute condition that caused the long-term impairment, such as a cerebral infarction

- A status post or late effect code, such as late effect of a cerebrovascular accident (CVA), category 438 code

Coders who have no experience with rehabilitation coding requirements or acute care hospital coders who had to adapt to the requirements for the rehabilitation PPS system for the hospital's rehabilitation unit often initially have difficulty conceptualizing the differences in coding for the IRF-PAI and coding for the UB-92/UB-04. The coder must focus on the IRF-PAI definitions to correctly identify the rehabilitation reasons for services. For example, if a patient had an acute CVA with resulting hemiparesis and dysphagia, both conditions would be coded in the acute care record, with the acute CVA listed as the principal diagnosis. This patient then is transferred to the inpatient rehabilitation unit or to a rehabilitation hospital. In the case of UB-92/UB-04 coding for this rehabilitation stay, the principal diagnosis would be a V57 category code, admitted for rehabilitation services. The secondary diagnoses would be the impairment, such as hemiparesis and dysphagia, followed by a diagnosis to describe the conditions as late effects of a cerebrovascular disease (category 438). However, in the case of the IRF-PAI, the acute codes for hemiparesis (code 787.2) and dysphagia (342.90) would be used because these are the conditions receiving the rehabilitative care and not the CVA.

Another difference is that "possible" or "probable" conditions are not coded on the IRF-PAI but can be coded for the UB-92/UB-04. Thus, the coder in the rehabilitation setting must balance two sets of coding reporting requirements.

Other Practice Opportunities for Coding Professionals

A number of alternative options exist for coders in addition to the many opportunities to be found in general acute care and the specialized care settings previously discussed. Coding positions have become increasingly available in third-party billing companies, insurance companies, and other settings. Professional roles are also being created for coders such as chargemaster coordinators, patient screeners, and referral assistants. Chapter 13 also discusses future and emerging roles for clinical coders.

Third-Party Billing Companies

Other more recent employers of credentialed clinical coders are the third-party billing companies for physicians or other healthcare providers. The billing company receives proper documentation from the service provider and translates the medical information into ICD-9-CM and CPT procedure codes and submits it with the patient demographics on a CMS-1500 professional claim form. In the past, billing companies hired and trained people to do both the technical aspects of the claims submission and the coding. Realizing that the coding required a different skill set, many billing companies have separated these two functions. The billing company coder evaluates the documentation received to determine if a code can be accurately assigned, and if not, requests additional information from the healthcare provider. The coder also may be involved with postpayment claims analysis to determine what has been paid and what was denied. The coder may be able to advise the healthcare provider on how documentation can be improved to support future claims or to appeal a recent denial.

Insurance Companies and Other Settings

Insurance companies are not typical employers of credentialed clinical coders. The coding of medical diagnoses and procedures is performed by the provider, not at the insurance company. The limited number of coders hired by insurance companies has been found to be a valuable asset to insurance companies for several reasons, including the following:

- They can interpret and classify clinically coded data for their nonclinical coworkers.

- They serve as data analysts by reviewing claims information from providers.

- They assist in linking coverage policy with codes.

- They analyze incoming claims data to identify trends for future benefits planning.

Coders who work in insurance companies, managed care organizations, research offices, or statistical agencies generally spend a good portion of their time analyzing and validating data that have already been coded. These coders validate data for the following purposes:

- To prepare data to be entered into a provider file or master database

- To use data to analyze a healthcare delivery system

- To adjudicate payment for services rendered

- To correct or remove coding errors, thus ensuring a clean batch of statistical data

After coders complete their initial tasks, the data are stored in data banks for future analysis of hospitals, physicians, or other providers. Institutions such as insurance companies use coded data to make assumptions about terms of coverage, benefits plans, and rate setting; to analyze methods of healthcare delivery; and to project future needs in patient care.

Sometimes coders at insurance companies recode data to meet the needs of their internal, standardized set of codes or coding methodology. In such instances, coders may be trained to use an internal coding system that is unique to the company in which they work.

Insurance companies, managed care firms, and statistical agencies are just beginning to realize the value of coding experts and may hire more credentialed coders in the future.

Coders as Chargemaster Coordinators

Chapter 6 discusses the chargemaster and the role that coders can play in the maintenance and auditing of chargemaster coding.

Coders as Patient Screening and Referral Assistants

According to some payer regulations, hospitals and ambulatory care centers must screen referral information from physicians when patients register for some types of ambulatory care. Certain payers require that their beneficiaries be notified in writing prior to receiving a service if that service is not covered by their benefits plan.

For example, a physician orders a complete blood count (CBC) serum test for a particular Medicare patient and writes a diagnosis on the referral form along with the test requisition. A registrar or technician at the hospital must review that requisition and compare it against Medicare coverage to determine whether the CBC serum test is considered a covered service with the diagnosis indicated. If the CBC serum test is not considered "covered," the registrar or technician issues a written notice to the patient stating that the clinical indication noted for the test is not covered by Medicare.

Because referral information is of such importance, some hospitals and ambulatory care centers place coders in or near the registration area. Coders then screen referrals before the patient receives the service. This action ensures proper coding of the diagnosis and supports the process of notifying patients of noncoverage. Such screening assistance is a new entry-level role for outpatient coders.

Conclusion

The practice of coding varies according to the type of healthcare facility involved and the services the facility offers. Numerous other factors also can have an impact on the practice of coding, including government reimbursement regulations, prospective payment rules and definitions, third-party payer guidelines, official coding guidelines, tools and technology, content of the health record, and the preferences of coding professionals. Table 3.1 presents a summary of the coding systems and billing forms used by different healthcare entities.

Hospitals have traditionally been the exclusive employers of credentialed clinical coders. However, other employers and healthcare settings now offer coders career opportunities in a variety of positions that allow coders to acquire specialty coding and reimbursement skills and to contribute to patient care outside the hospital environment.

Coders are in the unique position not only of understanding the clinical data needs of today's healthcare organizations, but also of piloting the emerging technology to support those needs. The perspective that coders bring to the healthcare environment is opening up new practice opportunities, expanding their leadership roles, and offering initiatives and incentives for their professional growth.

Table 3.1. Comparison of coding systems and billing formats used in various nonacute care treatment settings

Health Care Setting	Diagnosis Codes	Procedure Codes	Billing Format*
Physicians and Clinics	ICD-9-CM	CPT/HCPCS	CMS 1500
Ambulatory Surgery Centers	ICD-9-CM	CPT/HCPCS	CMS 1500 with modifier –SG attached to CPT code to indicate the facility fee
Behavioral Health Physicians	ICD-9-CM	CPT/HCPCS	CMS 1500
Behavioral Health Institutions	ICD-9-CM	CPT/HCPCS	CMS 1450 or UB-92/UB-04
Children's Hospitals	ICD-9-CM	ICD-9-CM for inpatient CPT/HCPCS for outpatient	CMS 1450 or UB-92/UB-04
Home Health	ICD-9-CM	ICD-9-CM	CMS 1450 or UB-92/UB-04
Hospice	ICD-9-CM	ICD-9-CM	CMS 1450 or UB-92/UB-04
LTC Units/ Skilled Nursing Facilities/ Intermediate Care Facilities	ICD-9-CM	ICD-9-CM	CMS 1450 or UB-92/UB-04
Long Term Acute Care Hospitals	ICD-9-CM	ICD-9-CM	CMS 1450 or UB-92/UB-04
Rehabilitation Units or Hospitals	ICD-9-CM	ICD-9-CM	CMS 1450 or UB-92/UB-04
Radiology Centers	ICD-9-CM	CPT/HCPCS	CMS 1500

*The UB-92 is being replaced by the UB-04 in March 1, 2007, with a transition period until May 22, 2007 (NUBC 2005). See chapter 4 for more information on the UB-04.

References and Resources

AHIMA Policy and Government Relations. 2004 (December). Summary of Final Rule for Medicare Prospective Payment System for Inpatient Psychiatric Facilities. Available online from http://www.ahima.org/dc/Analysis_IPF_PPS_reg.asp.

American Hospital Association. 1999 (Fourth Quarter). Long-term care issues. *Coding Clinic for ICD-9-CM*. Chicago: American Hospital Association.

American Hospital Association. 2002 (First Quarter). *Coding Clinic for ICD-9-CM*. Chicago: American Hospital Association.

American Hospital Association. 2003 (Fourth Quarter). *Coding Clinic for ICD-9-CM*. Chicago: American Hospital Association.

American Health Information Management Association. 2002. Data for decisions: the HIM workforce and workplace. 2002 member survey. Chicago: American Health Information Management Association.

American Psychiatric Association. 2000. *Diagnostic and Statistical Manual of Mental Disorders, Fourth Edition, Text Revision (DSM-IV-TR)*. Arlington, VA: American Psychiatric Publishing.

Centers for Medicare and Medicaid Services (CMS). 2006. Transmittal 899—Revised Health Insurance Claim Form CMS-1500. Available online from http://www.cms.hhs.gov/Transmittals/downloads/R899CP.pdf.

Centers for Medicare and Medicaid Services. 2004 (Nov. 15). Medicare Program; Prospective payment system for inpatient psychiatric facilities. *Federal Register* 69(219):66921–67015. Available online from http://www.access.gpo.gov/su_docs/fedreg/a041115c.html.

Gottschalk, Reesa. 2000. *ICD-9-CM Coding for Long-term Care.* Chicago: American Health Information Management Association.

Kuehn, Lynn. 2006. *CPT/HCPCS Coding and Reimbursement for Physician Services.* Chicago: American Health Information Management Association.

National Uniform Billing Committee. 2005 (June 21). NUBC announces approval of UB-04. Available online from http://www.nubc.org/INFORMATION_ON_UB-04.pdf.

Wing, Paul, Margie Langelier, Tracey Continelli, and David Armstrong. 2003 (May). Summary of the responses to the 2002 AHIMA member survey. Workforce research study funded through AHIMA's Foundation of Research and Education (FORE).

Chapter 4

Classifications and Terminologies

Ann H. Peden, MBA, RHIA, CCS

Over the years, coded data have become increasingly important in the delivery and reporting of healthcare services. In the 21st century, healthcare practitioners often view classification systems as either a method to facilitate the computerization of data or a mechanism to facilitate reimbursement. Although coding systems can serve both functions, healthcare data were maintained in coded form long before the introduction of computers or the inception of current reimbursement methods.

Data classification systems were first used for public health purposes, such as mortality reporting. The International Classification of Diseases (ICD) has its roots in the Bertillon Classification, or International List of Causes of Death, that dates back to 1893 (WHO 1992). In the 20th century, hospitals began using coding systems to index diseases and operations for research purposes. For many years, accrediting organizations, such as the Joint Commission on Accreditation of Healthcare Organizations (JCAHO), have promulgated standards requiring the coding and indexing of clinical information.

Coding systems are necessary to retrieve data for various purposes in healthcare organizations. Such purposes include provider credentialing, quality improvement, and utilization management. However, today's emphasis is on coding systems as they pertain to reimbursement and to the development of electronic health record systems. Numerous coding systems exist, and each system provides different functions. By understanding the wide range of systems available, individuals and organizations can select appropriate coding systems to achieve a variety of purposes.

This chapter discusses standards that have been established to manage healthcare data. It then defines classifications, nomenclature, and clinical terminologies before providing an overview of the most commonly used coding and classification systems used in the United States.

Standards for Healthcare Data

The increasing emphasis on electronic health records (EHRs) and electronic data interchange (EDI) has resulted in a quest for standards to facilitate data manipulation and transfer. Standards are important to coding professionals because the code sets themselves are standards and because other types of standards require the use of certain coding systems.

Examples of Standard-Setting Organizations

The American National Standards Institute (ANSI) facilitates the development of voluntary standards by accrediting the procedures of standard-setting organizations, including the health-related standards ASC X12, ASTM E1384, and HL7, which are described below (ANSI 2006; ANSI n.d.).

- Accredited Standards Committee (ASC) X12: ASC X12 develops, maintains, and publishes standards for EDI across industries (ASC X12 2006). The insurance subcommittee, X12N, develops standards and guidelines for the insurance industry, including health insurance and electronic submission of claims by providers (Rollins 2003). ASC X12N 837 standards apply to claims, encounters, and coordination of benefits (Amatayakul, Jorwic, and Scichilone 2003).

- ASTM International (originally known as the American Society for Testing and Materials): ASTM develops technical standards for materials, products, systems, and services. ASTM standard E1384-02a is the active version of the "Standard Guide for Content and Structure of the Electronic Health Record (EHR)" (ASTM International 2006).

- Health Level Seven (HL7): HL7 describes itself and its mission as to serve as "an international community of healthcare subject matter experts and information scientists collaborating to create standards for the exchange, management and integration of electronic healthcare information. HL7 promotes the use of such standards within and among healthcare organizations to increase the effectiveness and efficiency of healthcare delivery for the benefit of all." (Health Level Seven n.d.). The National Committee on Vital and Health Statistics endorsed HL7 as the standard for the electronic exchange of patient medical record information (Rollins 2003).

Standards under the Health Insurance Portability and Accountability Act

Many standards that were developed voluntarily are now mandatory as a result of the Health Insurance Portability and Accountability Act (HIPAA) of 1996. Under the Administrative Simplification (AS) provisions of HIPAA, the secretary of the Department of Health and Human Services (HHS) promulgates standards through the federal rule-making process. The first HIPAA rule, published on August 17, 2000, dealt primarily with electronic transactions, including standard code sets (Rode 2001). This rule also established several designated standards maintenance organizations, as follows (U.S. Government Printing Office 2000, 50373; 2003, 8382):

- Accredited Standards Committee X12N (ASC X12N) (http://www.x12.org)

- Health Level Seven, Inc. (HL7) (http://www.hl7.org)

- National Council for Prescription Drug Programs (NCPDP) (http://www.ncpdp.org)

- National Uniform Billing Committee (NUBC) (http://www.nubc.org)

- National Uniform Claim Committee (NUCC) (http://www.nucc.org)

- Dental Content Committee of the American Dental Association (http://www.ada.org)

In addition to previously mentioned ASC X12N and HL7, the NUBC and the NUCC are of interest to coding professionals. These two committees are responsible for the processes by which—and the forms on which—codes are submitted for payment.

The Centers for Medicare and Medicaid Services (CMS) adopted billing and claim forms originally developed by the American Hospital Association (AHA) and the American Medical Association (AMA). The NUBC maintains the UB-92 (also known as CMS-1450 and HCFA-1450) form that is used for hospital billing (NUBC 1999). The UB-92 has been in use for well over a decade, but is being replaced by the UB-04 in March 1, 2007; the UB-04 or the UB-92 can be used during the transition period until May 22, 2007 (NUBC 2005a). Reasons for revising the UB include creating consistency with data fields used in the X12 837 electronic transmission protocols, accommodating ICD-10, and supporting national provider and plan identifiers (Health Data Management 2004). Refer to figure 4.1 for examples of code submission using the UB-92. ICD-9-CM final diagnosis codes are included in Form Locators (FL) 67-67Q. FL 69 provides a field for the admitting diagnosis and FL 72 allows documentation of up to three E Codes. Up to six ICD-9-CM procedure codes and the dates the procedures were performed can be reported in FL 74-74e. Although not pictured in figure 4.1, which is an example of an inpatient bill, CPT or HCPCS codes for outpatients are reported in FL 44. The blank UB-04 form can be downloaded from http://www.nubc.org/public/whatsnew/UB-04Proofs.pdf (NUBC 2005b).

The NUCC maintains the CMS-1500 form used by the noninstitutional healthcare community, including physicians, for filing insurance claims (NUCC 2006). Figure 4.2 provides an example of code submission using this form. Up to four ICD-9-CM diagnosis codes may be entered in item 21 of the form. Item 24-D provides a column for submission of up to six CPT/HCPCS procedure codes and associated modifiers. Item 24-E allows the procedure code to be linked to the diagnosis for which the procedure was performed. For example, in figure 4.2, the number "1" in column 24-E indicates that this procedure relates to the first-listed diagnosis code. A revised version of the CMS-1500 form dated 08-05 will be implemented in 2007 (Medicare Learning Network 2006). Copies of both the UB-92 form (listed as HCFA-1450) and the CMS-1500 form, as well as many other forms, may be obtained from the CMS Web site at http://www.cms.hhs.gov/CMSForms/CMSForms/list.asp.

Before HIPAA implementation, billing or claims data were submitted electronically in the form of a flat file (that is, fixed-length records and fields). HIPAA rules now require that electronically submitted billing or claims data follow the ASC X12N 837 protocols (Amatayakul 2000). This means that information is formatted as streams of data rather than chunks of data submitted in fields as on paper forms. Codes and code sets are identified by qualifiers that appear in the data stream. As Amatayakul, Jorwic, and Scichilone (2003, 16D) explain:

> Each time a code set is used, a qualifier is needed to explain what type of code follows. For example, HI*BK:99762~ designates that this is the segment for Principal, Admitting, E-Code, and Patient Reason for Visit Diagnosis Information (HI) and that Principal Diagnosis (BK) follows, which is 997.62. 'BK' is the code list qualifier code. The (X12N 837) implementation guide specifies that this code must be from . . . ICD-9-CM.

Frequently asked questions (FAQs) about the HIPAA transaction standards may be found at the HHS Web site on administrative simplification (http://aspe.os.dhhs.gov/admnsimp/faqtx.htm).

Figure 4.1. Code submission example using UB-92 (CMS-1450) form

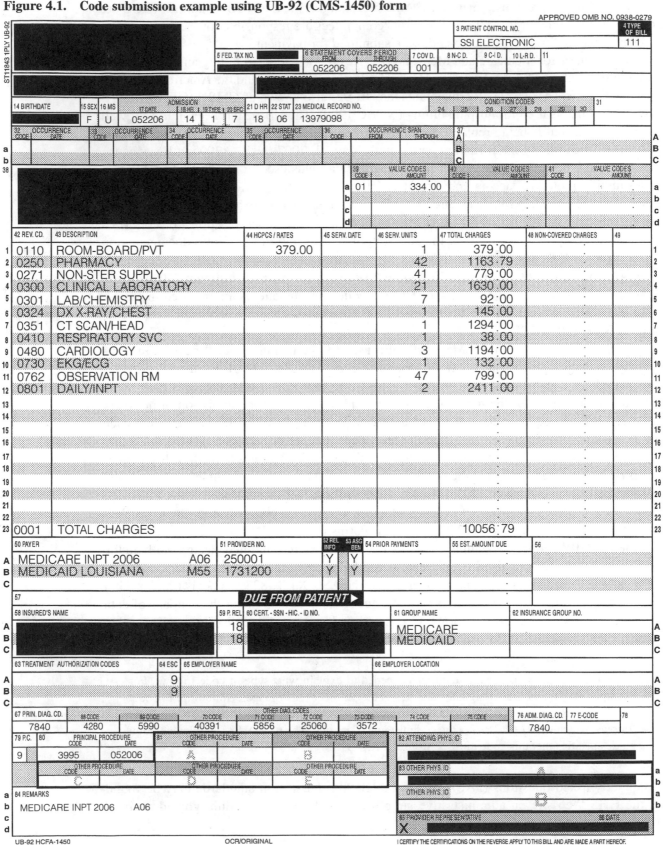

Source: NUBC 2005b.

Figure 4.2. Code submission example using CMS-1500 form

CASE ID: 00450168003   M01   4448   PAGE 1

1. MEDICARE [X] (Medicare #) MEDICAID (Medicaid #) CHAMPUS (Sponsor's SSN) CHAMPVA (VA File #) GROUP HEALTH PLAN (SSN or ID) FECA BLK LUNG (SSN) OTHER (ID)	1a. INSURED'S I.D. NUMBER (FOR PROGRAM IN ITEM 1)
2. PATIENT'S NAME (Last Name, First Name, Middle Initial)	3. PATIENT'S BIRTH DATE MM DD YY SEX M [ ] F [X]	4. INSURED'S NAME (Last Name, First Name, Middle Initial)
5. PATIENT'S ADDRESS (No., Street)	6. PATIENT RELATIONSHIP TO INSURED Self [ ] Spouse [ ] Child [ ] Other [ ]	7. INSURED'S ADDRESS (No., Street)
CITY STATE	8. PATIENT STATUS Single [X] Married [ ] Other [ ]	CITY STATE
ZIP CODE TELEPHONE (Include Area Code)	Employed [ ] Full-Time Student [ ] Part-Time Student [ ]	ZIP CODE TELEPHONE (INCLUDE AREA CODE) ( )

9. OTHER INSURED'S NAME (Last Name, First Name, Middle Initial)

10. IS PATIENT'S CONDITION RELATED TO:

11. INSURED'S POLICY GROUP OR FECA NUMBER

a. OTHER INSURED'S POLICY OR GROUP NUMBER

a. EMPLOYMENT? (CURRENT OR PREVIOUS) YES [ ] NO [X]

a. INSURED'S DATE OF BIRTH MM DD YY   SEX M [ ] F [ ]

b. OTHER INSURED'S DATE OF BIRTH MM DD YY   SEX M [ ] F [ ]

b. AUTO ACCIDENT?   PLACE (State) YES [ ] NO [X]

b. EMPLOYER'S NAME OR SCHOOL NAME

c. EMPLOYER'S NAME OR SCHOOL NAME

c. OTHER ACCIDENT? YES [ ] NO [X]

c. INSURANCE PLAN NAME OR PROGRAM NAME

d. INSURANCE PLAN NAME OR PROGRAM NAME

10d. RESERVED FOR LOCAL USE

d. IS THERE ANOTHER HEALTH BENEFIT PLAN? YES [ ] NO [ ] If yes, return to and complete item 9 a-d.

READ BACK OF FORM BEFORE COMPLETING & SIGNING THIS FORM.

12. PATIENT'S OR AUTHORIZED PERSON'S SIGNATURE I authorize the release of any medical or other information necessary to process this claim. I also request payment of government benefits either to myself or to the party who accepts assignment below.

SIGNED SIGNATURE ON FILE   DATE 03 03 06

13. INSURED'S OR AUTHORIZED PERSON'S SIGNATURE I authorize payment of medical benefits to the undersigned physician or supplier for services described below.

SIGNED SIGNATURE ON FILE

14. DATE OF CURRENT: MM DD YY ILLNESS (First symptom) OR INJURY (Accident) OR PREGNANCY(LMP)

15. IF PATIENT HAS HAD SAME OR SIMILAR ILLNESS. GIVE FIRST DATE MM DD YY

16. DATES PATIENT UNABLE TO WORK IN CURRENT OCCUPATION FROM MM DD YY TO MM DD YY

17. NAME OF REFERRING PHYSICIAN OR OTHER SOURCE

17a. I.D. NUMBER OF REFERRING PHYSICIAN

18. HOSPITALIZATION DATES RELATED TO CURRENT SERVICES FROM MM DD YY TO MM DD YY

19. RESERVED FOR LOCAL USE

20. OUTSIDE LAB? YES [ ] NO [X] $ CHARGES

21. DIAGNOSIS OR NATURE OF ILLNESS OR INJURY. (RELATE ITEMS 1,2,3 OR 4 TO ITEM 24E BY LINE)

1. V67 . 00   3. ___ . ___
2. ___ . ___   4. ___ . ___

22. MEDICAID RESUBMISSION CODE   ORIGINAL REF. NO.

23. PRIOR AUTHORIZATION NUMBER

24. A DATE(S) OF SERVICE					B Place of Service	C Type of Service	D PROCEDURES, SERVICES, OR SUPPLIES (Explain Unusual Circumstances) CPT/HCPCS	MODIFIER	E DIAGNOSIS CODE	F $ CHARGES	G DAYS OR UNITS	H EPSDT Family Plan	I EMG	J COB	K RESERVED FOR LOCAL USE
From MM	DD	YY	To MM	DD											
01	26	05			11		93923	26	1	484 50	1				020000398

25. FEDERAL TAX I.D. NUMBER   SSN EIN [X]

26. PATIENT'S ACCOUNT NO.

27. ACCEPT ASSIGNMENT? (For govt. claims, see back) [X] YES [ ] NO

28. TOTAL CHARGE $ 484 50

29. AMOUNT PAID $ 0 00

30. BALANCE DUE $

31. SIGNATURE OF PHYSICIAN OR SUPPLIER INCLUDING DEGREES OR CREDENTIALS (I certify that the statements on the reverse apply to this bill and are made a part thereof.) SIGNED   DATE

32. NAME AND ADDRESS OF FACILITY WHERE SERVICES WERE RENDERED (If other than home or office)

33. PHYSICIAN'S, SUPPLIER'S BILLING NAME, ADDRESS, ZIP CODE & PHONE # PIN#   GRP#

(APPROVED BY AMA COUNCIL ON MEDICAL SERVICE 8/88)   **PLEASE PRINT OR TYPE**   APPROVED OMB-0938-0008 FORM CMS-1500 (12-90), FORM RRB-1500, APPROVED OMB-1215-0055 FORM OWCP-1500, APPROVED OMB-0720-0001 (CHAMPUS)

PATIENT AND INSURED INFORMATION

PHYSICIAN OR SUPPLIER INFORMATION

Source: CMS 2006.

Code Set Standards under HIPAA

Of particular interest to coding professionals are the HIPAA standards for medical data code sets. The code sets are (U.S. Government Printing Office 2000, 50370):

- *International Classification of Diseases, Ninth Edition, Clinical Modification* (ICD-9-CM), Volumes 1 and 2

- *International Classification of Diseases, Ninth Edition, Clinical Modification* (ICD-9-CM), Volume 3 Procedures

- *National Drug Codes* (NDC)

- *Code on Dental Procedures and Nomenclature, Second Edition* (CDT-2)

- The combination of *Healthcare Common Procedure Coding System* (HCPCS) and *Current Procedural Terminology, Fourth Edition* (CPT)

HIPAA Standards for the Future

In future years, HIPAA could establish changes and additions to these initial code sets. For example, ICD-10-CM and ICD-10-PCS (Procedure Coding System) provide more specificity in coding than does ICD-9-CM. As part of its responsibilities under HIPAA, the National Committee on Vital and Health Statistics (NCVHS) monitors the continued effectiveness of the health data standards adopted. In 2003, the NCVHS recommended that the secretary of HHS begin the process of making ICD-10-CM and ICD-10-PCS standard code sets, replacing ICD-9-CM Volumes 1, 2, and 3. Implementation of these new systems as HIPAA standards would occur no earlier than 2 years after HHS publishes a final rule. As of June 2006, HHS had not issued any rules regarding replacement systems for ICD-9-CM.

HIPAA includes "tables of terms" and "medical concepts" in its definition of code sets, meaning that future implementations of HIPAA also could include standards for clinical terminologies, which are described in the next section of this chapter (HIPAA 1996).

Classifications, Nomenclatures, and Clinical Terminologies

A **classification** is a system that groups related entities to produce necessary statistical information. ICD-9-CM is an example of a classification system. The term **nomenclature** literally means "name calling." A nomenclature is a system of names used in any science or art. In medicine, a nomenclature presents preferred terminology for naming disease processes. An example of a nomenclature was the classic coding system of the mid-20th century, the *Standard Nomenclature of Diseases and Operations*.

The idea of a standardized **clinical terminology** is a newer concept than that of a classification or a nomenclature. The first National Conference on Terminology for Clinical Patient Description defined a clinical terminology as:

Standardized terms and their synonyms which record patient findings, circumstances, events and interventions with sufficient detail to support clinical care, decision support, outcomes research, and quality improvement; and can be efficiently mapped to broader classifications for administrative, regulatory, oversight, and fiscal requirements (CPRI 1999).

An example of a clinical terminology is the *Systematized Nomenclature of Human and Veterinary Medicine Clinical Terminology* (SNOMED CT). More information is provided on specific classifications, nomenclatures, and clinical terminologies later in this chapter.

Several structural terms are related to classifications, nomenclatures, and terminologies. For example, a **hierarchical system** is structured with broad groupings that can be further subdivided into more narrowly defined groupings or detailed entities. A **multiaxial system** can classify an entity in several different ways. For example, a neoplasm can be classified by site, by morphology, and by behavior—three axes. Many systems are both hierarchical and multiaxial. The **granularity** of a system refers to the level of detail the system is able to capture. A highly granular system captures finer details of data than a less granular system.

Overview of Coding Systems

The most commonly used coding systems in the United States are those used for reimbursement. These include the ICD-9-CM, HCPCS, and CPT coding systems.

ICD-9-CM Codes

ICD-9-CM Volumes 1 and 2 provide diagnosis codes for a variety of healthcare providers, including hospitals, home health providers, long-term care facilities, and physicians. ICD-9-CM Volume 3 provides procedure codes for hospital inpatient billing.

HCPCS and CPT Codes

HCPCS and CPT codes are used to bill physicians' procedures and services—both inpatient and outpatient. Hospitals use HCPCS/CPT codes to bill Medicare and other insurers for hospital outpatient procedures. (See table 4.1.) Traditionally, there have been three levels of HCPCS codes. (See table 4.2.)

Table 4.1. Typical reimbursement uses of ICD-9-CM and HCPCS/CPT

Coding System	Hospital Use	Physician Use
ICD-9-CM Volumes 1 and 2	Diagnoses for inpatients and outpatients	Diagnoses for inpatients and outpatients
ICD-9-CM Volume 3	Procedures for inpatients	None
HCPCS/CPT	Procedures for outpatients	Procedures for inpatients and outpatients

Table 4.2. Levels of HCPCS

Level	Name	Origin	Code Structure	Example
I	CPT Codes	AMA	Five numeric characters	00540
II	National Codes	CMS/HCFA	Alphanumeric codes beginning A–V	J0150
III*	Local Codes	Local Carriers	Alphanumeric codes beginning W–Z	W0001

*Note: HIPAA eliminated Level III (Local Codes) effective December 31, 2003. They are presented here because coding professionals who review data from 2003 and earlier may need to be aware of them.

Level I Codes

Level I codes are CPT codes developed by the American Medical Association (AMA). CPT codes contain five numeric characters (for example, 00540).

Level II Codes

Level II codes are national codes developed by CMS. They are alphanumeric codes that begin with the letters A–V (for example, J0150). In informal usage, the term "HCPCS codes" often refers to Level II codes.

Level III Codes

Level III codes were local codes developed by local carriers. Local codes were alphanumeric codes that began with the letters W–Z (for example, W0001). HIPAA rules eliminated Level III codes effective December 31, 2003. Coding professionals reviewing data from 2003 and earlier may need to reference Level III codes, even though they are no longer in use.

International Classification of Diseases

Volumes 1 and 2 of ICD-9-CM classify diseases and are based on ICD-9, which was developed and published by the World Health Organization (WHO). Because ICD-9 was designed primarily for mortality classification, it was clinically modified as ICD-9-CM for use in the United States for morbidity reporting as well. The National Center for Health Statistics (NCHS) maintains the disease classification in the United States.

Volume 3 of ICD-9-CM classifies procedures and was created for use in the United States. Therefore, it has no corresponding section in the WHO ICD-9. CMS maintains Volume 3.

Rules and Guidelines for Using ICD-9-CM

The Cooperating Parties develop coding rules and guidelines for correct use of ICD-9-CM. The Cooperating Parties are AHIMA, AHA, CMS, and the NCHS.

Coding Clinic

Coding Clinic is a publication that contains coding advice and decisions made by the Cooperating Parties. It is published quarterly by AHA's Central Office on ICD-9-CM. Because the Cooperating Parties agree to content and guidelines before publication, information appearing in *Coding Clinic* is considered to be authoritative advice on the correct use of ICD-9-CM.

Other Guidelines

The Cooperating Parties also have approved "Official ICD-9-CM Guidelines for Coding and Reporting." This document contains official coding guidelines and combines selected coding and reporting rules in one source (AHA 2005). It was named in the HIPAA regulations as part of the ICD-9-CM standard code set. The "Official ICD-9-CM Guidelines for Coding and Reporting" is available free of charge online at the Centers for Disease Control and Prevention (CDC) Web site under the NCHS classification of diseases initiative (http://www.cdc.gov/nchs/datawh/ftpserv/ftpicd9/icdguide05.pdf). See figure 4.3 for an excerpt from the official guidelines.

Figure 4.3.   Excerpt from *ICD-9-CM Official Guidelines,* December 1, 2005

---

14.   Chapter 14: Congenital Anomalies (740-759)

a.   Codes in categories 740-759, Congenital Anomalies

Assign an appropriate code(s) from categories 740-759, Congenital Anomalies, when an anomaly is documented. A congenital anomaly may be the principal/first listed diagnosis on a record or a secondary diagnosis.

When a congenital anomaly does not have a unique code assignment, assign additional code(s) for any manifestations that may be present.

When the code assignment specifically identifies the congenital anomaly, manifestations that are an inherent component of the anomaly should not be coded separately. Additional codes should be assigned for manifestations that are not an inherent component.

Codes from Chapter 14 may be used throughout the life of the patient. If a congenital anomaly has been corrected, a personal history code should be used to identify the history of the anomaly. **Although present at birth, a congenital anomaly may not be identified until later in life. Whenever the condition is diagnosed by the physician, it is appropriate to assign a code from codes 740-759.**

For the birth admission, the appropriate code from category V30, Liveborn infants, according to type of birth should be sequenced as the principal diagnosis, followed by any congenital anomaly codes, 740-759.

Source: CDC 2005, pp. 36–37.

ICD-10

WHO published the *International Statistical Classification of Diseases and Related Health Problems, Tenth Revision* (ICD-10), in 1992. ICD-10 is a more comprehensive and detailed classification than ICD-9. Unlike ICD-9, the main classification of ICD-10 is alphanumeric. Each code in the classification begins with an alphabetic character followed by numerals. For example, B15.9 is the code for hepatitis A without hepatic coma (WHO 1992, 152). This alphanumeric format expanded the number of codes available, allowing ICD-10 to capture greater detail than ICD-9. The United States uses ICD-10 for mortality reporting (on death certificates), but as of 2004, it is one of the few nations of the world that had not yet adopted ICD-10 or one of its modifications for morbidity (disease) reporting.

ICD-10-CM

The United States has developed ICD-10-CM, a clinical modification of ICD-10. Adopting ICD-10-CM would provide an expanded classification with more clinical detail and facilitate comparison of U.S. data with data from other countries. As previously explained, ICD-10-CM must be adopted as a HIPAA standard code set before it can be implemented in the United States. ICD-10-CM includes the following improvements over ICD-9-CM in content and format:

- "The addition of information relevant to ambulatory and managed care encounters;

- Expanded injury codes;

- The creation of combination diagnosis/symptom codes to reduce the number of codes needed to fully describe a condition;

- The addition of a sixth character;

- Incorporation of common fourth and fifth digit subclassifications;

- Laterality (that is, the ability to specify right or left side of the body); and Greater specificity in code assignment" (NCHS 2004b, 2).

Furthermore, ICD-10-CM provides for greater expansion of codes. It permits the coding of risk factors in addition to disease and injuries; it includes newly discovered diseases; it updates both clinical terminology and disease classification; and its greater detail can provide better data to decision makers, payers, and clinicians, resulting in improved delivery of high-quality healthcare and more appropriate resource utilization (Hazelwood and Venable 2003). Figure 4.4 is an excerpt from a draft of ICD-10-CM that illustrates some of its new features, such as the seventh character extension available in some categories (CDC 2003a). Just as there are guidelines for the use of ICD-9-CM, there are also draft guidelines that have been published for ICD-10-CM. Figure 4.5 is an excerpt from these draft guidelines (CDC 2003b).

ICD-10-PCS

Realizing that more detail was needed in the procedural classification as well as in the diagnostic classification, the United States developed ICD-10-PCS (Procedure Coding System) to replace Volume 3 of ICD-9-CM. ICD-10-PCS uses a seven-character, alphanumeric code structure. The classification is divided into 16 sections. The first character in each code is the letter or number designating the appropriate section (medical and surgical, obstetrics, imaging, and so on) within the classification. Within each section, each position in a code captures a specific concept and each character used in a position has a meaning specific to that position.

For example, "Open reduction internal fixation of left tibia with plate and screws" would be coded 0QQH04Z. The initial "0" in the code indicates the medical and surgical section; "Q," the body system, "lower bones"; "Q," the root operation, "repair"; "H," the body part, "left tibia"; "0," the approach, "open"; "4," the device, an "internal fixation device"; and "Z," there is "no qualifier" (Averill et al. 1998). Figure 4.6 contains an excerpt from the ICD-10-PCS tabular section (CMS 2005).

Current Procedural Terminology

Current Procedural Terminology (CPT) is copyrighted and maintained by the AMA. From the beginning, CPT was designed as a means of communication between physicians and third-party payers. CPT codes represent procedures and services performed by physicians in clinical practice. CPT comprises six major sections: evaluation and management, anesthesiology, surgery, radiology, pathology and laboratory, and medicine. These six sections comprise CPT's Category I codes. In addition, CPT includes Category II codes, which are available for performance measurement, and Category III codes, which are temporary codes for new procedures and services (AMA 2006). (Categories I, II, and III of CPT should not be confused with Levels I, II, and III of HCPCS, described in a previous section.)

Figure 4.4. Excerpt from *Draft ICD-10-CM Tabular*, June 2003

T22	**Burn and corrosion of shoulder and upper limb, except wrist and hand**

Excludes2: burn and corrosion of interscapular region (T21.-)
burn and corrosion of wrist and hand (T23.-)

The following 7th character extensions are to be added to each code for category T22:

    a initial encounter
    d subsequent encounter
    q sequela

T22.0 Burn of unspecified degree of shoulder and upper limb, except wrist and hand
Use additional external cause code to identify the source, place and intent of the burn
(X00–X19, X75–X77, X96–X98, Y92)

T22.00 Burn of unspecified degree of shoulder and upper limb, except wrist and hand, unspecified site

T22.01 Burn of unspecified degree of forearm
T22.011 Burn of unspecified degree of right forearm
T22.012 Burn of unspecified degree of left forearm
T22.019 Burn of unspecified degree of unspecified forearm

T22.02 Burn of unspecified degree of elbow
T22.021 Burn of unspecified degree of right elbow
T22.022 Burn of unspecified degree of left elbow
T22.029 Burn of unspecified degree of unspecified elbow

T22.03 Burn of unspecified degree of upper arm
T22.031 Burn of unspecified degree of right upper arm
T22.032 Burn of unspecified degree of left upper arm
T22.039 Burn of unspecified degree of unspecified upper arm

T22.04 Burn of unspecified degree of axilla
T22.041 Burn of unspecified degree of right axilla
T22.042 Burn of unspecified degree of left axilla
T22.049 Burn of unspecified degree of unspecified axilla

T22.05 Burn of unspecified degree of shoulder
T22.051 Burn of unspecified degree of right shoulder
T22.052 Burn of unspecified degree of left shoulder
T22.059 Burn of unspecified degree of unspecified shoulder

T22.06 Burn of unspecified degree of scapular region
T22.061 Burn of unspecified degree of right scapular region
T22.062 Burn of unspecified degree of left scapular region
T22.069 Burn of unspecified degree of unspecified scapular region

T22.09 Burn of unspecified degree of multiple sites of shoulder and upper limb, except wrist and hand
T22.091 Burn of unspecified degree of multiple sites of right shoulder and upper limb, except wrist and hand
T22.092 Burn of unspecified degree of multiple sites of left shoulder and upper limb, except wrist and hand
T22.099 Burn of unspecified degree of multiple sites of unspecified shoulder and upper limb, except wrist and hand

Source: CDC 2003a.

Figure 4.5.   Excerpt from *Draft ICD-10-CM Official Guideline*, June 2003

Excerpt from Draft ICD-10-CM Official Guidelines For Coding and Reporting for Acute Short-term and Long-term Hospital Inpatient and Physician Office and other Outpatient Encounters, p. 11. Accessed on-line from http://www.cdc.gov/nchs/data/icd9/draft_i10guideln.pdf

I.h Excludes notes
The ICD-10-CM has two types of excludes notes. Each note has a different definition for use but they are all similar in that they indicate that codes excluded from each other are independent of each other.

Excludes1

A type 1 Excludes note is a pure excludes. It means "NOT CODED HERE!" An Excludes1 note indicates that the code excluded should never be used at the same time as the code above the Excludes1 note. An Excludes1 is used when two conditions cannot occur together, such as a congenital form versus an acquired form of the same condition.

Excludes2

A type 2 excludes note represents "Not included here". An excludes2 note indicates that the condition excluded is not part of the condition represented by the code, but a patient may have both conditions at the same time. When an Excludes2 note appears under a code, it is acceptable to use both the code and the excluded code together.

Source: CDC 2003b.

Figure 4.6.   Excerpt from ICD-10-PCS tabular section

O: MEDICAL AND SURGICAL

Q: LOWER BONES

Q: REPAIR: Restoring, to the extent possible, a body part to its natural anatomic structure and function

Body Part Character 4	Approach Character 5	Device Character 6	Qualifier Character 7
0 Lumbar Vertebra 1 Sacrum 2 Pelvic Bone, Right 3 Pelvic Bone, Left 4 Acetabulum, Right 5 Acetabulum, Left 6 Upper Femur, Right 7 Upper Femur, Left 8 Femoral Shaft, Right 9 Femoral Shaft, Left B Lower Femur, Right C Lower Femur, Left D Patella, Right F Patella, Left G Tibia, Right H Tibia, Left J Fibula, Right K Fibula, Left L Tarsal, Right M Tarsal, Left N Metatarsal, Right P Metatarsal, Left Q Toe Phalanx, Right R Toe Phalanx, Left S Coccyx	0 Open 3 Percutaneous 4 Percutaneous Endoscopic X External	Z No Device	Z No Qualifier

Source: CMS 2005.

Implementation of the Category II and III codes has been part of the AMA's CPT-5 project, which expands the purposes of CPT beyond its traditional billing and administrative uses. More detail about the new CPT code categories is provided below:

- Category I codes are the five-digit codes traditionally found in the fourth edition of CPT.

- Category II codes are optional tracking codes used in performance measurement. These are five-character, alphanumeric codes with a letter in the last field (for example, 1234F).

- Category III codes are used to track new and emerging procedures and services that have clinical efficacy. In the past, such procedures may have been assigned local codes, which are no longer available under HIPAA. Like Category II codes, Category III codes are alphanumeric codes containing a letter in the last field (for example, 1234T).

Both Category II and III codes are located in separate sections of CPT, following the medicine section (Beebe 2001). Category II and III codes are updated twice a year by the AMA. The AMA publishes newly updated codes on its Web site (http://www.ama-assn.org) and in *CPT Assistant,* which is a monthly newsletter that provides authoritative guidance on the correct use of CPT. Transmittals and bulletins from CMS, Medicare carriers, and fiscal intermediaries are other sources of guidance on the use of CPT.

Single-Procedure Classification System

In 1993, the NCVHS recommended that the United States move to a single procedural coding system. In other words, it recommended abandoning the practice of using different coding systems in different settings, for example, using ICD for hospital inpatient coding and CPT for outpatient and physician coding. In the past, AHIMA has been a supporter of a single-procedure classification system but has testified to the NCVHS that the most important procedural coding issue in the current environment is the adoption of a replacement system for Volume 3 of ICD-9-CM, which is outdated and severely limited. AHIMA supports the adoption of ICD-10-PCS as the replacement system for Volume 3 of ICD-9-CM (Prophet 2002). Meanwhile, the AMA has been making improvements in CPT as a classification system, for example, by developing the Category II and III codes described previously. At the present time, more attention is being given to improving the two procedural coding systems that are currently mandated under HIPAA than to adoption of a single-procedure classification system in the United States.

Other Coding and Classification Systems

Numerous other coding and classification systems have significance in various arenas ranging from electronic transmittal of data to clinical research. The systems mentioned in the following paragraphs are not exhaustive. However, they do provide a glimpse of the many facets of classifications, nomenclatures, and clinical terminologies.

The Unified Medical Language System Metathesaurus and RxNorm

The Unified Medical Language System (UMLS) Metathesaurus is an ongoing project of the National Library of Medicine (NLM). The NLM describes the Metathesaurus as follows:

> "The Metathesaurus is a very large, multi-purpose, and multi-lingual vocabulary database that contains information about biomedical and health related concepts, their various names, and the relationships among them. Designed for use by system developers, the Metathesaurus is built from the electronic versions of many different thesauri, classifications, code sets, and lists of controlled terms used in patient care, health services billing, public health statistics, indexing and cataloging biomedical literature, and/or basic, clinical, and health services research. These are referred to as the 'source vocabularies' of the Metathesaurus. The term Metathesaurus draws on Webster's Dictionary third definition for the prefix 'Meta,' i.e., 'more comprehensive, transcending.' In a sense, the Metathesaurus transcends the specific thesauri, vocabularies, and classifications it encompasses" (NLM 2006, 1).

The Metathesaurus electronically links a broad range of clinical terminologies or vocabularies. It integrates those vocabularies by using a concept unique identifier that permits the source vocabularies to maintain their own definitions but links equivalent concepts across vocabularies (Campbell, Oliver, and Shortliffe 1998, 12–13). The UMLS includes many of the classification and terminology systems mentioned in this chapter and is licensed free of charge to both U.S. and international users (although there are some use restrictions on specific systems within the UMLS). Thus the UMLS can serve as a readily available distribution channel for various vocabulary systems.

RxNorm is a standardized terminology for clinical drugs. The National Library of Medicine developed the terms in RxNorm so that the name of a drug combines its ingredients, strengths, and form. "RxNorm links its names to many of the drug vocabularies commonly used in pharmacy management and drug interaction software, including those of First Databank, Micromedex, MediSpan, and Multum. By providing links between these vocabularies, RxNorm can mediate messages between systems not using the same software and vocabulary" (NLM 2005).

Diagnostic and Statistical Manual of Mental Disorders

The *Diagnostic and Statistical Manual of Mental Disorders, Fourth Edition, Text Revision* (DSM-IV-TR), published by the American Psychiatric Association (APA), is an example of a specialized coding system for mental health. DSM-IV-TR code numbers correspond to ICD-9-CM; however, its text and terminology are different (APA 2000a). In 2000, this classification was revised to update the text and any codes that had been updated in ICD-9-CM (APA 2000b). Before the 2000 revision, the classification had been known simply as DSM-IV. The APA has implemented a research agenda for the development of a fifth edition of DSM, although it does not anticipate publication of DSM-V before 2011 (APA Division of Research 2004).

The APA designed another version of DSM-IV for primary care clinician use. The DSM-IV-PC provides a standard approach to diagnosing mental health disorders, with an emphasis on disorders likely to be detected in the primary care setting (AHIMA 1998, 54). The system was designed to be useful in education, communication, and research. It facilitates collaboration between primary care and mental health specialists.

Systematized Nomenclature of Medicine Clinical Terms (SNOMED CT)

SNOMED International, a division of the College of American Pathologists, publishes Systematized Nomenclature of Human and Veterinary Medicine Clinical Terminology (SNOMED CT). SNOMED CT is available in multiple languages and has been voluntarily adopted by numerous organizations in more than 30 countries. It was created by merging an earlier version of SNOMED with the United Kingdom's National Health Service's (NHS) Clinical Terms Version 3 (CTV3). The merger of these two systems has resulted in the most comprehensive clinical terminology available because the primary care focus of CTV3 complements SNOMED's strength in specialty areas. (CTV3 has been known more commonly as the Read Codes or Read Thesaurus.) SNOMED CT is released twice a year in order to maintain its currency.

The three major elements in SNOMED CT are concepts, descriptions, and relationships. SNOMED CT contains more than 366,170 *concepts*, which are organized into categories such as clinical findings, body structure, organism, and so on (SNOMED International n.d.). Each concept has been assigned a unique identifier that is "nonsemantic" in nature, meaning that the identifier carries no meaning in and of itself. For example, in SNOMED CT the concept identifier for extrinsic asthma is 389146007 and the concept identifier for intrinsic asthma is 266361008. There is nothing in the two SNOMED concept identifiers (code numbers) themselves to indicate that there is any relationship between the terms. Contrast this with ICD-9-CM, where extrinsic asthma is coded 493.00 and intrinsic asthma is coded 493.10. In ICD-9-CM, the code number itself has a degree of meaning in that the category number 493 identifies both codes as representing a type of asthma.

The advantage of nonsemantic identifiers, as found in SNOMED CT, is that they provide both flexibility and consistency over time—flexibility because there is no need for concern about "running out" of numbers in a particular category (as has happened with some ICD-9-CM categories) and consistency in the event that new medical knowledge places the concept in a new category. If the concept changes categories because of new discoveries, there is no need for the concept identifier to change because it is not inherently tied to any particular category. It may help coding professionals who are accustomed to recognizing meanings in codes to remember that SNOMED CT is designed to operate in electronic systems; therefore, its codes or concept identifiers do not need to possess meanings that can be easily recognized or remembered by humans.

Because SNOMED CT codes themselves do not establish relationships between terms, how are relationships established? *Relationships* between codes are established apart from the concept identifier itself through various types of linkages. For example, the "is-a" hierarchical relationship links both extrinsic asthma and intrinsic asthma to the general concept of asthma. That is, extrinsic asthma "is a" type of asthma and intrinsic asthma "is a" type of asthma. Concepts can be linked hierarchically to more than one concept. For example, extrinsic asthma also "is a" type of allergic disorder. Attribute relationships provide links across hierarchies. For example, a disease can be linked to its anatomical location by a "finding site" relationship. In the case of extrinsic asthma, this disease concept can link by a "finding site" relationship to both lung structure and bronchial structure. There are around 1.46 million semantic relationships in SNOMED CT (SNOMED International n.d.).

Descriptions are the terms or text associated with each concept, including the fully specified name of the concept, the preferred term or name in common use, and synonyms (Brouch 2004). SNOMED CT contains more than 993,420 English-language descriptions or synonyms to express clinical concepts (SNOMED International n.d.). This combination of concepts, descriptions, and relationships enables SNOMED CT to capture rich clinical detail in electronic form to facilitate the indexing, storing, retrieving, and aggregating of patient data. (See figure 4.7 for a depiction of the various components of SNOMED CT.)

SNOMED CT is expected to play a significant role in the development of electronic health records. It has been recommended as a standard by several different organizations. In making recommendations to DHHS for uniform data standards for patient medical record information (PMRI), the NCVHS (2003, 3) recommended adoption of SNOMED CT as the "general terminology" standard, stating:

> The breadth of content, sound terminology model, and widely recognized value of SNOMED CT qualify it as a general-purpose terminology for the exchange, aggregation, and analysis of patient medical information.

As part of the move toward a national health information infrastructure, the DHHS has licensed SNOMED CT through the National Library of Medicine in order to make it available free of charge to healthcare facilities (SNOMED International 2003).

Figure 4.7.   SNOMED CT Components

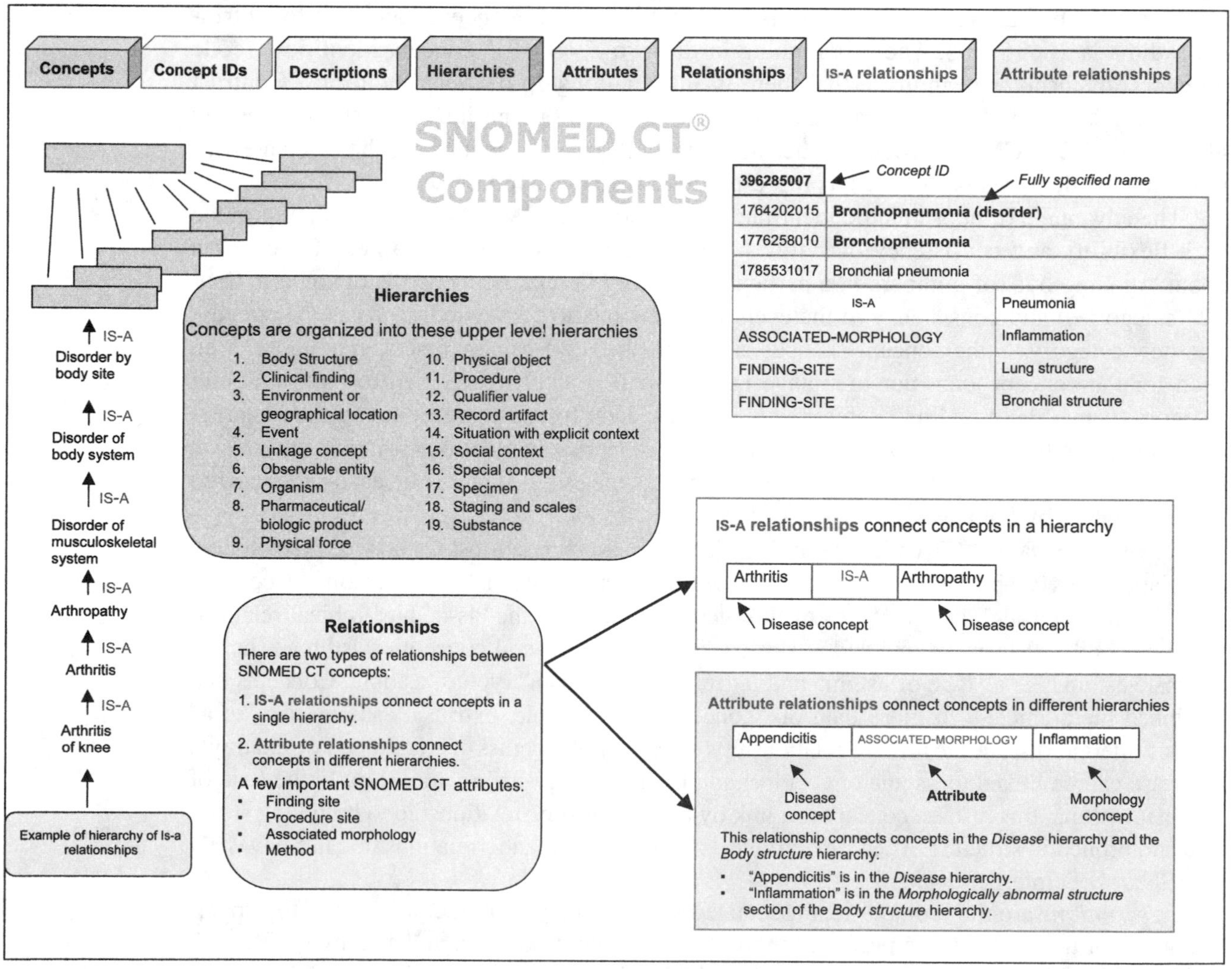

Source: 2006 College of American Pathologists. SNOMED and SNOMED CT are registered trademarks of the College. Available online from http://www.snomed.org/snomedct/what_is.html.

Code Sets Used in Preliminary Standards

Logical Observation Identifiers, Names, and Codes (LOINC) is a terminology and coding system for reporting laboratory results and other observations for electronic health records (Prophet 1997). The Regenstrief Institute maintains LOINC, which has been endorsed by numerous parties as a means of communicating laboratory and other observations (Stark 2006). It has been used in preliminary X12 standards, such as standards 277/275, Healthcare Claim Request for Additional Information and Response. Lab LOINC also has been designated as a PMRI standard by DHHS (NCVHS 2003). Figure 4.8 provides an example of how LOINC is used in a laboratory transaction.

Data Elements for Emergency Department Systems (DEEDS), developed by the National Center for Injury Prevention and Control (NCIPC), also is included as a code set in HL7 messages in preliminary ASC X12N standards for attachments. Those standards are expected to be included in future HIPAA rules (Washington Publishing Company 2001).

International Classification for Primary Care

The International Classification for Primary Care (ICPC-2) was developed by the World Organization of Family Doctors (WONCA) International Classification Committee (WICC). The World Organization of Family Doctors is the currently accepted short name for the World Organization of National Colleges, Academies, and Academic Associations of General Practitioners/Family Physicians (WONCA 2003).

ICPC-2 is a merger of the following three earlier classifications:

- Reason for Encounter Classification (RFEC)

- International Classification of Process in Primary Care (IC-Process-PC)

- *International Classification of Health Problems in Primary Care, Second Edition, Defined* (ICHPPC-2-D) (Jamoulle and Humbert 2001)

An electronic version of the ICPC classification, ICPC-2-E, was developed for use with electronic patient records. Both ICPC-2 and ICPC-2-E have been mapped to ICD-10 (Okkes et al. 2000, 101).

Figure 4.8.   Sample LOINC laboratory use case

- A laboratory order for a serum potassium is entered into an EHR system by a clinician.
- The test is ordered as a serum potassium and is translated to LOINC code 2697-1, the code for the method used in the laboratory performing the test.
- The EHR system generates a paper or electronic order that is sent to the laboratory (a commercial, hospital, or office laboratory). Information such as the patient identifier and test identifier is included. The LOINC code is added to pending orders on the patient record.
- The information from the order is transmitted to the laboratory information system (LIS).
- The LIS generates labels for ordered tests. The information regarding the specimen to draw and how to collect is associated with the LOINC code within the LIS.
- The specimen is collected or delivered to the lab.
- The lab performs the ordered tests.
- The status or results of the ordered tests are electronically sent to the EHR system that generated the order using LOINC code 2697-1, followed by the numerical result. The electronic message may be in a format similar to the following: OBX|3|ST|2697-1^POTASSIUM^LN^3.6^MG/DL|2006/04/14 09:06.24

Source: Stark 2006.

ABC Codes

The ABC codes are another interesting classification system. Copyrighted by ABC Coding Solutions (formerly Alternative Link, Inc.), ABC codes describe "what is said, done, ordered, prescribed, or distributed by providers of alternative medicine" (Prophet 1999, 65).

ABC codes were developed for electronic transactions that require a code for complementary and alternative medicine (CAM) services, as well as for services rendered by more conventional healthcare practitioners. They are available for acupuncture, chiropractic, holistic medicine, homeopathy, massage therapy, midwifery, naturopathy, and osteopathy, as well as for services provided by physician assistants, nurse practitioners, and others (ABC Coding Solutions n.d.). Moreover, the ABC codes have been incorporated into the NLM's UMLS Metathesaurus.

Classification Systems for Nursing

Several classification systems for nursing have been developed in North America. The American Nurses Association (ANA) established the Nursing Information and Data Set Evaluation Center (NIDSEC) to develop standards and to evaluate vendor products related to nursing information systems (Henry et al. 1998, 51). As of 2006, NIDSEC had recognized the following 13 data element sets and terminologies that meet ANA standards (ANA 2006):

Data Element Sets

1. NMDS—Nursing Minimum Data Set

2. NMMDS—Nursing Management Minimum Data Set

Interface Terminologies

3. CCC—Clinical Care Classification [formerly Home Healthcare Classification (HHCC)]

4. ICNP—International Classification of Nursing Practice

5. NANDA—NANDA (North American Nursing Diagnosis Association) International

6. NIC—Nursing Intervention Classification

7. NOC—Nursing Outcome Classification

8. OMAHA SYSTEM—Omaha System

9. PCDS—Patient Care Data Set

10. PNDS—Perioperative Nursing Data Set

Multidisciplinary Terminologies

11. ABC Codes—ABC Codes

12. LOINC—Logical Observation Identifiers Names and Codes

13. SNOMED CT—Systematized Nomenclature of Medicine Clinical Terms

Some of these systems have been discussed previously and apply to other areas of healthcare as well as to nursing. Of the systems that deal wholly with nursing, one of the first groups to formally identify and classify nursing diagnoses was NANDA (NANDA 2001), which primarily names and classifies conditions that nurses treat. NIC classifies nursing interventions or the treatments that nurses perform. NOC classifies the outcomes of those treatments. Both NIC and NOC are maintained by the University of Iowa's Center for Nursing Classification (University of Iowa College of Nursing 2001).

Other systems, such as the Omaha System, the Clinical Care Classification, and the International Classification for Nursing Practice (ICNP) provide ways to classify data in all three areas—diagnoses, interventions, and outcomes. The ICNP can map concepts from one nursing classification system to another, which should facilitate the description and comparison of nursing practices across nations (Henry et al. 1998, 50; ICN 2001; Clark 1998).

Other Special-Purpose Classifications and Terminologies

Also in the international arena are several other special-purpose classifications and terminologies. Some of these are discussed in the following sections.

The Universal Medical Device Nomenclature System (UMDNS) is a product of ECRI (formerly the Emergency Care Research Institute), a nonprofit health services research agency. UMDNS has been incorporated into the UMLS and has been adopted by nations and agencies around the world for classifying medical devices. In addition, the Committee on Data Standards for Patient Safety of the Institute of Medicine recommended UMDNS as one of the core terminologies for the electronic health record. UMDNS provides five-digit Universal Medical Device Codes (UMDC) for any type of medical device, equipment, supplies, and so on (ECRI 2006). In other words, almost any item other than a drug that is used in patient care can be coded in UMDNS (Giannangelo & Hull 2006).

Medical Dictionary for Drug Regulatory Affairs

The *Medical Dictionary for Drug Regulatory Affairs* (MedDRA) has been developed for the purpose of pharmaceutical regulation. Pharmaceutical companies use MedDRA internationally to report adverse drug reactions. As a standardized medical terminology, MedDRA includes terms for symptoms, signs, diseases, and the results of investigations rather than the names of drugs. MedDRA is both hierarchical and multiaxial and also incorporates other terminologies that were in use prior to its development (Rulon 2000).

International Classification of Diseases for Oncology

The International Classification of Diseases for Oncology (ICD-O) is used throughout the world for data collection and analysis in cancer registries. ICD-O is based on ICD-10 and uses codes for topography, morphology, and behavior of neoplasms (WHO 2001).

International Classification of Functioning, Disability and Health (ICF)

Another international classification system is WHO's Classification of Functioning, Disability, and Health (ICF), most recently revised in 2001. The ICF replaces the International Classification of Impairments, Disabilities, and Handicaps (ICIDH), first published in 1980. The components of the ICF are as follows:

- Body functions and structure

- Activities and participation

- Severity and environmental factors (NCHS 2004a)

Historical Coding Systems

Several 20th-century coding systems have historical importance. In some organizations, research databases that were begun using one of these historical systems have continued to be maintained under the same system for the sake of continuity, with the organization itself creating its own "updates" to the system. Even in organizations where historical systems are no longer in current use, health information managers assisting with research projects may occasionally have to retrieve data using one of the following legacy systems:

- The Standard Nomenclature of Diseases and Operations (SNDO) was a dual classification that used site and etiology as disease axes and site and procedure as operation axes. For example, the site "aorta" is represented by 461, and the procedure "biopsy" is represented by 16. Therefore, "Biopsy of the aorta" would be coded 461-16 (Cofer 1994, 324). The AMA last published SNDO in the 1960s.

- The AMA also published Current Medical Information and Terminology (CMIT), which used nonsemantic identifiers. In addition to codes, CMIT provided concise information, such as etiology, signs, symptoms, and laboratory findings for the diseases it listed.

- The Standard Nomenclature of Pathology (SNOP), published by the College of American Pathologists, was the forerunner to SNOMED. SNOP used four axes—topography, morphology, etiology, and function.

- The *International Classification of Diseases, Adapted for Use in the United States, Eighth Edition* (ICDA-8) was the forerunner to ICD-9-CM.

- The Hospital Adaptation of ICDA (H-ICDA), a contemporary of ICDA-8, was published by the Commission on Professional and Hospital Activities (Cofer 1994, 335).

Conclusion

The scope of services provided by various coding systems is far greater than the typical consumer of a given coding system may realize. Clinical concepts can be translated into a wide variety of codes. These codes can be used to manipulate and transmit data in a computerized system; map concepts from one coding system to another; and classify cases into broad groupings

Codes and their groupings can be used for many purposes, including for public health surveillance and epidemiology, research, maintenance of electronic health records, and reimbursement. The knowledgeable coding consumer keeps these many purposes in mind when compiling or using coded data.

References and Resources

ABC Coding Solutions. n.d. Coding and systems solutions for CAM and nursing. Available online from http://www.alternativelink.com/.

Accredited Standards Committee (ASC) X12. 2006. ASC X12 Vision and Mission. Available online from http://www.x12.org/x12org/about/VisionMission.cfm.

Accredited Standards Committee (ASC) X12. 2006. About ASC X12. Available online from http://www.x12.org/x12org/about/index.cfm

Amatayakul, M. 2000. Fundamentals for the newly initiated. 2000 *HIPAA Conference Presentation*. Available online from http://library.ahima.org.

Amatayakul, M., T. Jorwic, and R. Scichilone. 2003. Ready for the transactions rule? Get started with code sets (HIPAA on the job series). *Journal of American Health Information Management Association* 74(7): 16A–D.

American Health Information Management Association. 1998. DSM-IV gets a fresh look. *Journal of American Health Information Management Association* 69(5): 54.

American Hospital Association Central Office on ICD-9-CM. 2005. *Coding Clinic for ICD-9-CM*. Available online from http://www.aha.org/ahacentraloffice/coding/icd-9-cm.jsp.

American Medical Association. 2001a. CPT category III temporary codes. *CPT Assistant*, February, 5–6.

American Medical Association. 2006. *Current Procedural Terminology*. Chicago: American Medical Association.

American National Standards Institute. 1997. Supporting standards: Healthcare Informatics Standards Board inventory of healthcare information standards pertaining to the Health Insurance Portability and Accountability Act (HIPAA) of 1996 (P.L. 104–191). Available online from http://aspe.os.dhhs.gov/datacncl/hisbinv0.htm.

American National Standards Institute. 2006 (Sept. 29). ANSI Accredited Standards Developers. Available online from http://publicaa.ansi.org/sites/apdl/_layouts/1033/searchresults.aspx.

American National Standards Institute. n.d. Introduction. Available online from http://www.ansi.org/about_ansi/introduction/introduction.aspx?menuid=1.

American Nurses Association. 2006. Nursing Information and Data Set Evaluation Center (NIDSEC). Available online from http://www.ana.org/nidsec/index.htm.

American Psychiatric Association. 2000a. APA about to publish text revision of DSM-IV. *Psychiatric News*. Available online from http://www.psych.org/pnews/00-05-05/publish.html.

American Psychiatric Association. 2000b. *Diagnostic and Statistical Manual of Mental Disorders,* 4th ed. (DSM-IV), Primary Care Version. Available online from http://www.appi.org/book.cfm?id=2024.

American Psychiatric Association, Division of Research. 2004. DSM research planning. *Psychiatric Research Report* 20 (1): 1–3.

ASTM International. 2006. *E1381 02a Practice for Content and Structure of the Electronic Health Record (EHR)*. Available online from http://www.astm.org.

Averill, R. F., et al. 1998. Development of the ICD-10 procedure coding system (ICD-10-PCS). *Journal of American Health Information Management Association* 69(5): 65–72.

Beebe, M. 2001. Coding notes: CPT 5 supports performance measurement, technology. *Journal of American Health Information Management Association* 72(4).

Brouch, K. 2004. Speaker: SNOMED promises to change HIM practice (convention wrap-up). *Journal of American Health Information Management Association* 75(1): 66–67.

Campbell, K. E., D. E. Oliver, and E. H. Shortliffe. 1998. The unified medical language system: toward a collaborative approach for solving terminologic problems. *Journal of American Medical Informatics Association* 5(1): 12–16.

Centers for Disease Control and Prevention, National Center for Health Statistics. 2003a. *Draft ICD-10-CM Tabular List of Diseases and Injuries*. Available online from http://www.cdc.gov/nchs/data/icd9/draft_i10tabular.pdf.

Centers for Disease Control and Prevention, National Center for Health Statistics. 2003b. *Draft ICD-10-CM Official Guidelines for Coding and Reporting for Acute Short-term and Long-term Hospital Inpatient and Physician Office and other Outpatient Encounters*. Available online from http://www.cdc.gov/nchs/data/icd9/draft_i10guideln.pdf

Centers for Disease Control and Prevention, National Center for Health Statistics. 2005. *Official ICD-9-CM Guidelines for Coding and Reporting Effective December 1, 2005*. Available online from http://www.cdc.gov/nchs/datawh/ftpserv/ftpicd9/icdguide05.pdf.

Centers for Medicare and Medicaid Services. 2006 (Aug. 10). CMS forms. Available online from http://www.cms.hhs.gov/CMSForms/CMSForms/list.asp.

Centers for Medicare and Medicaid Services. 2005. ICD-10-PCS tabular section. Available online from http://www.cms.hhs.gov/ICD9ProviderDiagnosticCodes/Downloads/lowbone.pdf.

Clark, J. 1998. The international classification for nursing practice project. *Online Journal of Issues in Nursing.* Available online from http://www.nursingworld.org/ojin/tpc7/tpc7_3.htm.

Cofer, J., ed. 1994. *Health Information Management,* 10th ed. Berwyn, Ill.: Physicians' Record Company.

Computer-Based Patient Record Institute. 1999. National Conference on Terminology for Clinical Patient Description. Terminology II: Establishing the consensus, lessons from experience. Tysons Corner, Virginia, April 27–29.

ECRI. 2006. Universal Medical Device Nomenclature System™ (UMDNS™). Available online from http://www.ecri.org/Products_and_Services/Products/UMDNS/Default.aspx

Giannangelo, K., & Hull, S. 2006. Other and emerging vocabulary, terminology, and classification systems. In *Healthcare Code Sets, Clinical Terminologies, and Classification Systems.* Edited by K. Giannangelo. Chicago: American Health Information Management Association.

Hazelwood, A., and C. Venable. 2003. *ICD-10-CM Preview.* Chicago: American Health Information Management Association.

Health and Human Services. 2000 (Aug. 17). Health insurance reform: Standards for electronic transactions. *Federal Register* 65(160): 50312–373. 45 CFR Parts 160 and 162. Available online from http://aspe.os.dhhs.gov/admnsimp/final/txfinal.pdf

Health and Human Services. 2000. Frequently asked questions about code set standards adopted under HIPAA. Available online from http://aspe.os.dhhs.gov/admnsimp/faqcode.htm.

Health and Human Services. 2001. *Administrative Simplification.* Available online from http://aspe.os.dhhs.gov/admnsimp/.

Health Data Management. 2004 (Dec. 29). Comment sought on UB-04. Available online from http://www.healthdatamanagement.com/html/PortalStory.cfm?type=trend&DID=12221

Health Insurance Portability and Accountability Act of 1996. Public Law 104–191. Available online from http://aspe.os.dhhs.gov/admnsimp/pl104191.htm.

Health Level Seven. N.d. *About HL7.* Available online from http://www.hl7.org/about.

Henry, S. B., et.al. 1998. Nursing data, classification systems, and quality indicators: what every HIM professional needs to know. *Journal of American Health Information Management Association* 69(5): 48–55.

International Council of Nurses. 2001 (March). International Classification for Nursing Practice (ICNP) information sheet. Available online from http://www.icn.ch/icnp.htm.

Jamoulle, M., and J. Humbert. 2001. ICPC structure. Available online from http://www.ulb.ac.be/esp/wicc/structen.html.

Medicare Learning Network. 2006. Revised CMS-1500 Claim Form. *MLN Matters Number: MM4293.* Available online from http://www.cms.hhs.gov/MLNMattersArticles/downloads/MM4293.pdf

National Center for Health Statistics. 2004a. International Classification of Functioning, Disability and Health (ICF). Available online from http://www.cdc.gov/nchs/about/otheract/icd9/icfhome.htm.

National Center for Health Statistics. 2004b. *International Statistical Classification of Diseases, 10th Revision, Clinical Modification* (ICD-10-CM). Available online from http://www.cdc.gov/nchs/about/otheract/icd9/abticd10.htm.

National Committee on Vital and Health Statistics. 2003. Letter to the Honorable Tommy G. Thompson, Secretary, U. S. Department of Health and Human Services, November 5, 2003. Available online from http://www.ncvhs.hhs.gov/031105lt3.pdf.

National Library of Medicine. 2006. Fact sheet: UMLS metathesaurus. Available online from http://www.nlm.nih.gov/pubs/factsheets/umlsmeta.html.

National Library of Medicine. 2005. RxNorm. Available online from http://www.nlm.nih.gov/research/umls/rxnorm/index.html

National Uniform Billing Committee. 1999. About the NUBC. Available online from http://www.nubc.org/about.html.

National Uniform Billing Committee. 2005a (June 21). NUBC announces approval of UB-04. Available online from http://www.nubc.org/INFORMATION_ON_UB-04.pdf.

National Uniform Billing Committee. 2005b (April 19). UB-04 proofs. Available online from http://www.nubc.org/public/whatsnew/UB-04Proofs.pdf.

National Uniform Claim Committee. 2006. Who are we? Available online from http://www.nucc.org/.

North American Nursing Diagnosis Association. 2001. Available online from http://www.nanda.org/.

Okkes, I. M., M. Jamoulle, H. Lamberts, and N. Bentzen. 2000. ICPC-2-E: the electronic version of ICPC-2. Differences from the printed version and the consequences. *Family Practice* 17(2): 101–7.

Prophet, S. 1997. Classification systems: taking a broader look. *Journal of American Health Information Management Association* 68(5): 46–50.

Prophet, S. 1999. Alternative medicine: growing trend for the new millennium, part II. *Journal of American Health Information Management Association* 70(5): 65–71.

Prophet, S. 2002. Testimony of the American Health Information Management Association to the National Committee on Vital and Health Statistics on ICD-10-PCS, April 9, 2002. Available online from AHIMA.org.

Rode, D. 2001. Understanding HIPAA transactions and code sets. *Journal of American Health Information Management Association* 72(1): 26–33.

Rollins, Gina. 2003. HIM on the front lines of change: marching towards the health information infrastructure. *Journal of American Health Information Management Association* 74(1): 22–26.

Rulon, V. 2000. A global language for pharmaceutical regulation. *Journal of American Health Information Management Association* 71(1).

Stark, M. 2006 (July 2). Look at LOINC: The established standard for lab data gains visibility as data exchange increases. *Journal of American Health Information Management Association* 77(7): 52–55.

SNOMED International. 2003. U.S. healthcare industry moves toward the reality of electronic health records. News Release, July 1, 2003. Available online from http://www.snomed.org/news/pdfs/E-NLMPR.pdf.

SNOMED International. No date. What is SNOMED CT? Available online from http://www.snomed.org/snomedct/what_is.html.

University of Iowa College of Nursing. 2001. Center for Nursing Classification. Available online from http://www.nursing.uiowa.edu/cnc/.

U.S. Government Printing Office. 2003. Health insurance reform: modifications to electronic transaction standards and code sets; final rule. *Federal Register* 68(34): 8381–8399.

Washington Publishing Company. 2001. ANSI ASC X12N HIPAA implementation guides. Available online from http://hipaa.wpc-edi.com/HIPAA_40.asp.

WONCA. 2003. Global family doctor. Available online from http://www.globalfamilydoctor.com.

World Health Organization. 1992. *International Statistical Classification of Diseases and Related Health Problems, 10th revision* (ICD-10). Geneva: World Health Organization.

World Health Organization. 2001. Publications: disease classification, nomenclature. Available online from http://www.who.int/dsa/cat98/disease8.htm.

Chapter 5

Uses of Coded Data in Risk Adjustment and Payment Systems

Ann H. Peden, MBA, RHIA, CCS

As noted in chapter 4, there are many classification and terminology systems. These systems can be used for many purposes, including research, public health, accreditation, credentialing, quality improvement, utilization management, electronic health records, and reimbursement. This chapter deals primarily with the uses of coded data in risk adjustment and payment systems.

Case-Mix, Severity-of-Illness, or Risk-Adjustment Systems

Coded healthcare data are used in many ways in the United States, including in systems that attempt to account for increased risk of resource consumption, expenditures, and mortality. These systems are sometimes called case-mix, severity-of-illness, or risk-adjustment systems. Some of the systems are used to compare healthcare outcomes. For example, when two hospitals have different mortality rates, does this indicate that the quality of care was inadequate in the hospital with the higher death rate or does it mean that the patients in that hospital were more severely ill? Some risk-adjustment systems address this type of question so that comparisons can be made of mortality rates and other outcome indicators. Other systems are used more for internal data analysis and benchmarking purposes. Another important use of case-mix or risk-adjustment systems is in adjusting payments to providers in various healthcare settings.

Although the terms *case mix, severity of illness,* and *risk adjustment* are sometimes used interchangeably, shades of meaning can be distinguished. Case-mix systems are designed to group cases that are clinically similar and that ordinarily use similar resources. As the name implies, severity-of-illness systems attempt to measure the severity or seriousness of the patient's condition (Bowman 2001). Risk adjustment is a more general term that includes both case-mix and severity-of-illness systems (Iezzoni 2003).

Early Systems

Since the early 1980s when it was mandated as the prospective payment system (PPS) for Medicare, the diagnosis-related group (DRG) system has been the most widely used inpatient case-mix system. Because DRGs were based on the Medicare population, the first evolutions of this case-mix system were modified for use with other groups. Pediatric-modified DRGs

(PM-DRGs) were developed for use in children's hospitals; all-payer DRGs (AP-DRGs) evolved for use with the general population. Outpatient case-mix systems began receiving more attention when ambulatory patient groups (APGs) were developed as a possible PPS for hospital-based outpatient services. However, when the hospital outpatient prospective payment system (HOPPS or OPPS) was actually implemented, the system chosen was the ambulatory payment classification (APC) system.

Sampling of Risk Adjustment Methodologies

Numerous risk-adjustment systems are currently available. Some use coded data; others require more information than is ordinarily needed to assign standard ICD-9-CM codes. Examples of risk-adjustment systems include:

- The all-patient-refined DRG (APR-DRG) is a severity-of-illness system that can be used with all patients, including children. APR-DRGs adjust for severity of illness by considering the number of and severity of patient complications, comorbidities, and procedures coded. Birth weight also is a factor in some categories (Iezzoni 2003). APR-DRGs are the basis of a severity-adjusted case mix system proposed for implementation in Medicare's inpatient prospective payment system, which will be discussed later in the chapter.

- Disease staging (DS) is a severity-of-illness/risk-adjustment system that uses both coded data and information such as diagnostic test results. Stages range from no complications (Stage 1) to death (Stage 4) (Iezzoni 2003; MEDSTAT 2005).

- Cerner APACHE III for Critical Care (Acute Physiology Age Chronic Health Evaluation) is used to assess severity among patients treated in settings such as intensive care units. In addition to considering age and chronic health conditions, APACHE III is based on 17 acute physiologic findings (Iezzoni 2003).

- The episode treatment group (ETG) system facilitates analysis of resource consumption and clinical outcomes for clinically similar episodes of care as identified through inpatient, outpatient, and pharmaceutical claims data (Forthman, Dove, and Wooster 2000, 53).

- The Comprehensive Severity-of-Illness Index (CSI) (formerly Computerized Severity Index) calculates severity-of-illness scores based on the degree of abnormality of individual signs and symptoms, not just on coded diagnoses (International Severity Information Systems 2001).

- The Atlas System (formerly the MedisGroups System) uses key clinical findings abstracted from the patient record rather than diagnoses to adjust for severity (Iezzoni 2003).

This list is far from exhaustive, but it does provide a sampling of various risk-adjustment systems currently available. Other systems are discussed in more detail in the following sections.

Medicare Risk-Adjustment for Managed Care Providers

The Medicare program has evaluated several different risk-adjustment proposals for payments to its managed care providers in the Medicare Advantage (formerly Medicare+Choice [M+C]) program. The concept behind risk adjustment is to pay higher premiums to managed care providers who care for "sicker" patients.

Principal inpatient diagnostic cost groups (PIP-DCGs) comprised the interim system implemented in 2000 for risk adjustment of payments to M+C plans (HCFA 2000a, 40306).

The diagnosis codes used to adjust payment rates were taken only from inpatient admissions. Because patients who have been hospitalized increase costs for managed care organizations, the PIP-DCG system provided a measure of clinically based risk adjustment. For example, the risk-adjustment factor for a patient who has been hospitalized for a kidney infection might be twice that of an unhospitalized individual. Another example would be a patient with two hospitalizations, including one for lung cancer. Such a patient might have four times the risk-adjustment factor of the "healthy" patient (Tully and Rulon 2000, 64).

However, the PIP-DCG system was found to be limited in comparison with more comprehensive systems. Therefore, the Centers for Medicare and Medicaid Services implemented the CMS-HCC risk-adjustment model for health plans in 2004. This model uses a limited number of ICD-9-CM diagnosis codes to place patients into disease groups called hierarchical condition categories (HCCs). The CMS-HCC system contains more than 70 disease groups, each of which comprises clinically similar conditions that also are similar in costs. Each group has an associated coefficient that is used to calculate per person, per month payments to Medicare Advantage plans. In addition to the adjustments based on disease groups, the CMS-HCC model uses variables based on age, sex, Medicaid eligibility, disability status, and so on. The CMS-HCC models are additive in nature and are derived from a broader base of data sources than were PIP-DCGs. For example, PIP-DCGs placed a person in a single cost group based on his or her most costly inpatient diagnosis. However, the CMS-HCC model is additive, meaning that it results in increased payment amounts for each of the person's disease groups. As a general rule, an enrollee with three different diseases falling into three separate disease groups would trigger increases in CMS's payment to the health plan for each of the three groups. The CMS-HCC model considers diagnosis codes from physician and hospital outpatient visits in addition to inpatient diagnoses (CMS 2004a). Since its initial implementation in 2004, the CMS-HCC model has continued to be refined for specific subgroups of Medicare beneficiaries (Kautter, Pope and Olmstead 2005, CMS 2006a).

Prospective Payment Systems

Coded data also are used in the variety of prospective payment systems (PPS) initiated by the federal government. Information about these systems can be found at the CMS Web site under Medicare (http://www.cms.hhs.gov/home/medicare.asp).

PPS regulations for hospitals include the DRG system for hospital inpatients and the APC system for hospital outpatients. PPS regulations also are in place for home health providers, skilled nursing facilities, inpatient rehabilitation programs, long-term care hospitals, and inpatient psychiatric facilities.

Diagnosis-Related Groups

DRGs were originally implemented as a payment mechanism for Medicare inpatients. Currently, they are used for many purposes, including:

- Reimbursement by other insurers

- Data analysis in negotiating managed care contracts

- Utilization management

There are approximately 500 DRGs, and each inpatient admission is assigned to only one DRG. Updates to the DRG system are published each year in the *Federal Register.*

Calculating DRGs

A computer program called a grouper calculates DRGs. (See table 5.1 for basic DRG vocabulary.) Decision-tree diagrams depict grouper logic in assigning DRGs. (See figure 5.1 for an example of a DRG decision tree.) The grouper uses coded data—ICD-9-CM codes and other information from the UB-92/UB-04—to categorize cases into DRGs. Grouper logic ordinarily uses the following pattern or algorithm:

1. In assigning a DRG, the grouper uses the principal diagnosis to place the case in a major diagnostic category (MDC).

2. If the patient had a procedure normally done in an operating room (an OR procedure), the grouper places the case in the surgical partition of the decision tree. If the patient did not undergo an OR procedure, the grouper places the case in the medical partition of the decision tree.

Table 5.1. Vocabulary related to diagnosis-related groups (DRGs)

Term	Definition
Case-Mix Index (CMI)	The average of the relative weights of all cases treated at a given hospital. The case-mix index can be used to make comparisons between hospitals. The theoretical "average" case-mix index is 1.0000.
CC	A complication or comorbidity
Comorbidity	An additional diagnosis that exists at the time of admission and extends the length of stay in most cases
Complication	An additional diagnosis that arises during hospitalization and extends the length of stay in most cases
Decision Tree	A diagram depicting grouper logic in assigning DRGs
Diagnosis-Related Group (DRG)	A grouping of cases that are similar with respect to diagnoses and treatment
Grouper	A computer program that uses coded data to categorize cases into DRGs
Major Diagnostic Category (MDC)	An initial category into which the grouper places the patient based (usually) on the principal diagnosis
Medical Partition	A branch of a decision tree for cases without OR procedures
Medicare Code Editor	Computer program designed to detect errors in Medicare claims, such as invalid codes, age and gender conflicts, nonspecific and questionable principal diagnoses, nonspecific and noncovered procedures
OR Procedure	A procedure normally done in an operating room
PPS Rate or Blended Rate	A dollar amount that is based on an individual hospital's costs of operating and that is multiplied by the DRG relative weight to calculate that hospital's reimbursement for a given DRG
Principal Diagnosis (PDx)	The condition established after study to be chiefly responsible for occasioning the admission of the patient to the hospital
Relative Weight	A number that is assigned to each DRG and that is used as a multiplier to determine reimbursement
Surgical Hierarchy	An arrangement of surgical procedures in order of resource consumption
Surgical Partition	The branch of a decision tree for cases with OR procedures

Figure 5.1. Example of a DRG decision tree

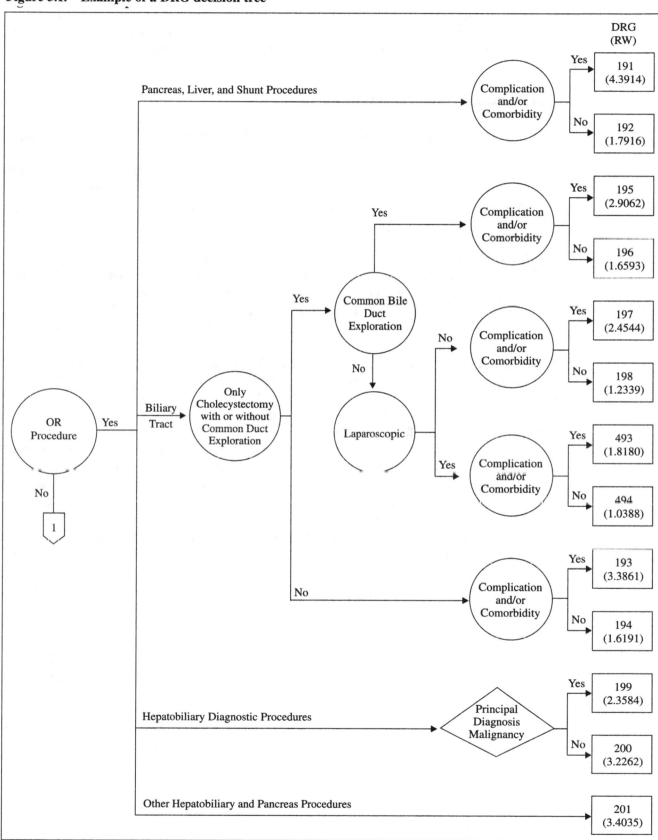

3. Within the surgical partition, the surgical hierarchy determines the next branch of the decision tree taken by the grouper. The surgical hierarchy is an arrangement of surgical procedures in order of resource consumption. If the patient underwent more than one surgical procedure, the procedure highest in the hierarchy would control the choices of DRGs available for that case.

Complications and Comorbidities

Complications and comorbidities (CCs) also play a part in determining the DRG. CCs are additional, or secondary, diagnoses that ordinarily extend the length of stay. A **complication** is a secondary condition that arises during hospitalization; a **comorbidity** is one that exists at the time of admission. Some DRGs are paired, with one DRG including cases with a CC and the other DRG including the same type of cases, but without a CC. The DRG with the CC is the higher-paying DRG in each pair. Other factors, such as the patient's age and discharge disposition, also can affect DRG assignment.

Relative Weight of DRGs

Each DRG is assigned a relative weight. The **relative weight** is a multiplier that determines reimbursement. For example, a DRG with a relative weight of 2.0000 would pay twice as much as a DRG with a relative weight of 1.0000. The hospital's PPS rate, or blended rate, makes up the other component of the DRG payment calculation. Each hospital's PPS rate is a dollar amount based on its operating costs as determined by several blended factors. This blended rate is multiplied by the DRG's relative weight to calculate the hospital's reimbursement for a given DRG. For example, a hospital with a PPS rate of \$4,000 would receive \$6,000 for a case in a DRG with a relative weight of 1.5000 ($1.5000 \times \$4000 = \$6000$).

Case-Mix Index and DRG System

A hospital can monitor its performance under the DRG system by monitoring its **case-mix index** (CMI). The CMI is the average of the relative weights of all cases treated at a given hospital. The Medicare CMI for every participating hospital is published annually in the *Federal Register.* The CMI can be used to make comparisons between hospitals and to assess the quality of documentation and coding at a particular hospital. The theoretical average case-mix index is 1.0000. Thus, a hospital with a CMI of 1.5000 theoretically has a more severely ill patient population than the average hospital. On the other hand, a hospital with a CMI of 0.9500 theoretically has a less severely ill patient population than the average hospital. If a hospital's CMI seems low compared with the perceived severity of the patient population, coding staff may be failing to document and code all relevant diagnoses and procedures. (See chapter 12.)

DRG Creep

As hospitals have striven to improve their CMIs year after year, the phenomenon of **DRG creep** has appeared. DRG creep is the rise in the CMI through the coding of higher-paying principal diagnoses and of more complications and comorbidities, even though the actual severity level of the patient population did not change. Because an improved CMI could be viewed as an indication of fraud or abuse, coders must adhere to established coding guidelines and ethical principles in code assignment. Legitimate improvements in the quality of coding and documentation can lead to a legitimate rise in the CMI.

DRG Payment in Patient Transfer

When a patient is transferred from one acute hospital to another, "full payment is made to the final discharging hospital and each transferring hospital is paid a per diem rate for each day of the stay, not to exceed the full DRG payment that would have been made if the patient had been discharged without being transferred" (CMS 2003a, 45404). This transfer policy generally results in a reduced payment to the transferring facility. A similar policy is in effect for patients transferred to certain post–acute care settings when the hospital stay falls into certain DRGs. In 2006, 182 DRGs were subject to the postacute transfer policy (Leary & D'Amato 2005). When the DRG is covered by the post–acute care transfer policy and when the patient is transferred to a psychiatric hospital/unit, a rehabilitation hospital/unit, a children's hospital, a long-term care hospital, a cancer hospital, a skilled nursing facility, or home health services, payment to the transferring facility is a based on a per diem rate (CMS 2003a). To avoid allegations of fraudulent billing, it is important to ensure that discharge dispositions submitted on claims are accurate.

All Patient Refined Diagnosis Related Group System (APR DRGs)

The All Patient Refined Diagnosis Related Group (APR DRG) System is a severity-adjusted DRG system designed by 3M Health Information Systems. APR DRGs differ from traditional or CMS DRGs in several ways. CMS DRGs recognize only two levels of severity for a given diagnosis grouping—one level with a CC and one level without a CC. In contrast, the APR DRG system recognizes four levels of severity for each diagnosis grouping. The result is that there are more than twice as many APR DRGs as there are CMS DRGs. Also, in the CMS DRG system, the number of CCs does not affect the severity level; for example, a case with seven CCs can fall into the same DRG as a case with only one CC. In addition, the grouper logic for APR DRGs is much more complex, involving multiple steps to determine severity and sometimes rerouting to a different MDC based on codes other than the principal diagnosis. The differences between the two systems are summarized in table 5.2.

In searching for a more refined severity-adjusted payment system for the Medicare IPPS, CMS noted, "More than a third of the hospitals in the United States are already using APR DRG software to analyze comparative hospital performance. Many major health information system vendors have integrated this system into their products. Several State agencies utilize the APR DRGs for the public dissemination of comparative hospital performance reports. APR

Table 5.2. Comparison of the CMS DRG System and the APR DRG System

Element	CMS DRG System	APR DRG System
Number of base DRGs	367	314
Total number of DRGs	526	1,258
Number of CC (severity) subclasses	2	4
Multiple CCs recognized	No	Yes
CC assignment specific to base DRG	No	Yes
Logic of CC subdivision	Presence or absence	18-step process
Logic of MDC assignment	Principal diagnosis	Principal diagnosis with rerouting
Death used in DRG definitions	Yes	No
Data requirements	Hospital claims	Hospital claims

Source: CMS 2006b, 80.

DRGs have been widely applied in policy and health services research" (CMS 2006b, 72). The state of Maryland also began using APR DRGs for payment for hospital inpatient services by all payers, including Medicare, Medicaid, and third-party insurers in 2005 (3M n.d.). CMS provided the data in table 5.3 to illustrate how payments to hospitals could be more effectively refined using the APR DRG system.

In 2006, CMS proposed implementing a modified version of the APR DRG system—Consolidated Severity-Adjusted DRGs (CS DRGs)—as the basis of the inpatient prospective payment system. Because APR DRGs were designed for all-payer patient populations, certain APR DRGs would have very low volume for the Medicare population, If CMS were to establish weights in the many categories that would have few cases, this could result in instability in the system. The solution that CMS proposed was to consolidate the APR-DRGs into a smaller number of categories. Through the consolidation process, CMS was able to reduce the number of severity-adjusted DRGs from over 1,200 to fewer than 900, which would also have the advantage of maintaining a three-character field in databases and information systems that had been designed to capture the CMS DRGs. See table 5.4 for examples of Consolidated Severity-Adjusted DRGs excerpted from the CMS proposed rule. Note that in the "Type" column, the "S" indicates a surgical DRG and "M" indicates a medical DRG. In the last column, the number following "SOI" indicates the severity of illness classification.

The final rule for Fiscal Year 2007 (FY 2007) did not commit CMS to the implementation of Consolidated Severity-Adjusted DRGs, but did state that CMS will implement some type of severity-adjusted DRG system no later than October 2007 (FY 2008) (CMS 2006d).

Ambulatory Payment Classifications

The APC system was created as a result of provisions in the Balanced Budget Act of 1997. Its purpose was to implement a PPS for hospital outpatient services for Medicare

Table 5.3   Example of sample cases assigned under the CMS DRG system and under the APR DRG system

Principal Diagnosis Code: 562.11 Procedure Code 45.71	CMS DRG System		APR DRG System	
	DRG Assigned	Average Charge	DRG Assigned	Average Charge
Case 1— Secondary Diagnosis: 569.41	149 without CC	$25,147	221 with severity of illness subclass 1	$25,988
Case 2— Secondary Diagnoses: 569.41 560.9	148 without CC	$59,519	221 with severity of illness subclass 2	$38,209
Case 3— Secondary Diagnoses: 569.41 560.9 422.99 426.0	148 without CC	$59,519	221 with severity of illness subclass 3	$66,597
Case 4— Secondary Diagnoses: 569.41 560.9 422.99 426.0 584.9	148 without CC	$59,519	221 with severity of illness subclass 4	$130,750

Table 5.4. Examples of Consolidated Severity-Adjusted DRGs

Type	MDC	Consolidated Severity-Adjusted DRG	Consolidated Severity-Adjusted DRG Description
S	1	20	NERVOUS SYSTEM PROCEDURES SOI 4
S	1	21	CRANIOTOMY FOR TRAUMA SOI 1
S	1	22	CRANIOTOMY FOR TRAUMA SOI 2
S	1	23	CRANIOTOMY FOR TRAUMA SOI 3
M	1	39	NERVOUS SYSTEM MEDICAL DIAGNOSES EXCEPT INFECTIONS SOI 4
M	1	40	INFECTIONS OF NERVOUS SYSTEM SOI 4
M	1	41	SPINAL DISORDERS & INJURIES SOI 1
M	1	42	SPINAL DISORDERS & INJURIES SOI 2
M	1	43	SPINAL DISORDERS & INJURIES SOI 3

Source: CMS 2006b, 1076.

patients. APCs were implemented in August 2000. Numerous updates and corrections to the APC system have been published in the years since its implementation, through either the annual updates in the *Federal Register* or through CMS program memoranda and transmittals.

The APC system groups procedures that have similar clinical characteristics with similar costs based on the CPT/HCPCS codes assigned. Diagnosis codes do not affect APC assignment per se; however, diagnostic codes may affect reimbursement by indicating (or failing to indicate) the medical necessity of the services provided. There are approximately 1,000 APCs, which include the following groupings:

- Significant procedures, therapies, or services

- Medical visits

- Ancillary tests and procedures

- Partial hospitalization

- Drugs and biologicals

- Devices

APC System versus DRG System

One major difference between the APC and DRG systems is that an outpatient may be assigned more than one APC per hospital encounter whereas an inpatient is assigned only one DRG per hospital admission. For example, a patient's emergency department visit includes evaluation and management (E/M), x-ray diagnosis of a fracture, and treatment of the fracture. This encounter will generate several APCs. The payment to the hospital would include amounts for each APC as indicated in table 5.5.

Table 5.5.   Example of APC reimbursement for an emergency department visit

Code	Procedure	Payment *
APC 0043	Closed treatment fracture finger/toe/trunk	$105
APC 0260	Level I plain film except teeth	$45
APC 0611	Mid-level emergency visit	$130
		Total $280

* Dollar amounts are for illustrative purposes only and do not represent actual payments.

Evaluation and Management Codes

Medical visits present several interesting aspects of the APC. For the most part, APCs follow the CPT coding rules as set forth by the AMA. However, for medical visits, hospitals have been able to develop their own criteria for assigning E/M codes that determine the level of the visit. In addition, hospitals do not follow the same guidelines as physicians. When APCs were first implemented, the American Hospital Association (AHA) recommended that hospitals develop a system for E/M code assignment that (1) reasonably reflects the medical necessity of services provided and (2) is based on documentation found in the patient record (Holbrook et al. 2001). In 2003, the Hospital Evaluation and Management Coding Panel of the American Hospital Association and American Health Information Management Association developed a "Recommendation for Standardized Hospital Evaluation and Management Coding of Emergency Department and Clinic Services" (AHA and AHIMA 2003). In 2006, CMS published a modification of these AHA and AHIMA guidelines as a draft proposal to standardize the method of determining the level of visit to any hospital clinic or emergency department (CMS 2006e).

From the implementation of the APC system, hospital clinic or emergency department visits have been classified according to one of three levels of service—low level, midlevel, or high level—based on E/M coding. However, the proposed rule issued by CMS in 2006 for calendar year 2007 used five levels of service for clinic and emergency department visits (CMS 2006f).

Discounted Payment for Multiple Procedures

Although the example in table 5.5 indicates full payment for each APC, there are actually several situations in which the payment could be reduced or discounted. One such situation is when multiple procedures are performed during a single encounter. The APC system recognizes that when several procedures are performed at the same time, certain efficiencies occur that reduce costs. For example, only one operating room is used and the patient is prepared only once.

Use of APC Status Indicators in Discounted Payments

The APC status indicator of the given service determines whether the service will be discounted in such a situation. If the status indicator is "T," multiple-procedure reductions apply. For example, the surgery or procedure with the highest APC rate may be paid at 100 percent, but any other surgical procedures performed may be paid at 50 percent. However, if the status indicator is "S," each procedure is paid at full APC value. In addition to "T" and "S" status indicators, several other status indicators provide information about each APC. (See table 5.6.)

Use of Modifiers in Discounted Payments

Another type of discounting may occur when procedures are terminated or discontinued. A CPT modifier indicates that a procedure was terminated or discontinued. For example, modifier –74 indicates that surgery was terminated after induction of anesthesia had started. Hospital costs are essentially the same when a procedure is discontinued after induction of anesthesia as when the procedure is completed. Therefore, a procedure discontinued after induction of anesthesia is paid at

Table 5.6. Payment Status Indicators for the Hospital Outpatient Prospective Payment System as of 2006

Indicator	Item/Code/Service	Explanation
A	Services furnished to a hospital outpatient that are paid under a fee schedule/payment system other than OPPS, for example: • Ambulance services • Clinical diagnostic laboratory services • Nonimplantable prosthetic and orthotic devices • EPO for ESRD patients • Physical, occupational, and speech therapy • Routine dialysis services for ESRD patients provided in a certified dialysis unit of a hospital • Diagnostic mammography • Screening mammography	Not paid under OPPS. Paid by fiscal intermediaries under a fee schedule/payment system other than OPPS
B	Codes that are not recognized by OPPS when submitted on an outpatient hospital Part B bill type (12x, 13x, and 14x)	Not paid under OPPS • May be paid by intermediaries when submitted on a different bill type (for example, 75x [CORF]), but not paid under OPPS • An alternate code that is recognized by OPPS when submitted on an outpatient hospital Part B bill type (12x, 13x, and 14x) may be available.
C	Inpatient procedures	Not paid under OPPS. Admit patient; bill as inpatient
D	Discontinued codes	Not paid under OPPS
E	Items, codes, and services: • That are not covered by Medicare based on statutory exclusion • That are not covered by Medicare for reasons other than statutory exclusion • That are not recognized by Medicare, but for which an alternate code for the same item or service may be available • For which separate payment is not provided by Medicare	Not paid under OPPS
F	Corneal tissue acquisition; certain CRNA services and Hepatits B Vaccines	Not paid under OPPS; paid at reasonable cost
G	Pass-through drugs and biological	Paid under OPPS; separate APC payment includes pass-through amount
H	(1) Pass-through device categories (2) Brachytherapy sources (3) Radiopharmaceutical agents	(1) Separate cost-based pass-through payment; not subject to coinsurance (2) Separate cost-based non-pass-through payment (3) Separate cost-based non-pass-through payment
K	Non-pass-through drugs and biologicals	Paid under OPPS; separate APC payment
L	Influenza vaccine; Pneumococcal pneumonia vaccine	Not paid under OPPS; paid at reasonable cost; not subject to deductible or coinsurance
M	Items and services not billable to the fiscal intermediary	Not paid under OPPS.
N	Items and services packaged into APC rates	Paid under OPPS. Payment is packaged into payment for other services, including outliers. Therefore, there is no separate APC payment.
P	Partial hospitalization	Paid under OPPS; per diem APC payment
Q	Packaged services subject to separate payment under OPPS payment criteria	Paid under OPPS; Addendum B displays APC assignments when services are separately payable. (1) Separate APC payment based on OPPS payment criteria. (2) If criteria are not met, payment is packaged into payment for other services, including outliers. Therefore, there is no separate APC payment.
S	Significant Procedure, not discounted when multiple	Paid under OPPS; separate APC payment
T	Significant Procedure, multiple-procedure reduction applies	Paid under OPPS; separate APC payment
V	Clinic or emergency department visit	Paid under OPPS; separate APC payment
Y	Nonimplantable durable medical equipment	Not paid under OPPS. All institutional providers other than home health agencies bill to DMERC.
X	Ancillary service	Paid under OPPS; separate APC payment

100 percent of the APC rate. However, if the procedure is terminated after the patient is prepared, but before anesthesia is started, modifier –73 is used and 50 percent of the APC rate is paid.

When for any reason the procedure or service performed is less than that ordinarily indicated by the CPT code, the hospital can indicate this situation by using modifier –52 with the CPT code. The hospital will then receive a discounted payment for the reduced services.

OPPS and APC Payments

The OPPS provides transitional pass-through payments. The purpose of these payments is to cover additional costs of innovative medical devices, drugs, and biologicals. Transitional pass-through payments provide separate payments in addition to APC payments. Payments for a given drug, device, or biological can be made on a pass-through basis for at least 2, but not more than 3, years. CMS Web site explains the process for submitting a new item for consideration for pass-through payments (HCFA 2000b, 18438).

OPPS and Provider-Based Clinics

Another issue in the OPPS is that of provider-based hospital clinics. When a Medicare patient is seen in a provider-based hospital clinic, the clinic receives an APC payment and the physician receives a reduced payment for services. The rationale for the reduction in the payment to the physician is that his or her practice expense has been shifted to the hospital. However, the total of the two payments in this situation is greater than the full-fee schedule payment that a physician in a freestanding clinic would receive. Therefore, CMS is very cautious about awarding provider-based status to a clinic that has not previously held that status.

APC Coding Edits

The outpatient code editor (OCE) operates in the systems of fiscal intermediary (FI) contractors. The OCE provides a series of flags that can affect APC payments because it identifies coding errors in claims. National Correct Coding Initiative (NCCI or CCI) edits also apply to the APC system. The main purpose of CCI edits is to prohibit unbundling of procedures. CCI edits are updated quarterly.

Physicians Fee Schedule and Resource-Based Relative Value Scale

Medicare reimburses physician outpatient services on a different basis from that of hospital outpatient services. As previously explained, hospitals receive APC payments from Medicare for their outpatient services. Physicians, on the other hand, receive fee schedule payments based on a resource-based relative value scale (RBRVS) for their services. Both systems are based on CPT/HCPCS codes.

The physicians fee schedule (PFS) system has been in effect for physicians since 1992. The RBRVS system is used by Medicare to develop fee schedules for Part B payments to physicians. Although RBRVS is the name commonly used for this mechanism, CMS regulations use the term relative value units (RVUs) when describing this methodology. RVUs function in a manner similar to relative weights in the DRG system, with an RVU of 2.00 paying twice as much as an RVU of 1.00.

The components that make up the total RVU for a given procedure are physician work, practice expense, and malpractice expense. The RVUs for each of these three components and the total for each CPT/HCPCS procedure code are listed annually in the *Federal Register.* An oversimplified example of RVUs is provided in table 5.7. (For a complete table, see the annual Medicare physician fee schedule in the *Federal Register.*) To arrive at a fee schedule amount for each procedure, the RVUs are multiplied by a national conversion factor and adjusted by a geographic practice-cost index (GPCI) (Bowman 2005).

Table 5.7.   Examples of relative value units (RVUs)

CPT/ HCPCS Code	Description	Physician Work RVUs	Practice Expense RVUs	Malpractice RVUs	Total RVUs
10040	Acne surgery	1.18	1.01	0.05	2.24
10060	Drainage of skin abscess	1.17	1.21	0.12	2.50
93000	Electrocardiogram, complete	0.17	0.51	0.03	0.71
99201	Office/outpatient visit, new (Level 1)	0.45	0.49	0.03	0.97
99205	Office/outpatient visit, new (Level 5)	2.67	1.78	0.15	4.60

CPT five-digit codes and/or nomenclature are copyrighted by the American Medical Association.

Skilled Nursing Facility Prospective Payment System

Federal data collection in skilled nursing facilities (SNFs) is based on the resident assessment instrument (RAI) process. A key component of this process is the periodic completion of a comprehensive resident assessment. This assessment is included as part of the Minimum Data Set (MDS) form. (See figure 5.2.)

Although the PPS for SNFs was implemented July 1, 1998, the RAI/MDS process has been in effect for all nursing home residents since 1991. If the data abstracted on the MDS indicate that the resident is affected by any of 18 conditions that correlate with the functional well-being of the patient, a resident assessment protocol (RAP) is generated or "triggered." Examples of conditions that can trigger an RAP include:

- Cognitive impairment
- Pressure ulcers
- Delirium
- Feeding tubes
- Falls
- Urinary incontinence
- Use of physical restraints

The RAP summary provides guidelines for further assessment of the patient. RAP concepts are incorporated into the resident's care plan (Hawes et al. 1995).

Identification of diagnoses and ICD-9-CM coding is a part of the MDS process. One section of the MDS form captures diagnoses of diseases relating to the resident's activities of daily living (ADL) status. (See section I in figure 5.2.) Although some diagnoses can be reported using the check boxes in parts one and two of section I, the third part of this section provides space for reporting more detailed diagnoses with ICD-9-CM codes.

The SNF PPS system uses a case-mix adjustment based on the MDS. For each resident, the SNF receives per diem payments that are case-mix adjusted using the resident classification system, or **resource utilization group, version III** (RUG-III). RUGs are based on data from resident assessments (MDS 2.0), and relative weights are developed from staff-time data (King and Gorenflo 2005).

Figure 5.2. Portion of MDS 2.0 form

Resident_____   Numeric Identifier_____

2.	BATHING	How resident takes full-body bath/shower, sponge bath, and transfers in/out of tub/shower (EXCLUDE washing of back and hair.) *Code for most dependent in self-performance and support.* (A) BATHING SELF-PERFORMANCE codes appear below	(A)	(B)
		0. Independent—No help provided		
		1. Supervision—Oversight help only		
		2. Physical help limited to transfer only		
		3. Physical help in part of bathing activity		
		4. Total dependence		
		8. Activity itself did not occur during entire 7 days *(Bathing support codes are as defined in Item 1, code B above)*		

3.	TEST FOR BALANCE (see training manual)	*(Code for ability during test in the last 7 days)* 0. Maintained position as required in test 1. Unsteady, but able to rebalance self without physical support 2. Partial physical support during test; or stands (sits) but does not follow directions for test 3. Not able to attempt test without physical help	
		a. Balance while standing	
		b. Balance while sitting—position, trunk control	

4.	FUNCTIONAL LIMITATION IN RANGE OF MOTION (see training manual)	*(Code for limitations during last 7 days that interfered with daily functions or placed resident at risk of injury)* (A) RANGE OF MOTION (B) VOLUNTARY MOVEMENT 0. No limitation 0. No loss 1. Limitation on one side 1. Partial loss 2. Limitation on both sides 2. Full loss	(A)	(B)
		a. Neck		
		b. Arm—Including shoulder or elbow		
		c. Hand—Including wrist or fingers		
		d. Leg—Including hip or knee		
		e. Foot—Including ankle or toes		
		f. Other limitation or loss		

5.	MODES OF LOCOMOTION	*(Check all that apply during last 7 days)*	
		Cane/walker/crutch a.	Wheelchair primary mode of locomotion d.
		Wheeled self b.	
		Other person wheeled c.	NONE OF ABOVE e.

6.	MODES OF TRANSFER	*(Check all that apply during last 7 days)*	
		Bedfast all or most of time a.	Lifted mechanically d.
		Bed rails used for bed mobility or transfer b.	Transfer aid (e.g., slide board, trapeze, cane, walker, brace) e.
		Lifted manually c.	NONE OF ABOVE f.

7.	TASK SEGMENTATION	Some or all of ADL activities were broken into subtasks during last 7 days so that resident could perform them 0. No 1.Yes	

8.	ADL FUNCTIONAL REHABILITATION POTENTIAL	Resident believes he/she is capable of increased independence in at least some ADLs a.	
		Direct care staff believe resident is capable of increased independence in at least some ADLs b.	
		Resident able to perform tasks/activity but is very slow c.	
		Difference in ADL Self-Performance or ADL Support, comparing mornings to evenings d.	
		NONE OF ABOVE e.	

9.	CHANGE IN ADL FUNCTION	Resident's ADL self-performance status has changed as compared to status of 90 days ago (or since last assessment if less than 90 days) 0. No change 1. Improved 2. Deteriorated	

SECTION H. CONTINENCE IN LAST 14 DAYS

1.	CONTINENCE SELF-CONTROL CATEGORIES *(Code for resident's PERFORMANCE OVER ALL SHIFTS)*
	0. *CONTINENT*—Complete control [includes use of indwelling urinary catheter or ostomy device that does not leak urine or stool]
	1. *USUALLY CONTINENT*—BLADDER, incontinent episodes once a week or less; BOWEL, less than weekly
	2. *OCCASIONALLY INCONTINENT*—BLADDER, 2 or more times a week but not daily; BOWEL, once a week
	3. *FREQUENTLY INCONTINENT*—BLADDER, tended to be incontinent daily, but some control present (e.g., on day shift); BOWEL, 2-3 times a week
	4. *INCONTINENT*—Had inadequate control BLADDER, multiple daily episodes; BOWEL, all (or almost all) of the time

a.	BOWEL CONTINENCE	Control of bowel movement, with appliance or bowel continence programs, if employed	
b.	BLADDER CONTINENCE	Control of urinary bladder function (if dribbles, volume insufficient to soak through underpants), with appliances (e.g., foley) or continence programs, if employed	

2.	BOWEL ELIMINATION PATTERN	Bowel elimination pattern regular—at least one movement every three days a.	Diarrhea c.
		Constipation b.	Fecal impaction d.
			NONE OF ABOVE e.

3.	APPLIANCES AND PROGRAMS	Any scheduled toileting plan a.	Did not use toilet room/ commode/urinal f.
		Bladder retraining program b.	Pads/briefs used g.
		External (condom) catheter c.	Enemas/irrigation h.
		Indwelling catheter d.	Ostomy present i.
		Intermittent catheter e.	NONE OF ABOVE j.

4.	CHANGE IN URINARY CONTINENCE	Resident's urinary continence has changed as compared to status of 90 days ago (or since last assessment if less than 90 days) 0. No change 1.Improved 2. Deteriorated	

SECTION I. DISEASE DIAGNOSES

Check only those diseases that have a relationship to current ADL status, cognitive status, mood and behavior status, medical treatments, nursing monitoring, or risk of death. (Do not list inactive diagnoses)

1.	DISEASES	*(If none apply, CHECK the NONE OF ABOVE box)*			
		ENDOCRINE/METABOLIC/ NUTRITIONAL		Hemiplegia/Hemiparesis	v.
				Multiple sclerosis	w.
		Diabetes mellitus	a.	Paraplegia	x.
		Hyperthyroidism	b.	Parkinson's disease	y.
		Hypothyroidism	c.	Quadriplegia	z.
		HEART/CIRCULATION		Seizure disorder	aa.
		Arteriosclerotic heart disease (ASHD)	d.	Transient ischemic attack (TIA)	bb.
				Traumatic brain injury	cc.
		Cardiac dysrhythmias	e.	**PSYCHIATRIC/MOOD**	
		Congestive heart failure	f.	Anxiety disorder	dd.
		Deep vein thrombosis	g.	Depression	ee.
		Hypertension	h.	Manic depression (bipolar disease)	ff.
		Hypotension	i.		
		Peripheral vascular disease	j.	Schizophrenia	gg.
		Other cardiovascular disease	k.	**PULMONARY**	
		MUSCULOSKELETAL		Asthma	hh.
		Arthritis	l.	Emphysema/COPD	ii.
		Hip fracture	m.	**SENSORY**	
		Missing limb (e.g., amputation)	n.	Cataracts	jj.
		Osteoporosis	o.	Diabetic retinopathy	kk.
		Pathological bone fracture	p.	Glaucoma	ll.
		NEUROLOGICAL		Macular degeneration	mm.
		Alzheimer's disease	q.	**OTHER**	
		Aphasia	r.	Allergies	nn.
		Cerebral palsy	s.	Anemia	oo.
		Cerebrovascular accident (stroke)	t.	Cancer	pp.
				Renal failure	qq.
		Dementia other than Alzheimer's disease	u.	NONE OF ABOVE	rr.

2.	INFECTIONS	*(If none apply, CHECK the NONE OF ABOVE box)*			
		Antibiotic resistant infection (e.g., Methicillin resistant staph)	a.	Septicemia	g.
				Sexually transmitted diseases	h.
		Clostridium difficile (c. diff.)	b.	Tuberculosis	i.
		Conjunctivitis	c.	Urinary tract infection in last 30 days	j.
		HIV infection	d.	Viral hepatitis	k.
		Pneumonia	e.	Wound infection	l.
		Respiratory infection	f.	NONE OF ABOVE	m.

3.	OTHER CURRENT OR MORE DETAILED DIAGNOSES AND ICD-9 CODES	a. _____	·
		b. _____	·
		c. _____	·
		d. _____	·
		e. _____	·

SECTION J. HEALTH CONDITIONS

1.	PROBLEM CONDITIONS	*(Check all problems present in last 7 days unless other time frame is indicated)*			
		INDICATORS OF FLUID STATUS		Dizziness/Vertigo	f.
				Edema	g.
		Weight gain or loss of 3 or more pounds within a 7 day period	a.	Fever	h.
				Hallucinations	i.
				Internal bleeding	j.
		Inability to lie flat due to shortness of breath	b.	Recurrent lung aspirations in last 90 days	k.
		Dehydrated; output exceeds input	c.	Shortness of breath	l.
				Syncope (fainting)	m.
		Insufficient fluid; did NOT consume all/almost all liquids provided during last 3 days	d.	Unsteady gait	n.
				Vomiting	o.
		OTHER		NONE OF ABOVE	p.
		Delusions	e.		

The Home Health PPS

The home health PPS (HH PPS) became the basis for Medicare payments to home healthcare providers on October 1, 2000. The case-mix system used in home health is called home health resources groups (HHRGs). The unit of payment is a 60-day episode, paid in two payments. The amount received by the home healthcare provider is adjusted according to the level of the HHRG for that case.

Data for the HH PPS come from a comprehensive patient assessment in a manner similar to the MDS assessment process for residents of SNFs. The comprehensive assessment used for home health is the outcomes and assessment information set (OASIS), which, in addition to its uses in patient care and quality improvement, captures data needed to group cases to the appropriate HHRG. Of interest to coding professionals are the different types of diagnoses that can be captured on the OASIS form. The primary diagnosis is the condition that represents the chief reason for providing home care. *Other* or *secondary diagnoses* are those that existed at the time the plan of care was developed or that arose later during the home health episode. The *case-mix diagnosis* determines the Medicare PPS case-mix group and ordinarily is found in the primary diagnosis field. However, when a V code is reported in the primary diagnosis field, separate *payment diagnoses* should be submitted in fields designed for this purpose. Two fields are provided for payment diagnoses so that both etiology and manifestation codes may be submitted when necessary. Because V codes are unacceptable as case-mix diagnoses, the OASIS instrument allows data collection to follow standard coding guidelines, using V codes as primary diagnoses when appropriate while providing payment diagnosis fields to capture the data necessary to determine the HHRG (CMS 2002c).

On claims, HHRGs are represented by health insurance prospective payment system (HIPPS) codes. HIPPS codes for HH PPS are five-position alphanumeric codes that represent specific patient characteristics from which Medicare payment determinations are made. The second, third, and fourth characters of an HIPPS code are alpha characters that represent the three domains of the HHRG system—clinical, functional, and service. See table 5.8 for examples of HHRGs, their corresponding HIPPS codes, and the three HHRG domains.

Inpatient Rehabilitation Facility PPS

On August 7, 2001, the final rule describing the inpatient rehabilitation facility PPS (IRF PPS) was published in the *Federal Register.* The IRF PPS uses a patient assessment instrument to classify patients into 1 of 100 different case-mix groups (CMGs). Determination of the CMG for a given case depends on rehabilitation impairment codes (RICs), motor admission score, cognitive admission score, age, and comorbidities. Most of the CMGs will be subject to four weights depending on the patient's comorbidities. ICD-9-CM coding is important under the IRF PPS because ICD-9-CM codes determine the RICs and the comorbidities, both of which influence the CMG payment (CMS 2003b). Figure 5.3 shows the placement of the ICD-9-CM codes on the Inpatient Rehabilitation Facility Patient Assessment Instrument (IRF-PAI), which serves purposes similar to the MDS for long-term care and the OASIS for home health.

Table 5.8. Examples of HHRGs with corresponding HIPPS codes and domain levels

HHRG	HIPPS Code	Clinical Domain	Functional Domain	Service Domain
C0F0S0	HAEJ1	Min	Min	Min
C0F0S1	HAEK1	Min	Min	Low
C0F0S2	HAEL1	Min	Min	Mod

Figure 5.3. Inpatient rehabilitation facility patient assessment instrument

APPENDIX BB Patient_____ Numeric Identifier_____

4.	**BOWEL CONTINENCE** (Code for last 7-14 days)	0. *CONTINENT*— Complete control, does not use ostomy device 1. *CONTINENT WITH OSTOMY*—Complete control with use of an ostomy device that does not leak stool 2. *BI/WEEKLY INCONTINENCE*—Incontinent episodes less than once a week (i.e., once in last 2 weeks) 3. *WEEKLY INCONTINENCE*—Incontinent episodes once a week 4. *OCCASIONALLY INCONTINENT*—2-3 times a week 5. *FREQUENTLY INCONTINENT*—4+ times a week but not all of time 6. *INCONTINENT*—All of time 8. *DID NOT OCCUR*— No bowel movement during the entire 14 day assessment period
5.	**BOWEL APPLIANCES** (Code for last 3 days)	CODE: 0. No 1. Yes a. Bedpan c. Medication for control b. Enema d. Ostomy
6.	**BOWEL APPLIANCE SUPPORT** (Code for last 24 hours)	0. No appliances (**in item F5**) 1. Use of appliances, did not require help or supervision 2. Use of appliances, required supervision or setup 3. Minimal contact assistance (light touch only) 4. Moderate assistance; patient able to do 50% or more of tasks 5. Maximal assistance; patient able to do 25-49% of all sub-tasks 6. Total dependence

4.	**OTHER CURRENT OR MORE DETAILED DIAGNOSES AND ICD-9-CM CODES** (Any new diagnosis at reassessment or discharge is to be recorded here)	A. *CODE ICD-9-CM diagnosis code* B. *CODE:* 1. Other primary diagnosis/diagnoses for current stay (not primary impairment) 2. Diagnosis present, receiving active treatment 3. Diagnosis present, monitored but no active treatment A ICD-9-CM B a. | | | • | | b. | | | • | | c. | | | • | | d. | | | • | | e. | | | • | |
5.	**COMPLICA-TIONS/ COMOR-BIDITIES**	*Code the ICD-9-CM diagnostic code. Refer to manual to code comorbidities.* DIAGNOSIS ICD-9-CM a. | | | • | | b. | | | • | | c. | | | • | | d. | | | • | |

SECTION G. DIAGNOSES

1.	**IMPAIRMENT GROUP**	*Refer to manual for coding of impairment group* | | | • | | |
2.	**OTHER DISEASES**	CODE [Blank] Not present 1. Other primary diagnosis/diagnoses for current stay (not primary impairment) 2. Diagnosis present, receiving active treatment 3. Diagnosis present, monitored but no active treatment [If no disease in list, check G2aq *None of Above* item]

ENDOCRINE
a. Diabetes mellitus (250.00)
b. Hypothyroidism (244.9)

HEART/CIRCULATION
c. Cardiac arrythmias (427.9)
d. Congestive heart failure (428.0)
e. Coronary artery disease (746.85)
f. Deep vein thrombosis (451.1)
g. Hypertension (401.9)
h. Hypotension (458.9)
i. Peripheral vascular disease (arteries) (443.9)
j. Post acute MI (within 30 days) (410.92)
k. Post heart surgery (e.g., valve, CABG) (V45.81)
l. Pulmonary embolism (415.1)
m. Pulmonary failure (518.8)
n. Other cardiovascular disease (429.2)

MUSCULOSKELETAL
o. Fracture - hip (V43.64)
p. Fracture - lower extremity (812.40)
q. Fracture(s) - other (829.0)
r. Osteoarthritis (715.90)
s. Osteoporosis (733.00)
t. Rheumatoid arthritis (714.0)

NEUROLOGICAL
u. Alzheimer's disease (331.0)

v. Aphasia or Apraxia (784.3, 784.69)
w. Cerebral palsy (343.9)
x. Dementia other than Alzheimer's disease (290.0)
y. Hemiplegia/hemiparesis — left side (342.90)
z. Hemiplegia/hemiparesis — right side (342.90)
aa. Multiple sclerosis (340)
ab. Parkinson's disease (332.0)
ac. Quadriplegia (344.00 - 344.09)
ad. Seizure disorder (780.39)
ae. Spinal cord dysfunction— non-traumatic (336.9)
af. Spinal cord dysfunction— traumatic (952.9)
ag. Stroke (CVA) (436)

PSYCHIATRIC/MOOD
ah. Anxiety disorder (300.00)
ai. Depression (311)
aj. Other psychiatric disorder (300.9)

PULMONARY
ak. Asthma (493.9)
al. COPD (496)
am. Emphysema (492.8)

OTHER
an. Cancer (199.1)
ao. Post surgery - non-orthopedic, non-cardiac (V50.9)
ap. Renal failure (586)
aq. *NONE OF ABOVE*

3.	**INFECTIONS**	CODE: [Blank] Not present 1. Other primary diagnosis/diagnoses for current stay (not primary impairment) 2. Diagnosis present, receiving active treatment 3. Diagnosis present, monitored but no active treatment (If no infections, check *NONE OF ABOVE* item G3l)

a. Antibiotic resistant infection (e.g., methicillin resistant staph - (041.11), VRE - (041.9))
b. Cellulitis (682.9)
c. Hepatitis (070.9)
d. HIV/AIDS (042)
e. Pneumonia (486)
f. Osteomyelitis (730.2)
g. Septicemia (038.9)
h. Staphylococcus infection (other than item "G3a") (041.10)
i. Tuberculosis (active) (011.90)
j. Urinary tract infection (599.0)
k. Wound infection (958.3, 998.59,136.9)
l. *NONE OF ABOVE*

SECTION H. MEDICAL COMPLEXITIES

1.	**VITAL SIGNS**	*Vital signs (pulse, BP, respiratory rate, temperature)* **Score for the most abnormal vital sign** 0. All vital signs were normal/standard (i.e., when compared to standard values) 1. Vital signs abnormal, but not on all days during assessment period 2. Vital signs consistently abnormal (on all days)
2.	**PROBLEM CONDITIONS** (In last 3 days)	(CHECK all problems present in the **last 3 days** unless otherwise noted)

FALLS/BALANCE
a. Dizziness/vertigo/light-headedness
b. Fell (since admission or last assessment)
c. Fell in **180 days** prior to admission

CARDIAC/PULMONARY
d. Advanced cardiac failure (ejection fraction < 25%)
e. Chest pain/pressure on exertion
f. Chest pain/pressure at rest
g. Edema - generalized
h. Edema - localized
i. Edema - pitting

j. Impaired aerobic capacity/endurance (tires easily, poor task endurance)

FLUID STATUS
k. Constipation
l. Dehydrated; output exceeds input; or BUN/Creat ratio > 25
m. Diarrhea
n. Internal bleeding
o. Recurrent nausea/vomiting
p. Refusal/inability to take liquids orally

OTHER
q. Delusions/hallucinations
r. Fever
s. Hemi-neglect (inattention to one side)
t. Cachexia (severe malnutrition)
u. Morbid obesity
v. End-stage disease, life expectancy of **6 or fewer months**
w. *NONE OF ABOVE*

3.	**RESPIRATORY CONDITIONS** (In last 3 days)	(CHECK all problems present in the **last 3 days**)

a. Inability to lie flat due to shortness of breath
b. Shortness of breath with exertion (e.g., taking a bath)
c. Shortness of breath at rest
d. Oxygen saturation < 90%

e. Difficulty coughing and clearing airway secretions
f. Recurrent aspiration
g. Recurrent respiratory infection
h. *NONE OF ABOVE*

4.	**PRESSURE ULCERS** (Code for last 24 hours)	a. *Highest current pressure ulcer stage* 0. No pressure ulcer (**if no, skip to H5**) 1. Any area of persistent skin redness (**Stage 1**) 2. Partial loss of skin layers (**Stage 2**) 3. Deep craters in the skin (**Stage 3**) 4. Breaks in skin exposing muscle or bone (**Stage 4**) 5. Not stageable (necrotic eschar predominant; no prior staging available) b. *Number of current pressure ulcers* SELECT THE CURRENT LARGEST PRESSURE ULCER TO CODE THE FOLLOWING—calculate three components (c through e) and code total score in f c. Length multiplied by width (open wound surface area) 0. 0.0 cm² 4. 1.1–2.0 cm² 8. 8.1–12.0 cm² 1. <0.3 cm² 5. 2.1–3.0 cm² 9. 12.1–24.0 cm² 2. 0.3–0.6 cm² 6. 3.1–4.0 cm² 10. > 24 cm² 3. 0.7–1.0 cm² 7. 4.1–8.0 cm² d. Exudate amount 0. None 1. Light 2. Moderate 3. Heavy

Two kinds of coding are required for the IRF PPS. The IRF-PAI requires the coding of the "etiologic" diagnosis, which is the original diagnosis from the acute admission that led to the rehabilitation referral (for example, cerebrovascular accident). The etiologic diagnosis determines the RIC, which is a factor in determining the CMG. On the other hand, the UB-92/UB-04 follows standard inpatient coding guidelines for principal and additional diagnoses. For the UB-92/UB-04, the principal diagnosis (the reason for admission) for the rehabilitation facility is usually a V code (Grzybowski and Draper 2002).

Long-Term Care Hospital PPS

Medicare implemented a PPS for long-term care hospitals (LTCHs) on October 1, 2002. LTCHs are acute care hospitals having an average inpatient length of stay of more than 25 days. The inpatient PPS developed for short-term acute care hospitals does not apply to LTCHs (CMS 2005). The long-term care hospital PPS (LTC-PPS) is based on DRGs; however, the long-term care diagnosis-related groups (LTC-DRGs) are not the same as Medicare's inpatient DRGs. The numbers and titles of the LTC-DRGs are the same as those of inpatient DRGs, but the relative weights and the associated lengths of stay are different to reflect the resources that are required to treat the medically complex patients who are seen in LTCHs. Like inpatient DRGs, LTC-DRGs are based on the patient's principal diagnosis, additional diagnoses, procedures performed during the stay, age, sex, and discharge status and serve as the basis of a per case payment to the facility (CMS 2002b). In a manner similar to the inpatient PPS, relative weights for the LTC-DRGs reflect resource utilization for each LTC-DRG and determine the payment that the LTCH receives for each Medicare patient discharged. The relative weight is multiplied times a standard rate to determine the payment amount (CMS n.d.). See Table 5.9 for examples of LTC-DRGs.

Inpatient Psychiatric Facility PPS

CMS first published a proposed rule for creation of an inpatient psychiatric facility prospective payment system (IPF PPS) in 2003. After a lengthy comment period, the final rule became effective on January 1, 2005 (CMS 2004b). For claims with a psychiatric principal diagnosis (Chapter Five of ICD-9-CM), the IPF PPS uses a standard per diem payment that is adjusted higher or lower by patient and other factors, some of which are based on ICD-9-CM codes assigned. For example, one of the adjustment factors is based on the DRG assigned as listed in table 5.10. Only those claims that group to one of these 15 DRGs will receive this DRG payment adjustment. For DRGs not included in this list, the IPF will still receive the federal

Table 5.9.　Examples of LTC-DRGs and their relative weights and average lengths of stay (FY 2007)

LTC-DRG	DRG Description	Relative Weight	Geometric ALOS	5/6ths Geometric ALOS
1	CRANIOTOMY AGE >17 W CC	1.6835	37.1	30.9
2	CRANIOTOMY AGE >17 W/O CC	1.6835	37.1	30.9
3	CRANIOTOMY AGE 0–17	1.6835	37.1	30.9

Source: CMS 2005.

Table 5.10. DRG adjustments in the inpatient psychiatric facility prospective payment system (IPF-PPS)

DRG	DRG Definition	Adjustment Factor
DRG 424	OR Procedure with Principal Diagnosis of Mental Illness	1.22
DRG 425	Acute Adjustment Reaction & Psychosocial Dysfunction	1.05
DRG 426	Depressive Neurosis	0.99
DRG 427	Neurosis, Except Depressive	1.02
DRG 428	Disorders of Personality & Impulse Control	1.02
DRG 429	Organic Disturbances & Mental Retardation	1.03
DRG 430	Psychoses	1.00
DRG 431	Childhood Mental Disorders	0.99
DRG 432	Other Mental Disorder Diagnoses	0.92
DRG 433	Alcohol/Drug Abuse or Dependence, Leave Against Medical Advice (LAMA)	0.97
DRG 521	Alcohol/Drug Abuse or Dependence with Comorbid Conditions	1.02
DRG 522	Alcohol/Drug Abuse or Dependence with Rehabilitation Therapy without Comorbid Conditions	0.98
DRG 523	Alcohol/Drug Abuse or Dependence without Rehabilitation Therapy without Comorbid Conditions	0.88
DRG 12	Degenerative Nervous System Disorders	1.05
DRG 23	Nontraumatic Stupor & Coma	1.07

Source: CMS 2006c.

per diem base rate and other applicable adjustments. For example, there are adjustments for certain comorbidities, listed in table 5.11. "These categories include ICD-9-CM diagnosis codes for medical and psychiatric conditions that the Centers for Medicare and Medicaid Services (CMS) believe require comparatively more costly treatment during an IPF stay than other comorbid conditions. IPFs may only receive one adjustment factor for each comorbidity category. However, if a patient has multiple diagnoses in several categories, the adjustment factors for each applicable category are multipled by the federal per diem base rate. The comorbidity adjustments are applied to each day of the stay" (AHIMA Policy and Government Relations 2004, p. 2). There is also an adjustment factor for electroconvulsive therapy, which is reported with an ICD-9-CM procedure code (CMS 2006c). An adjustment is made for each ECT treatment provided during hospitalization, because CMS has determined that ECT increases the costliness of the stay. "In order for an IPF to receive this payment adjustment, it must indicate the revenue and procedure codes for ECT and the number of units of ECT (the number of ECT treatments the patient received during the IPF stay)" (AHIMA Policy and Government Relations 2004). Accurate and complete ICD-9-CM coding is necessary for appropriate payment under the IPF PPS.

Table 5.11.   Comorbidity adjustments in the IPF PPS

Comorbidity	Adjustment Factor
Developmental Disabilities	1.04
Coagulation Factor Deficit	1.13
Tracheostomy	1.06
Eating and Conduct Disorders	1.12
Infectious Diseases	1.07
Renal Failure, Acute	1.11
Renal Failure, Chronic	1.11
Oncology Treatment	1.07
Uncontrolled Diabetes Mellitus with or without Complications	1.05
Severe Protein Calorie Malnutrition	1.13
Drug/Alcohol Induced Mental Disorders	1.03
Cardiac Conditions	1.11
Gangrene	1.10
Chronic Obstructive Pulmonary Disease	1.12
Artificial Openings – Digestive & Urinary	1.08
Severe Musculoskeletal & Connective Tissue Diseases	1.09
Poisoning	1.11

Source. CMS 2006c.

Conclusion

Coded data play an important role in many risk-adjustment systems and in the payment systems that use them. Medicare uses various risk-adjustment systems in its PPSs for hospital inpatient and outpatient, skilled nursing, home health, and inpatient rehabilitation settings. Coders should be aware of the coding issues that affect payment in these settings as well as in physician reimbursement and managed care organizations.

References and Resources

AHIMA Policy and Government Relations. 2004. Summary of final rule for Medicare prospective payment system for inpatient psychiatric facilities. Available online from http://www.ahima.org/dc/Analysis_IPF_PPS_reg.asp.

American Hospital Association and American Health Information Management Association. 2003 (June 24). Recommendation for Standardized Hospital Evaluation and Management Coding of Emergency Department and Clinic Services. Available online from ahima.org.

Bowman, E.D. 2001. Coding and classification systems. In *Health Information: Management of a Strategic Resource,* 2nd ed. Edited by M. Abdelhak et al. Philadelphia: W.B. Saunders Company.

Bowman, E.D. 2005. Freestanding ambulatory care. In *Comparative Health Information Management,* 2nd ed. Edited by A. Peden. Clifton Park, NY: Thomson Delmar Learning.

Centers for Medicare and Medicaid Services. 2002a. Case-mix prospective payment for SNFs: Balanced Budget Act of 1997. Available online from http://www.cms.hhs.gov/providers/snfpps/snfpps_overview.asp.

Centers for Medicare and Medicaid Services. 2002b. Long-term care hospital PPS. Available online from http://cms.hhs.gov/providers/longterm/background.asp.

Centers for Medicare and Medicaid Services. 2002c. OASIS in detail. Chapter 8 in *Outcome and Assessment Information Set Implementation Manual: Implementing OASIS at a Home Health Agency to Improve Outcomes, Revised.* Available online from http://www.cms.hhs.gov/oasis/usermanu.asp.

Centers for Medicare and Medicaid Services. 2003a (Aug. 1). Medicare program: Changes to the hospital inpatient prospective payment systems and fiscal year 2004 rates; Final rule. *Federal Register,* 68(148):45345–672.

Centers for Medicare and Medicaid Services. 2003. *Medicare Inpatient Rehabilitation Facility Prospective Payment System Training Manual.* Available online from http://cms.hhs.gov/medlearn/inpatref.asp.

Centers for Medicare and Medicaid Services. 2004a. *45 Day Notice for 2004 M+C Rates.* Available online from http://www.cms.hhs.gov/healthplans/rates/2004/45day-section-a.asp.

Centers for Medicare and Medicaid Services. 2004b (Nov. 15). Medicare Program; Prospective Payment System for Inpatient Psychiatric Facilities. *Federal Register* 69(219):66922–67015.Available online from http://www.cms.hhs.gov/quarterlyproviderupdates/downloads/cms1213f.pdf.

Centers for Medicare and Medicaid Services. 2005 (Dec. 14). Elements of LTCHPPS. Available online from http://www.cms.hhs.gov/LongTermCareHospitalPPS/02_elements_ltch.asp.

Centers for Medicare and Medicaid Services. 2006a. Announcement of Calendar Year (CY) 2007 Medicare Advantage Capitation Rates and Medicare Advantage and Part D Payment Policies. Available online from http://www.cms.hhs.gov/MedicareAdvtgSpecRateStats/Downloads/Announcement2007.pdf.

Centers for Medicare and Medicaid Services. 2006b. Medicare Program; Proposed Changes to the Hospital Inpatient Prospective Payment Systems and Fiscal Year 2007 Rates, Available online from http://www.cms.hhs.gov/AcuteInpatientPPS/downloads/cms1488p.pdf.

Centers for Medicare & Medicaid Services. 2006c. Medicare Program; Inpatient Psychiatric Facilities Prospective Payment System Payment Update for Rate Year Beginning July 1, 2006 (RY 2007). Available online from http://www.cms.hhs.gov/InpatientPsychFacilPPS/Downloads/CMS-1306-F_5-01-06.pdf.

Centers for Medicare & Medicaid Services. 2006d. Medicare Program; Changes to the Hospital Inpatient Prospective Payment Systems and Fiscal Year 2007 Rates. Available online from http://www.cms.hhs.gov/AcuteInpatientPPS/downloads/cms1488f.pdf.

Centers for Medicare & Medicaid Services. 2006e. Draft Visit Guidelines for Hospital Outpatient Care. Available online from http://www.cms.hhs.gov/HospitalOutpatientPPS/Downloads/CMS1506P_Draft_AHA_AHIMA_Guidelines.pdf.

Centers for Medicare & Medicaid Services. 2006f. Proposed Changes to the Hospital Outpatient PPS and CY 2007 Rates; Proposed CY 2007 Update to the ASC Covered Procedures List; and Proposed Changes to the ASC Payment System and CY 2008 Payment Rates. Available online from http://www.cms.hhs.gov/HospitalOutpatientPPS/Downloads/CMS1506P.pdf.

Forthman, M. T., H. G. Dove, and L. D. Wooster. 2000. Episode treatment groups (ETGs): a patient classification system for measuring outcomes performance by episode of illness. *Topics in Health Information Management* 21(2): 51–61.

Grzybowski, D., and S. Draper. 2002. Here comes rehab PPS! Journal of the *American Health Information Management Association* 73(1): 54–55.

Hawes, C., et al. 1995. Reliability estimates for the Minimum Data Set for nursing home resident assessment and care screening (MDS). *The Gerontologist* 35(2): 172–78. Available online from http://www.rti.org/publications/RAI_gerontologist.cfm.

Health Care Financing Administration. 2000a (June 29). Medicare+Choice program: final rule with comment period. *Federal Register* 65(126):40170–332.

Health Care Financing Administration. 2000b (April 7). Hospital outpatient services: prospective payment system. 42 CFR Parts 409. *Federal Register* 65(68): 18433–18820. Available online from http://www.access.gpo.gov/su_docs/fedreg/a000407c.html.

Holbrook, J., et al. 2001. APC coding for facility levels. Available online from http://www.hospitalconnect.com/aha/key_issues/opps/resources/APPCoding700.html.

Iezzoni, L.I. 2003. *Risk Adjustment for Measuring Health Care Outcomes.* Chicago: Health Administration Press.

International Severity Information Systems, Inc. 2001. Description of the CSI software system. *Comprehensive Severity Index.* Available online from http://www.isisicor.com.

Kautter, J., G. Pope, and E. Olmstead. 2005. Refinements to the CMS-HCC Model for Risk Adjustment of Medicare Capitation Payments Available online from http://www.academyhealth.org/2005/ppt/kautterj.ppt.

King, K., and B.A. Gorenflo. 2005. Long-term care. In *Comparative Health Information Management,* 2nd ed. Edited by A. Peden. Clifton Park, NY: Thomson Delmar Learning.

Leary, R., and D'Amato, C. 2005. DRG Changes for FY 2006. *Journal of American Health Information Management Association* 76(10):66–68.

MEDSTAT. 2005. Risk adjustment: Severity stages. *Disease Staging.* Ann Arbor, MI: Thomson MEDSTAT.

3M Health Information Systems. n.d. 3M APR DRG classification system and the state of Maryland. Available online from http://www.3m.com/us/healthcare/his/products/performance/apr_drg_maryland.jhtml.

Tully, L., and V. Rulon. 2000. Evolution of the uses of ICD-9-CM coding: Medicare risk adjustment methodology for managed care plans. *Topics in Health Information Management* 21(2):62–67.

Chapter 6

The Charge Description Master

Erica M. Leeds, MIS, RHIA, CCS, CCS-P

The **charge description master (CDM)** is known by various names, including:

- Chargemaster
- Charge compendium
- Service master
- Price compendium
- Service item master
- Charge list

Basically, the CDM is a translation table that puts the appropriate codes on the UB-92/UB-04 claim form or the X12N 837 Institutional Claims (837I) transaction, the electronic version of the UB-92/UB-04 billing form, used to categorize services and supplies for accounting purposes. The following statement explains the importance of the CDM for reimbursement:

> The various supplies and services listed on the chargemaster for the average facility drives reimbursement for approximately 73 percent of the UB-92/UB04 claims for outpatient services alone.... A current and accurate chargemaster is vital to any healthcare provider seeking proper reimbursement. Without it, the facility would not receive proper reimbursement. Among the negative impacts that may result from an inaccurate chargemaster are:
>
> - Overpayment
> - Underpayment
> - Undercharging for services
> - Claims rejections
> - Fines
> - Penalties
>
> Because a chargemaster is an automated process that results in billing numerous services for a high volume of patients—often without human intervention—there is a high risk that a single coding or mapping error could spawn error after error before it is identified and corrected (AHIMA 1999).

This chapter explains the purposes and elements of the CDM and describes how service or supply items on the CDM are transferred to claim forms for payment. It also explains how specific codes are attached to the CDM. Finally, the process of adding or deleting items from the CDM is discussed.

Purposes and Elements of the Charge Description Master

The CDM is a list of supplies and services with corresponding charges for each of those items. Usually, items are grouped together by the departments and nursing units of the healthcare facility. The patient accounting department and each of the other departments generally maintain those items that apply to charges they have generated. In some institutions, the HIM department assists with assigning the correct CPT/HCPCS codes to items on the CDM.

Purposes of the CDM

The principal purpose of the CDM is to allow the healthcare facility to efficiently charge routine services and supplies to the patient's bill. In addition, the CDM provides:

- Departmental workload statistics

- CPT/HCPCS codes for repetitive high-volume services and supplies

- Methods to group services

Department Workload Statistics

Department managers frequently use the CDM as a tool to accumulate workload statistics and to track resources. Workload statistics can assist managers with the tasks of monitoring productivity and forecasting budgets. The statistics can provide data regarding resources used, such as equipment, personnel, services, and supplies.

Soft Coding of CPT/HCPCS Codes

When a HIM coder reviews medical documentation and provides a CPT/HCPCS code to billing, this is referred to as **"soft coding."** These types of encounters require a skilled coder to analyze and justify the highest level of specificity from the documentation provided by healthcare providers. Depending on the size of your facility, most CPT/HCPCS codes can either be soft-coded by HIM or hard coded in the CDM. Most facilities have a blend of both.

For example, removal of a lesion requires the coder to identify the location of the lesion, the diameter, the type of closure, and apply the coding guidelines. Although all the codes for removal of a lesion could be hard-coded in the CDM, there is no guarantee the medical staff choosing the codes would be educated on all the elements required to choose the correct code(s). Most facilities would send these types of encounters to HIM for soft coding.

Hard Coding of CPT/HCPCS Codes

The CDM relieves the HIM department of repetitive coding that does not require documentation analysis. For frequently performed procedures, CPT/HCPCS codes may be hard-coded into the CDM to be included automatically on the UB-92/UB-04 billing form or its electronic equivalent, the 837I transaction. **Hard coding** is the process of attaching a HCPCS code to a procedure so that the code will be included automatically on the patient's bill. For example, a complete blood count is one of the tests most frequently performed by healthcare laboratories. Hard coding ensures that the code is reproduced accurately each time that test is ordered. Other areas of the healthcare facility that have tests or services hard-coded into the CDM include:

- Radiology

- Electrocardiogram and other cardiology services

- Electroencephalogram

- Respiratory therapy and pulmonary function

- Rehabilitation services (including physical therapy, occupational therapy, audiology, and speech therapy)

- Emergency department

Radiology services, cardiac catheterizations, and endoscopic procedures may be either hard-coded into the CDM or manually coded by HIM department staff. This is a joint decision that must be made by the HIM staff and the patient accounting departments based on the quality, workload, and productivity of the facility's outpatient coders. In some instances, it may be appropriate to have technicians in various areas assist with coding at the point of service. For example, radiology special procedure technicians have in-depth knowledge regarding interventional radiology procedures and the accompanying injection procedures.

Grouped Items on the CDM

The CDM also can provide a method for grouping items that are frequently reported together. Items that must be reported separately but that are used together, such as interventional radiology imaging and injection procedures, are called **exploding charges.** When grouped together, those items will be included on the bill automatically. This happens because the CDM uses a **pointer**— an item that has no dollar value and no code attached and that is mapped to two or more items with separate charges. When the pointer is charged, all of the grouped charges are added to the bill.

Each software program uses different terminology. Other names for pointers and exploding charges are **drivers and passengers** and **parents and children.** In the former, the driver is the item that explodes into other items; in the latter, the parent is the item that explodes into other items.

In the following example, codes 76932 and 93505 are added to the bill automatically when the charge for an ultrasonic endomyocardial biopsy is entered into the CDM:

Pointer   **Ultrasonic endomyocardial biopsy**
  Driver
  Parent

    Exploding charge 1   76932 Ultrasonic guidance for endomyocardial biopsy
      Passenger
      Child

    Exploding charge 2   93505 Endomyocardial biopsy
      Passenger
      Child

Elements of the CDM

Each service or supply item on the CDM has the following seven elements, as shown in figure 6.1:

- Charge code
- Item description
- General ledger (G/L) key
- Revenue code
- Insurance code mapping (Code A, Code B, Code C, Code D)
- Charges
- Activity date

Charge Code

The **charge code** is the numerical identification of the service or supply. Each item has a unique number with a prefix that indicates the department or revenue center in which the service or supply is provided. The charge code links the item to a particular department for revenue tracking, budget analysis, and cost-accounting reasons. Charge codes are issued in numerical order per department or nursing unit. As activity is posted to the item, the service and finance departments accumulate data on services and supplies on a monthly, quarterly, and annual basis. As a general rule, if an item has had no activity within the recent fiscal year, it should be considered for deletion or inactivation.

Item Description

The **item description** is the actual name of the service or supply. Because space is limited on the CDM, only a certain number of characters can be used to describe each item. The department or nursing unit chooses the item description. When describing a service or supply, the department or nursing unit should remember that this description appears on the patient's detailed bill. Within the constraints of space, the item description should be as clear as possible so that the patient can understand what the charge represents. When linked to a CPT code, the item description should match the CPT code descriptor as closely as possible.

General Ledger Key

The **general ledger (G/L) key** is the two- or three-digit number that assigns each item to a particular section of the general ledger in the healthcare facility's accounting section. Each time the item is chosen, it is tracked into the accounting system. Financial reporting on departmental activities is then possible at the end of each month, quarter, or year.

Revenue Code

The **revenue code** is the four-digit number used for Medicare billing. It totals all items and their charges for printing on the UB-92/UB-04 (or entering into the 837I). A complete list of revenue codes appears in appendix 6.1 (pp. 172–180). Medicare regulations require that items billed to the federal program be identified with a revenue code and, in some instances, with a

Figure 6.1.   Sample CDM

Charge Code	Item Description	CPT/HCPCS Code				G/L Key	Activity Date
		INS Code A	Rev Code A	INS Code B	Rev Code B		
52526944	FILGRASTIM INJ 300MCG/1ML (IV)		250	J1440	636	3	8/1/2006
52511730	CALCITONIN INJ 400UNITS/2ML		250	J0630	636	3	7/26/2006
52528239	CYTOMEGALOVIRUS IMM GLOB 2.5GM		250	J0850	636	3	6/25/2006
54600663	EXERCISE OXIMETRY EVALUATION	94761	460	94761	460	3	5/24/2006
54600325	FLUTTER VALVE TRAINING SEC CLR	94667	460	94667	460	3	4/25/2006
56208903	BENTSON GUIDWIRE 035/145		272	C1769	621	2	7/3/2006
56208846	ROSEN GUIDWIRE 035/145/1.5		272	C1769	621	2	8/14/2009
54001284	ECHO ENCEPHALOGRAM	76506	402	76506	402	3	7/21/2006
53200168	SINUSES; PARANASAL, COMPLT	70220	320	70220	320	3	7/13/2006
53002010	BILIRUBIN TOTAL	82247	301	82247	301	3	8/8/2006
53002127	CALCIUM TOTAL	82310	301	82310	301	3	7/15/2006
57100117	RECOVERY PHASE .5 HR		710		710	3	3/12/2006
56221609	WALLSTENT ILIAC 12MM/90MM		272	C1876	278	2	7/8/2006
53700035	MODERATE SEDN >5YRS 1ST 30MIN	99144	371	99144	371	3	6/15/2006
59200071	US; DUPLEX, ABDM/PELVC, LMTD	93976	921	93976	921	3	5/16/2006
52502341	VARICELLA VACCINE INJ 0.5ML		250	90716	636	3	8/1/2006
52502390	PNEUMOCOCCAL VACCINE 0.5ML		250	90732	636	3	7/26/2006
52502549	TOPOTECAN INJ 4MG		250	J9350	636	3	6/25/2006
52502556	ARGATROBAN INJ 250MG/2.5ML IV		250	C9121	636	3	5/24/2006
53101549	MORPH ANALY TUMOR IMMUNO QN	88360	310	88360	310	3	4/25/2006
53100004	INSHU LYBRID EACH PROBE	88365	310	88365	310	3	7/3/2006
53101143	EM DIAGNOSTIC	88348	312	88348	312	3	8/14/2009
53101150	MORPHOMETRIC ANALY SKEL MUSCLE	88355	312	88355	312	3	7/21/2006
53101168	MORPHOMETRIC ANALY TUMOR	88358	312	88358	312	3	7/13/2006
53101176	TISSUE IN SITU HYBRIDIZATION	88365	312	88365	312	3	8/8/2006
53600540	INJ WRIST ARTHROGRAM-SUR	25246	360	25246	360	3	7/15/2006
53600557	INJ WRIST ARTHROGRAM-SUR-BL	25246–50	360	25246–50	360	3	3/12/2006
54100144	MDI TREATMENT, INITIAL	94640	410	94640	410	3	7/8/2006
54100128	CONTINUOUS SPAG	94640	410	94640	410	3	6/15/2006
54100060	IPPB TX SUBSEQUENT	94640	410	94640	410	3	5/16/2006
54100037	IPPB THERAPY, INITIAL	94640	410	94640	410	3	8/1/2006
54100011	PENTAMADINE AEROSOL TX	94640	410	94640	410	3	7/26/2006
54100540	PR STRNGT/ENDURANCE PER 15 MIN	97535	410	G0237	410	3	6/25/2006
54100243	PULM REHAB 1 ON 1 PER 15 MIN	97110	410	G0238	410	3	5/24/2006
54100250	PULM REHAB THERAP PROC GRP	97150	410	G0239	410	3	4/25/2006
54100458	PR BREATHING RETRAINING	97535	419	G0237	419	3	7/3/2006
55400139	ALS AMBULANCE; GROUND PER MILE	A0425	540	A0425	540	3	8/14/2009
55400014	BLS AMBULANCE; GROUND PER MILE	A0425	540	A0425	540	3	7/21/2006
57400186	SIMP/COMP PL GEN W/O REPROGRAM	95970	740	95970	740	3	7/13/2006
57400194	SIMP PL GEN W/REPROGRAM	95971	740	95971	740	3	8/8/2006
57400202	CX BRAIN PL GEN W/RPG 1ST HR	95978	740	95978	740	3	7/15/2006
58000068	HEMOPERFUSION	90997	801	90997	801	3	3/12/2006
58200015	INCENTER DIALYSIS-PED OP <12KG	90999	821	90999	821	3	7/8/2006
58200023	INCENTER DIALYSIS-PED OP >24KG	90999	821	90999	821	3	6/15/2006
58200031	INCENTER DIALYSIS-PED OP 12–24	90999	821	90999	821	3	5/16/2006
58500000	HOME CCPD DAILY CHARGE-PED	90947	851	90947	851	3	8/1/2006
59201780	ELECTRONIC ANALY OF CI 1ST HR	95974	920	95974	920	3	7/26/2006
59201772	ELECTRONIC ANALY CI ADDL 30 MIN	95975	920	95975	920	3	6/25/2006

specific CPT/HCPCS code. For all outpatient claims, every line item must contain a date or dates of service for each revenue code or it will be rejected. (See appendix 6.2 [pp. 181–183] for revenue codes identified with specific CPT/HCPCS codes.)

The revenue code also tracks Medicare costs by revenue centers for the Medicare cost report. In most healthcare facilities, the entire billing process is electronic and an actual hard copy of the bill is not issued. The electronic 837I transaction should contain the same information that a hard copy of the UB-92/UB-04 billing form contains.

Insurance Code Mapping

Insurance code mapping allows a healthcare facility to hold more than one CPT/HCPCS code per CDM item. As many as five columns may be available for mapping specific codes to one item. Typically, CPT codes are listed in the first column because most payers accept one CPT/HCPCS code. However, some state Medicaid programs—such as those in Michigan, New York, Ohio, Pennsylvania, and California—use different HCPCS codes than Medicare does. In those states, healthcare facilities might have one column for Medicare, a second column for Medicaid, and a third column for certain Blue Cross/Blue Shield programs, if the state requires multiple codes for the same item on the CDM.

Code selection is based on the patient's financial class, which is verified when the patient presents for admission or an encounter for outpatient services. The Health Insurance Portability and Accountability Act (HIPAA) requirements are expected to standardize coded transactions so that coding by financial class of the patient will no longer be required.

Charges

Charges represent the dollar amounts owed by patients to the healthcare facility for specific services or supplies. The charges are set by the facility based on either fee schedules, contractual arrangements with healthcare plans, or the organization's cost-accounting system. Each budget year, charges are adjusted based on available information. Each facility determines the method of increasing its charges—a flat dollar amount increase, a percentage across-the-board increase, or an increase based on contracts.

Typically, each item has only one charge. However, the charge is adjusted based on contractual arrangements with certain payers or groups of payers.

Activity Date/Status

The **activity date/status** element indicates the most recent activity of an item. This may be coded or given a date of activity. Different accounting systems use the activity date to denote a variety of activities. It can indicate whether an item is active. Many accounting systems never delete items; they just inactivate them.

The activity date also can indicate whether an item has had any charges made or whether there has been any activity in the current fiscal year. For budgetary reasons, if an item has had activity during the current fiscal year, it is better to "turn it off" (deactivate it) rather than delete it. The activity then can be reactivated and used in the budget and workload indicator process.

Type of Coding Required for the CDM

For Medicare reporting, Levels I and II of HCPCS codes are used on the CDM. (See chapter 4 for discussion of the three levels of CPT codes and how HIPAA has eliminated the use of

Level III.) The CDM should have the capability to hold more than one CPT/HCPCS code per item. It is possible that the same item may appear in more than one department on the CDM. For example, the code for venipuncture may appear in the laboratory, clinic, and emergency department sections of the CDM.

Transitioning of Items from the CDM to Charges on the Claim Form

The completion of a UB-92/UB-04 claim form (or 837I transaction) begins with the registration process for an inpatient admission or an outpatient encounter. At the time of registration, the patient provides basic demographic information as well as insurance information. At or before the time of admission, the insurance information is verified and an insurance code is assigned. This code indicates how the items charged to the patient during the stay will be categorized.

Posting Charges to the Patient's Account

As services and supplies are used for the patient, charges are posted to the patient's account by CDM item number, using a variety of methods. In an electronic system, when the item number is entered into the order-entry software, several actions take place. The department involved with the service or supply receives notification that an order has been placed. At the same time, the accounting system is notified that a particular order has been placed. With order-entry software, electronic charges are posted to the account as soon as the item is ordered. Tests are added to the account at the time service is provided or at the time of order. Charges may be grouped together (batched) and transferred from the order-entry system to the accounting system at a designated time, such as midnight, to capture the correct date the service or supply was ordered or provided.

If the facility does not have order-entry software, the charges may be posted by hand each night at midnight. Departments complete manual "charge tickets" for each patient seen during the course of the day. At the end of the business day, the charge tickets are forwarded for data entry into the accounting system.

For outpatient services and supplies, charges are posted at the time of the order. The coding manager must make sure that posted items were actually provided and that items actually provided are posted to the correct account.

Preparing the Preliminary Bill

When a patient is discharged, the accounting system is notified of the patient's discharge status and the preliminary bill is prepared. The actual process of submitting a claim to the payer may be delayed for the bill hold period of 3 to 5 days for inpatients; 7 to 10 days for outpatients. The **bill hold period** is the time that a bill is suspended in the billing system awaiting late charges, diagnosis/procedure codes, insurance verification, and so on.

Under the ambulatory payment classification (APC) system, Medicare does not accept separate bills for late charges. As a result, many healthcare facilities experience a rise in outpatient accounts receivable balances because late charges must be processed with the rest of the patient's bill or an adjusted claim must be filed. Those actions delay payment and create extra work.

Inpatient Bills

No CPT/HCPCS codes are required by Medicare on bills for inpatients. Charges are accumulated and posted on the UB-92/UB-04 (837I) by revenue codes only. For inpatients, separate charges for certain departments do not have to be reported on a line-item basis. The charges are accumulated according to the nursing units and other services provided to the patient, as shown in figure 6.2.

Outpatient Bills

The 837I protocol requires that CPT/HCPCS codes be printed in segment SV2, element 02 (field locator 44 on the UB-92 claim form), on bills for outpatients. In addition, ancillary departments must identify charges separately with the appropriate CPT/HCPCS codes. Many of those codes, with the exception of surgical CPT codes, come from the CDM. Surgical CPT codes are assigned by the HIM department and entered into the billing software. The codes then appear on the UB-92/UB-04 claim form or 837I transaction, as shown in figure 6.3.

Coding and the CDM

The process for attaching specific codes to items on the CDM can be accomplished in the following ways:

- Department managers may identify codes and attach them to the services or supplies.

- A designated individual, committee, or workgroup within the department may identify and attach the codes.

Figure 6.2. Partial UB-92 form for an inpatient

	42 REV. CD.	43 DESCRIPTION	44 HCPCS / RATES	45 SERV. DATE	46 SERV. UNITS	47 TOTAL CHARGES	48 NON-COVERED CHARGES	49	
1	0120	ROOM-BOARD/SEMI	821.75		10	8217 50			1
2	0250	PHARMACY			1303	5591 25			2
3	0272	STERILE SUPPLY			1	192 31			3
4	0274	PROSTH/ORTH DEV			1	263 34			4
5	0301	LAB/CHEMISTRY			62	1580 75			5
6	0305	LAB/HEMATOLOGY			1	61 75			6
7	0312	PATHOL/HISTOL			1	149 75			7
8	0320	DX X-RAY			2	574 50			8
9	0360	OR SERVICES			1	3146 50			9
10	0370	ANESTHESIA			1	361 00			10
11	0444	SPEECH PATH/EVAL			1	557 75			11
12	0710	RECOVERY ROOM			1	824 00			12
13									13
14									14
15									15
16									16
17									17
18									18
19									19
20									20
21									21
22									22
23	001	TOTAL CHARGES				21520 40			23

Figure 6.3.   Partial UB-92 form for an outpatient

	42 REV. CD.	43 DESCRIPTION	44 HCPCS / RATES	45 SERV. DATE	46 SERV. UNITS	47 TOTAL CHARGES	48 NON-COVERED CHARGES	49	
1	0250	PHARMACY		011106	21	752 : 10			1
2	0278	SUPPLY/IMPLANTS		011106	2	316 : 80			2
3	0301	LAB/CHEMISTRY	82150	011106	1	59 : 50			3
4	0301	LAB/CHEMISTRY	82948	011106	2	64 : 00			4
5	0305	LAB/HEMATOLOGY	85025	011106	1	71 : 50			5
6	0305	LAB/HEMATOLOGY	85610	011106	1	37 : 50			6
7	0320	DX X-RAY	74010	011106	1	160 : 75			7
8	0320	DX X-RAY	74330	011106	1	761 : 25			8
9	0360	OR SERVICES	43269	011106	1	1055 : 00			9
10	0360	OR SERVICES	43262	011106	1	527 : 50			10
11	0360	OR SERVICES	43271	011106	1	527 : 50			11
12	0360	OR SERVICES	43204	011100	1	527 : 50			12
13	0360	OR SERVICES	50590	011106	1	527 : 50			13
14	0370	ANESTHESIA		011106	3	270 : 75			14
15	0371	ANESTHE/INCIDENT RAD		011106	4	238 : 00			15
16	0710	RECOVERY ROOM		011106	12	1250 : 75			16
17	0730	EKG/ECG	93005	011106	1	112 : 25			17
18	0750	GASTR-INTS SVS		011106	5	6904 : 25			18
19									19
20									20
21									21
22									22
23	001	TOTAL CHARGES				14164 : 40			23

- A particular facility employee may be responsible for coding and maintaining the CDM that attaches the code. (See appendix 6.3 [pp. 184–185] for a sample job description for the chargemaster coordinator.)

- A consulting firm may be used to review and update the codes for each item in the CDM when the required skills are not available within the staff.

Assigning Revenue Codes under the APC System

Recent requirements for the APC system indicate that the service or supply item should be assigned the revenue code for the department in which the item is provided. However, in some instances, specific revenue codes are assigned to specific CPT/HCPCS codes. (See appendix 6.2 [pp. 181–183] for specific revenue code and CPT/HCPCS requirements.)

Under the APC system, certain revenue codes have been packaged into the procedure code. That is, when charges for items using the packaged revenue codes appear on a Medicare bill, they are not paid separately. For example, the following revenue codes are packaged into an APC procedure:

0250   Pharmacy
0258   Intravenous Solutions
0370   Anesthesia
0710   Recovery Room
0762   Observation Room

A list of packaged revenue codes is updated annually in the *Federal Register* (2005, 68541) and in the Medicare Claims Processing Manual, Ch 4 Sec 20.5.1.1. They also may be obtained through the healthcare facility's fiscal intermediary (FI). A complete list has been provided in appendix 6.4 (pp. 186–187).

Assigning the Most Specific Revenue Code

Medicare requires providers to assign the most specific revenue code for their services. For example, providers have the following CT scan revenue codes to choose from:

CT Scan—General	0350
CT Scan—Head Scan	0351
CT Scan—Body Scan	0352
CT Scan—Other CT Scans	0359

For CPT code 70450, Computerized axial tomography, head or brain; without contrast material, the appropriate revenue code is 0351, CT Scan—Head Scan. That code is the specific revenue code required by Medicare, as opposed to the generic revenue code (0350, CT Scan—General). Revenue code 0359, CT Scan—Other CT Scans, is not used by Medicare but is reserved for state use in local billing requirements.

Use of revenue codes ending in "0" (General) and "9" (Other) may cause delays in payment from Medicare. In the event that a specific revenue code is unavailable, Medicare will accept the general revenue code. For example, pulmonary function has only two revenue codes, 0460 and 0469. In that instance, 0460 would be the only acceptable code to use on a UB-92/UB-04 billing form or 837I transaction for Medicare claims filed for Medicare beneficiaries.

Editing Programs for Revenue Codes

A healthcare facility's computer system should have an editing program that reviews revenue codes and any CPT/HCPCS code assignments prior to issuing the UB-92/UB-04 billing form or 837I transaction to Medicare. The latest version of the Medicare outpatient code editor (OCE) should be installed to review claims prior to releasing information to the Medicare program. OCE software contains the National Correct Coding Initiative (NCCI) edits for CPT. The NCCI edits were created to evaluate the relationships between CPT codes on the bill and to control improper coding leading to inappropriate payment on the Part B claims. They also identify component codes that were used instead of the appropriate comprehensive code, as well as other types of coding errors.

To learn more and to stay abreast of the latest updates on the NCCI edits, check the CMS and National Technical Information Service (NTIS) Web sites regularly. (See the annotated list of additional references at the end of this chapter.)

Keeping Current with Federal Requirements

With increased federal requirements for information on hospital outpatient services, the CDM has become a major communication tool not only with federal programs, but also with commercial insurance payers. Keeping this communication tool current is a challenging task.

To keep current with federal programs, Web sites and intermediary bulletins serve as the best resources. The annotated list of additional references at the end of this chapter includes federal government Web sites with information on changes in HCPCS Level II codes, revenue code requirements, and so on. Coding managers should consult those Web sites on a regular basis.

CDM Data Quality and Reimbursement

The CDM provides a database for chargeable services within healthcare facilities. As departmental activity is accumulated, a database of information becomes available. When department managers begin to accumulate information on current charges, management reports from the CDM system will be useful. Some reports that may be available include:

- Charge activity report, which summarizes volume activity for each item in the department CDM

- CDM budget report, which identifies summary charge and reimbursement by CDM item

- Inactive charges report, which lists items currently considered inactive

- CDM zero activity report, which identifies items with no activity for the current fiscal year and provides the department manager with information for inactivating/deleting items

For compliance purposes, it is important to track all changes made to the CDM over time. It is recommended that a copy of the CDM be printed or a file be maintained electronically with all major changes listed in chronological order. Should the need arise to establish which charges were in effect during a specific time period, the documentation would be available for reference.

Software CDM Maintenance Assistance

Several software packages allow users to download their CDMs. The software provides a basic level of maintenance control, change control, tracking of CDM changes, and a variety of executive reports. These software programs can quickly find obvious errors such as inappropriate links between revenue codes and CPT/HCPCS codes. Most of these software packages use the most updated CMS changes and quickly identify all the service codes that are in violation of the CMS and AHA changes.

Reimbursement Systems

The systems of reimbursement for inpatients and outpatients differ between Medicare and Medicaid. Other insurance plans reimburse for inpatients based on the terms of contracts signed with a healthcare facility and reimburse for outpatients on the basis of fee schedules or percentage of charges.

Medicare and Medicaid Inpatient Bills

On Medicare inpatient bills, most items included in the CDM are reimbursed through the diagnostic-related group (DRG) system.

Medicaid reimbursement varies from state to state. In some states, Medicaid payments are made through a DRG system. In other states, Medicaid pays on a per diem rate based on the patient's length of stay.

Medicare and Medicaid Outpatient Bills

Reimbursement for Medicare outpatients depends on the type of item on the CDM: service, procedure, or supply. If the item is a supply, it is either packaged as part of the APC reimbursement or identified on the pass-through list with a separate reimbursement based on the pass-through codes or categories. (See the annotated list of additional references at the end of this chapter.) If the item is a service or procedure in one of the following areas, it is paid based on a fee schedule:

- Laboratory

- Occupational therapy

- Physical therapy

- Speech therapy

The remaining diagnostic and therapeutic procedures identified on the CDM are paid under the APC system.

Medicaid pays for outpatient diagnostic testing on a fee-schedule basis. It pays for outpatient surgical procedures on the basis of an APC type of system or by CPT code on a fee-schedule basis.

The Reimbursement Process

The reimbursement process begins upon the payer's receipt of an electronic (837I) or paper (UB-92/UB-04) claim form. If all of the information on the form is correct, payment is issued for the services covered under the patient's policy or program.

Frequently, the payment (check) is returned to the provider in a batch format with an explanation of payment called a remittance advice. The check to the provider represents the total payment for all the patients processed on a given remittance advice.

The level of detail on the remittance advice varies from payer to payer. Some payers provide CPT/HCPCS code-level detail and identify each payment for each item. Other payers just list the patients' names with payment amounts. In either case, the patient accounting department enters the payment information into the accounting system and adjusts the balance for each patient's visit or encounter. If a balance remains, it is written off completely, resulting in a **zero balance,** or the patient is billed for the remaining amount due.

Detailed Medicare reimbursement information can be found on the Medicare Reimbursement Reference Grid Web site. (See the annotated list of additional references at the end of this chapter.)

CDM Maintenance

Although the principal owner of the CDM is the finance department in most instances, maintaining the CDM is a joint responsibility. Ideally, updating and maintaining the CDM is the work of a team, or committee, that includes members from the finance, patient accounting, information systems, and HIM departments. Managers of clinical departments, such as laboratory or radiology, should serve on the CDM maintenance committee on a rotating basis. The interdepartmental approach exposes the clinical departments to the issues faced by the nonclinical departments. This approach also promotes a greater understanding throughout the facility of the reporting and reimbursement process.

Adding a New Item to the CDM

The process for adding a new item to the CDM is as follows:

1. A request to add a new item (service, procedure, or supply) to the CDM originates in the department requesting the change. The department should use a form similar to the one in figure 6.4 to request a new item.

2. The request then should be circulated to the CDM maintenance committee for review. Committee members from the finance or patient accounting departments review the request to evaluate any potential financial impact and to assign the new item's revenue code, insurance code, and charge number. A committee member from the information system department also might be responsible for those tasks.

3. A qualified coder should review the suggested CPT/HCPCS code to ensure the accuracy of the new item's description.

4. The committee should exercise caution if the new item represents new technology or new services. Items covered by Medicare must have FDA approval for use with Medicare patients.

5. When the item is a supply, it may qualify for pass-through payment on APC claims.

6. When the supply is accompanied by a manufacturer-recommended CPT/HCPCS code, the code should be reviewed for appropriateness.

7. After the item has received all the appropriate approvals, the requesting department is notified of the new item information—charge number, item description, charge, CPT/HCPCS codes, revenue code, and insurance code. The item then is made available for use by the department. (See figure 6.5 for a flowchart illustrating the process for requesting a new item on the CDM.)

Changing an Existing Item on the CDM

Requests for changes to existing items on the CDM should follow a process similar to that of adding a new item to the CDM. If the change is a different CPT/HCPCS code, the HIM department member of the CDM maintenance committee should verify the correctness of the change.

The Role of Chargemaster Coordinator

Coders sometimes are placed in the role of **chargemaster coordinator.** As such, they are responsible for mentoring other staff and assisting each department with its line-item updates each year. In addition, they are responsible for maintaining their own level of expertise in HCPCS coding throughout the year.

Coders responsible for the chargemaster document may be given a title such as chargemaster coordinator so that all staff members know the focus of their position. The chargemaster coordinator meets routinely with departments to discuss issues such as:

*   New technology or equipment

*   Changes in procedure codes

*   Changes in reimbursement methodologies that require a revision of charges or text descriptions associated with the department's business

Figure 6.4. New charge request form

New Charge Form	
Routing Dates	
TBS Date	07/26/2006
TDS Date	07/28/2006
CDM Date	07/31/2006
S/M Date	08/01/2006

CDM Data	
Charge Number	401-9917-9
Description (30 char. max)	GUIDE WIRE 292.40
CPT/HCPCS Codes	A B C D M N O S W Z
Item Type	N
Charge Price	$76.50
Ins. Code	27
UB-92 Rev. Code	A 0272 B 0272 C 0272 D 0272 M 0272 N O S W 0272 Z

Requestor Info	
Contact Person (Requestor)	Janice X. Jones
Phone Number	14714

Figure 6.5. New charge request process

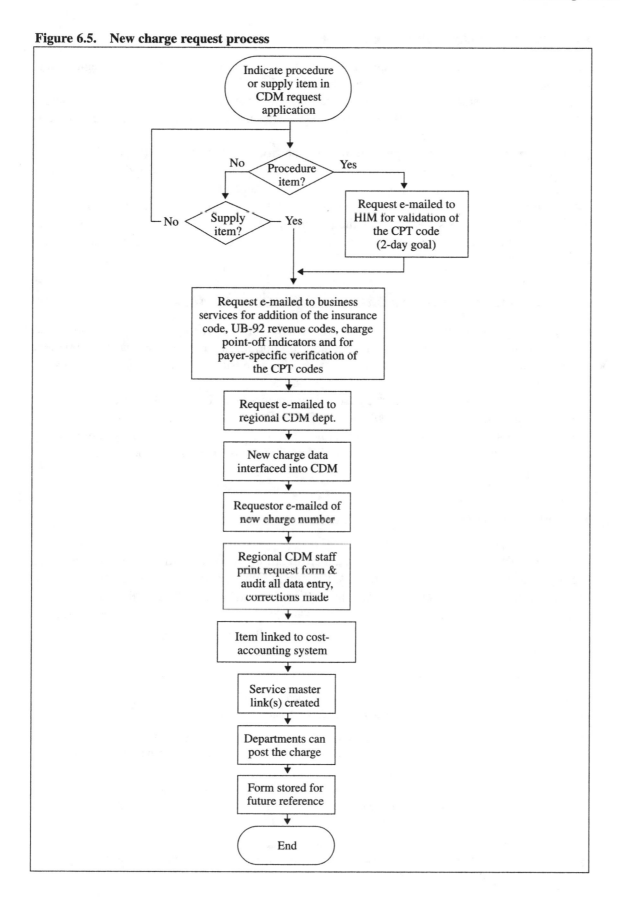

Chargemaster Coordinators and Medical Review Policies

The Medicare medical review policy is a composite of statutory provisions, federal regulations, CMS national coverage determinations (NCDs), and local coverage determinations (LCDs). In the absence of statutes, regulations, or national coverage decisions, Medicare contractors (including AdminaStar Federal) develop LCDs to describe when and under what circumstances Medicare will cover a service.

Chargemaster coordinators pass on information from published LCDs that outline diagnoses considered medically necessary for a certain test or procedure and is updated frequently. Chargemaster coordinators review LCDs with departments and registration personnel to ensure the proper administration of benefits for Medicare patients. LCDs generally list CPT/HCPCS and ICD-9-CM diagnosis codes within their memoranda. Chargemaster coordinators share this information with each department affected because revisions to line items in the chargemaster may be necessary.

Other Responsibilities of Chargemaster Coordinators

Chargemaster coordinators also may be responsible for reconciling any billing issues that arise from chargemaster-driven coding. If claims do not pass to a designated payer, the patient accounts/business office staff may look to the chargemaster coordinator for assistance in resolving the claim in order to complete the billing process.

Another responsibility of chargemaster coordinators may be that of conducting random internal audits. Such audits occur when procedure codes are generated from the chargemaster to ensure the integrity of data within the healthcare system. Outcomes from this type of auditing merge nicely with internal audits from the HIM coding areas, making the coding audit process more comprehensive.

Conclusion

Effective CDM management requires a team effort among many departments of the healthcare facility. The various medical departments, the nursing units, and the financial department all depend on the coding expertise of HIM professionals to avoid incorrect coding and potential compliance issues. Only through the use of a variety of experts can healthcare organizations master the complexities and reap the benefits of chargemaster technology.

References and Resources

American Health Information Management Association. 1999 (August). Practice Brief: The care and maintenance of charge masters. *Journal of American Health Information Management Association* 70(7).

Centers for Medicare and Medicaid Services. 2005a (July 22). Medicare Claims Processing Manual. Chapter 23: Fee schedule administration and coding requirements, Rev. 614. Available online from http://www.cms.hhs.gov/manuals/downloads/clm104c23.pdf.

Centers for Medicare and Medicaid Services. 2005b (Nov. 10) Medicare program; Changes to the hospital outpatient prospective payment system and calendar year 2006 payment rates. *Federal Register* 70(217):68516–980. Available online from http://www.access.gpo.gov/su_docs/fedreg/a051110c.html.

Centers for Medicare and Medicaid Services. 2006 (April 14). Medicare Claims Processing Manual. Chapter 4: Part B Hospital (Including Inpatient Hospital Part B and OPPS), Rev. 903. Available online from http://www.cms.hhs.gov/manuals/downloads/clm104c04.pdf.

Clarian Health Partners. n.d. Coordinator-Charge Integrity. Available online from http://www.clarian.org/.

The University of Utah. 1998 (March). Job title: CDM coordinator (charge description master). Available online from http://www.hr.utah.edu/comp/jobdescriptions/viewjd.php?id=144.

Annotated List of Additional References

To locate your local fiscal intermediary (FI), go to http://www.cms.hhs.gov/about/regions/professionals.asp and follow the instructions for Medicare intermediaries. Most FIs have bulletins available at their Web sites that can be downloaded. Some state Medicaid programs have Web sites that will provide access to state manuals, as well as Medicaid bulletins that have coding guidance for the Medicaid program in that state. To locate your Medicaid information and link to your state, go to http://www.cms.hhs.gov/states.

Web site address for program transmittals: http://www.cms.hhs.govTransmittals/01_Overview.asp

Web site address for frequently asked questions: http://questions.cms.hhs.gov/cgi-bin/cmshhs_cfg/php/enduser/std_alp.php

Web site address for OPPS Guidance: http://www.cms.hhs.gov/HospitalOutpatientPPS/05_OPPSGuidance.asp

Medicare reimbursement reference grid: http://www.ahima.org/infocenter/rgrid_nav.html

Web site address for CMS annual HCPCS update: http://www.cms.hhs.gov/providers/pufdownload/anhcpcdl.asp

Web site address for CMS Pass-Through Status and New Technology Ambulatory Payment Classification: http://www.cms.hhs.gov/HospitalOutpatientPPS/04_passthrough_payment.asp

Web site address for CMS: National Correct Coding Initiatives Edits (NCCI): http://www.cms.hhs.gov/NationalCorrectCodInitEd/

Web site address for National Technical Information Service (NTIS): http://www.ntis.gov/products/families/cci/

Web site address for the table of contents to the CMS Medicare Claims Processing Manual: http://www.cms.hhs.gov/Manuals/IOM/itemdetail.asp?filterType=none&filterByDID=-99&sortByDID=1&sortOrder=ascending&itemID=CMS018912

Appendix 6.1

List of Medicare Revenue Codes

Segment SV2, Element 01 revenue codes for outpatient ancillary services

Pharmacy   **25X**

Pharmacy—General	0250
Pharmacy—Generic Drugs	0251
Pharmacy—Nongeneric Drugs	0252
Pharmacy—Take-Home Drugs	0253
Pharmacy—Drugs Incident to Other Diagnostic Services	0254
Pharmacy—Drugs Incident to Radiology	0255
Pharmacy—Experimental Drugs	0256
Pharmacy—Nonprescription	0257
Pharmacy—IV Solutions	0258
Pharmacy—Other Pharmacy	0259

IV Therapy   **026X**

IV Therapy—General	0260
IV Therapy—Infusion Pump	0261
IV Therapy—IV Therapy/Pharmacy Services	0262
IV Therapy—IV Therapy/Drug/Supply Delivery	0263
IV Therapy—IV Therapy/Supplies	0264
IV Therapy—Other IV Therapy	0269

Medical/Surgical Supplies and Devices   **027X**

Medical/Surgical Supplies and Devices—General	0270
Medical/Surgical Supplies and Devices—Nonsterile Supply	0271
Medical/Surgical Supplies and Devices—Sterile Supply	0272
Medical/Surgical Supplies and Devices—Take-Home Supplies	0273
Medical/Surgical Supplies and Devices—Prosthetic/Orthotic Devices	0274
Medical/Surgical Supplies and Devices—Pacemaker	0275
Medical/Surgical Supplies and Devices—Intraocular Lens	0276
Medical/Surgical Supplies and Devices—Oxygen—Take-Home	0277
Medical/Surgical Supplies and Devices—Other Implants	0278
Medical/Surgical Supplies and Devices—Other Supplies/Devices	0279

Oncology   **028X**

Oncology—General	0280
Oncology—Other	0289

Durable Medical Equipment (Other than Renal)   **029X**

DME (Other than Renal)—General	0290
DME (Other than Renal)—Rental	0291
DME (Other than Renal)—Purchase of New DME	0292
DME (Other than Renal)—Purchase of Used DME	0293
DME (Other than Renal)—Supplies/Drugs for DME Effectiveness (HHAs Only)	0294
DME (Other than Renal)—Other Equipment	0299

Source: CMS 2005a.

Laboratory   **030X**

Laboratory—General	0300
Laboratory—Chemistry	0301
Laboratory—Immunology	0302
Laboratory—Renal Patient (Home)	0303
Laboratory—Nonroutine Dialysis	0304
Laboratory—Hematology	0305
Laboratory—Bacteriology and Microbiology	0306
Laboratory—Urology	0307
Laboratory—Other Laboratory	0309

Laboratory Pathological   **031X**

Laboratory Pathological—General	0310
Laboratory Pathological—Cytology	0311
Laboratory Pathological—Histology	0312
Laboratory Pathological—Biopsy	0314
Laboratory Pathological—Other	0319

Radiology—Diagnostic   **032X**

Radiology—Diagnostic—General	0320
Radiology—Diagnostic—Angiocardiography	0321
Radiology—Diagnostic—Arthrography	0322
Radiology—Diagnostic—Arteriography	0323
Radiology—Diagnostic—Chest X-ray	0324
Radiology—Diagnostic—Other	0329

Radiology—Therapeutic   **033X**

Radiology—Therapeutic—General	0330
Radiology—Therapeutic—Chemotherapy—Injected	0331
Radiology—Therapeutic—Chemotherapy—Oral	0332
Radiology—Therapeutic—Radiation Therapy	0333
Radiology—Therapeutic—Chemotherapy—IV	0335
Radiology—Therapeutic—Other	0339

Nuclear Medicine   **034X**

Nuclear Medicine—General	0340
Nuclear Medicine—Diagnostic	0341
Nuclear Medicine—Therapeutic	0342
Nuclear Medicine---Diagnostic Radiopharmaceuticals	0343
Nuclear Medicine---Therapeutic Radiopharmaceuticals	0344
Nuclear Medicine—Other	0349

CT Scan   **035X**

CT Scan—General	0350
CT Scan—Head Scan	0351
CT Scan—Body Scan	0352
CT Scan—Other CT Scans	0359

Operating Room Services   **036X**

Operating Room Services—General	0360
Operating Room Services—Minor Surgery	0361
Operating Room Services—Organ Transplant—Other than Kidney	0362
Operating Room Services—Kidney Transplant	0367
Operating Room Services—Other Operating Room Services	0369

Anesthesia   **037X**

Anesthesia—General	0370
Anesthesia—Anesthesia Incident to Radiology	0371
Anesthesia—Anesthesia Incident to Other Diagnostic Services	0372
Anesthesia—Acupuncture	0374
Anesthesia—Other Anesthesia	0379

Blood   **038X**

Blood—General	0380
Blood—Packed Red Cells	0381
Blood—Whole Blood	0382
Blood—Plasma	0383
Blood—Platelets	0384
Blood—Leukocytes	0385
Blood—Other Components	0386
Blood—Other Derivatives (Cryoprecipitates)	0387
Blood—Other Blood	0389

Blood Storage and Processing   **039X**

Blood Storage and Processing—General	0390
Blood Storage and Processing—Blood Administration	0391
Blood Storage and Processing—Other Blood Processing and Storage	0399

Other Imaging Services   **040X**

Other Imaging Services—General	0400
Other Imaging Services—Diagnostic Mammography	0401
Other Imaging Services—Ultrasound	0402
Other Imaging Services—Screening Mammography	0403
Other Imaging Services—Positron Emission Tomography	0404
Other Imaging Services—Other Imaging Services	0409

Respiratory Services   **041X**

Respiratory Services—General	0410
Respiratory Services—Inhalation Services	0412
Respiratory Services—Hyperbaric Oxygen Therapy	0413
Respiratory Services—Other Respiratory Services	0419

Physical Therapy   **042X**

Physical Therapy—General	0420
Physical Therapy—Visit Charge	0421
Physical Therapy—Hourly Charge	0422
Physical Therapy—Group Rate	0423
Physical Therapy—Evaluation or Reevaluation	0424
Physical Therapy—Other Physical Therapy	0429

Occupational Therapy   **043X**

Occupational Therapy—General	0430
Occupational Therapy—Visit Charge	0431
Occupational Therapy—Hourly Charge	0432
Occupational Therapy—Group Rate	0433
Occupational Therapy—Evaluation or Reevaluation	0434
Occupational Therapy—Other Occupational Therapy	0439

Speech-Language Pathology   **044X**

Speech-Language Pathology—General	0440
Speech-Language Pathology—Visit Charge	0441

Speech-Language Pathology—Hourly Charge   0442
Speech-Language Pathology—Group Rate   0443
Speech-Language Pathology—Evaluation or Reevaluation   0444
Speech-Language Pathology—Other Speech-Language Pathology   0449

Emergency Room   **045X**

Emergency Room—General   0450
Emergency Room—EMTALA Emergency Medical Screening Services   0451
Emergency Room—ER Beyond EMTALA Screening   0452
Emergency Room—Urgent Care   0456
Emergency Room—Other Emergency Room   0459

Pulmonary Function   **046X**

Pulmonary Function—General   0460
Pulmonary Function—Other Pulmonary Function   0469

Audiology   **047X**

Audiology—General   0470
Audiology—Diagnostic   0471
Audiology—Treatment   0472
Audiology—Other Audiology   0479

Cardiology   **048X**

Cardiology—General   0480
Cardiology—Cardiac Cath Lab   0481
Cardiology—Stress Test   0482
Cardiology—Echocardiology   0483
Cardiology—Other Cardiology   0489

Ambulatory Surgical Care   **049X**

Ambulatory Surgical Care—General   0490
Ambulatory Surgical Care—Other Ambulatory Surgical Care   0499

Outpatient Services   **050X**

Outpatient Services—General   0500
Outpatient Services—Other Outpatient Services   0509

Clinic   **051X**

Clinic—General   0510
Clinic—Chronic Pain Center   0511
Clinic—Dental Clinic   0512
Clinic—Psychiatric Clinic   0513
Clinic—OB/GYN Clinic   0514
Clinic—Pediatric Clinic   0515
Clinic—Urgent Care Clinic   0516
Clinic—Family Practice Clinic   0517
Clinic—Other Clinic   0519

Freestanding Clinic   **052X**

Freestanding Clinic—General   0520
Freestanding Clinic—Clinic visit by member to RHC/FQHC   0521
Freestanding Clinic—Home visit by RHC/FQHC practitioner   0522
Freestanding Clinic—Family Practice Clinic   0523
Freestanding Clinic—Visit by RHC/FQHC Practitioner to a Member
  in a Covered Part A Stay at SNF   0524

Freestanding Clinic—Visit by RHC/FQHC Practitioner to a member in an SNF (Not in a Covered Part A stay) or NF or ICF MR or Other Residential Facility	0525
Freestanding Clinic—Urgent Care Clinic	0526
Freestanding Clinic—Visit Nurse Service to a Member's Home in a Home Health Shortage Area	0527
Freestanding Clinic—Visit by RHC/FQHC Practitioner to other non-RHC/FQHC site (e.g. Scene of Accident)	0528
Freestanding Clinic—Other Freestanding Clinic	0529

Osteopathic Services   **053X**

Osteopathic Services—General	0530
Osteopathic Services—Osteopathic Therapy	0531
Osteopathic Services—Other Osteopathic Services	0539

Ambulance   **054X**

Ambulance—General	0540
Ambulance—Supplies	0541
Ambulance—Medical Transport	0542
Ambulance—Heart Mobile	0543
Ambulance—Oxygen	0544
Ambulance—Air Ambulance	0545
Ambulance—Neonatal Ambulance Services	0546
Ambulance—Pharmacy	0547
Ambulance—Telephone Transmission EKG	0548
Ambulance—Other Ambulance	0549

Magnetic Resonance Technology (MRT)   **061X**

Magnetic Resonance Imaging—General	0610
Magnetic Resonance Imaging—Brain (Including Brain Stem)	0611
Magnetic Resonance Imaging—Spinal Cord (Including Spine)	0612
Reserved	0613
Magnetic Resonance Imaging—Other MRI	0614
Magnetic Resonance Angiography—Head and Neck	0615
Magnetic Resonance Angiography—Lower Extremities	0616
Reserved	0617
Magnetic Resonance Angiography—Other MRA	0618
Magnetic Resonance Technology—Other MRT	0619

Medical/Surgical Supplies—Extension of 027X   **062X**

Medical/Surgical Supplies (Extension of 027X)—Supplies Incident to Radiology	0621
Medical/Surgical Supplies (Extension of 027X)—Supplies Incident to Other Diagnostic Services	0622
Medical/Surgical Supplies (Extension of 027X)—Surgical Dressings	0623
Medical/Surgical Supplies (Extension of 027X)—FDA Investigational Devices	0624

Pharmacy—Extension of 025X   **063X**

Reserved	0630
Pharmacy- (Extension of 025X)—Single Source Drug	0631
Pharmacy- (Extension of 025X)—Multiple Source Drug	0632
Pharmacy- (Extension of 025X)—Restrictive Prescription	0633
Pharmacy- (Extension of 025X)—Erythropoietin (EPO) Less than 10,000 Units	0634
Pharmacy- (Extension of 025X)—Erythropoietin (EPO) 10,000 or More Units	0635
Pharmacy- (Extension of 025X)—Drugs Requiring Detailed Coding	0636
Pharmacy- (Extension of 025X)—Self-Administrable Drugs	0637

Cast Room   **070X**

    Cast Room—General   0700
    Cast Room—Other Cast Room   0709

Recovery Room   **071X**

    Recovery Room—General   0710
    Recovery Room—Other Recovery Room   0719

EKG/ECG (Electrocardiogram)   **073X**

    EKG/ECG (Electrocardiogram)—General   0730
    EKG/ECG (Electrocardiogram)—Holter Monitor   0731
    EKG/ECG (Electrocardiogram)—Telemetry   0732
    EKG/ECG (Electrocardiogram)—Other EKG/ECG   0739

EEG (Electroencephalogram)   **074X**

    EEG (Electroencephalogram)—General   0740
    EEG (Electroencephalogram)—Other EEG   0749

Gastrointestinal Services   **075X**

    Gastrointestinal Services—General   0750
    Gastrointestinal Services—Other Gastrointestinal   0759

Treatment or Observation Room   **076X**

    Treatment or Observation Room—General   0760
    Treatment or Observation Room—Treatment Room   0761
    Treatment or Observation Room—Observation Room   0762
    Treatment or Observation Room—Other Treatment/Observation Room   0769

Preventive Care Services   **077X**

    Preventive Care Services—General   0770
    Preventive Care Services—Vaccine Administration   0771
    Preventive Care Services—Other Preventive Care Services   0779

Extracorporeal Shock Wave Therapy (formerly Lithotripsy)   **079X**

    Extracorporeal Shock Wave Therapy (formerly Lithotripsy)—General   0790
    Extracorporeal Shock Wave Therapy (formerly Lithotripsy)—Other Lithotripsy   0799

Organ Acquisition   **081X**

    Organ Acquisition—General   0810
    Organ Acquisition—Living Donor   0811
    Organ Acquisition—Cadaver Donor   0812
    Organ Acquisition—Unknown Donor   0813
    Organ Acquisition—Unsuccessful Organ Search—Donor Bank Charges   0814
    Organ Acquisition—Other Donor   0819

Hemodialysis—Outpatient or Home   **082X**

    Hemodialysis—Outpatient or Home Dialysis—General   0820
    Hemodialysis—Outpatient or Home Dialysis—Hemodialysis/Composite or Other Rate   0821
    Hemodialysis—Outpatient or Home Dialysis—Home Supplies   0822
    Hemodialysis—Outpatient or Home Dialysis—Home Equipment   0823
    Hemodialysis—Outpatient or Home Dialysis—Maintenance/100%   0824
    Hemodialysis—Outpatient or Home Dialysis—Support Services   0825
    Hemodialysis—Outpatient or Home Dialysis—Other Outpatient Hemodialysis   0829

Peritoneal Dialysis—Outpatient or Home   **083X**

Peritoneal Dialysis—Outpatient or Home—General	0830
Peritoneal Dialysis—Outpatient or Home—Peritoneal/Composite or Other Rate	0831
Peritoneal Dialysis—Outpatient or Home—Home Supplies	0832
Peritoneal Dialysis—Outpatient or Home—Home Equipment	0833
Peritoneal Dialysis—Outpatient or Home—Maintenance/100%	0834
Peritoneal Dialysis—Outpatient or Home—Support Services	0835
Peritoneal Dialysis—Outpatient or Home—Other Outpatient Peritoneal Dialysis	0839

CAPD (Dialysis)—Outpatient or Home   **084X**

CAPD (Dialysis)—Outpatient or Home—General	0840
CAPD (Dialysis)—Outpatient or Home—CAPD/Composite or Other Rate	0841
CAPD (Dialysis)—Outpatient or Home—Home Supplies	0842
CAPD (Dialysis)—Outpatient or Home—Home Equipment	0843
CAPD (Dialysis)—Outpatient or Home—Maintenance/100%	0844
CAPD (Dialysis)—Outpatient or Home—Support Services	0845
CAPD (Dialysis)—Outpatient or Home—Other Outpatient CAPD	0849

CCPD (Dialysis)—Outpatient or Home   **085X**

CCPD (Dialysis)—Outpatient or Home—General	0850
CCPD (Dialysis)—Outpatient or Home—CCPD/Composite or Other Rate	0851
CCPD (Dialysis)—Outpatient or Home—Home Supplies	0852
CCPD (Dialysis)—Outpatient or Home—Home Equipment	0853
CCPD (Dialysis)—Outpatient or Home—Maintenance/100%	0854
CCPD (Dialysis)—Outpatient or Home—Support Services	0855
CCPD (Dialysis)—Outpatient or Home—Other Outpatient CCPD	0859

Reserved for Dialysis (National Assignment)   **086X**

Reserved for Dialysis (National Assignment)   **087X**

Miscellaneous Dialysis   **088X**

Miscellaneous Dialysis—General	0880
Miscellaneous Dialysis—Ultrafiltration	0881
Miscellaneous Dialysis—Home Dialysis Aid Visit	0882
Miscellaneous Dialysis—Other Miscellaneous Dialysis	0889

Reserved for National Assignment   **089X**

Behavioral Health Treatments/Services (also see 091X, an extension of 090X)   **090X**

Behavioral Health Treatments/Services (also see 091X, an extension of 090X)—General	0900
Behavioral Health Treatments/Services (also see 091X, an extension of 090X)—Electroshock Treatment	0901
Behavioral Health Treatments/Services (also see 091X, an extension of 090X)—Milieu Therapy	0902
Behavioral Health Treatments/Services (also see 091X, an extension of 090X)—Play Therapy	0903
Behavioral Health Treatments/Services (also see 091X, an extension of 090X)—Activity Therapy	0904
Behavioral Health Treatments/Services (also see 091X, an extension of 090X)—Intensive Outpatient Services—Psychiatric	0905
Behavioral Health Treatments/Services (also see 091X, an extension of 090X)—Intensive Outpatient Services –Chemical Dependency	0906

Behavioral Health Treatments/Services (also see 091X, an extension of 090X)—Community Behavioral Health Program (Day Treatment)	0907
Behavioral Health Treatments/Services (also see 091X, an extension of 090X)—Reserved for National Use	0908
Behavioral Health Treatments/Services (also see 091X, an extension of 090X)—Reserved for National Use	0909
Behavioral Health Treatments/Services—Extension of 090X	091X
Behavioral Health Treatments/Services—Extension of 090X—Reserved for National Use	0910
Behavioral Health Treatments/Services—Extension of 090X—Rehabilitation	0911
Behavioral Health Treatments/Services—Extension of 090X—Partial Hospitalization—Less Intensive	0912
Behavioral Health Treatments/Services—Extension of 090X—Partial Hospitalization—Intensive	0913
Behavioral Health Treatments/Services—Extension of 090X—Individual Therapy	0914
Behavioral Health Treatments/Services—Extension of 090X—Group Therapy	0915
Behavioral Health Treatments/Services—Extension of 090X—Family Therapy	0916
Behavioral Health Treatments/Services—Extension of 090X—Biofeedback	0917
Behavioral Health Treatments/Services—Extension of 090X—Testing	0918
Behavioral Health Treatments/Services—Extension of 090X—Other	0919

Other Diagnostic Services   092X

Other Diagnostic Services—General	0920
Other Diagnostic Services—Peripheral Vascular Lab	0921
Other Diagnostic Services—Electromyelogram	0922
Other Diagnostic Services—Pap Smear	0923
Other Diagnostic Services—Allergy Test	0924
Other Diagnostic Services—Pregnancy Test	0925
Other Diagnostic Services—Other Diagnostic Service	0929

Not Assigned   093X

Other Therapeutic Services   094X

Other Therapeutic Services—General	0940
Other Therapeutic Services—Recreational Therapy	0941
Other Therapeutic Services—Education/Training	0942
Other Therapeutic Services—Cardiac Rehabilitation	0943
Other Therapeutic Services—Drug Rehabilitation	0944
Other Therapeutic Services—Alcohol Rehabilitation	0945
Other Therapeutic Services—Complex Medical Equipment—Routine	0946
Other Therapeutic Services—Complex Medical Equipment—Ancillary	0947
Other Therapeutic Services—Other Therapeutic Services	0949

Other Therapeutic Services (extension of 094X)   095X

Reserved	0950
Other Therapeutic Services – Athletic Training	0951
Other Therapeutic Services – Kinesiotherapy	0952

Professional Fees   096X

Professional Fees—General	0960
Professional Fees—Psychiatric	0961
Professional Fees—Ophthalmology	0962
Professional Fees—Anesthesiologist (MD)	0963
Professional Fees—Anesthetist (CRNA)	0964
Professional Fees—Other Professional Fees	0969

Professional Fees (extension of 096X)   **097X**

Professional Fees—Laboratory	0971
Professional Fees—Radiology—Diagnostic	0972
Professional Fees—Radiology—Therapeutic	0973
Professional Fees—Radiology—Nuclear Medicine	0974
Professional Fees—Operating Room	0975
Professional Fees—Respiratory Therapy	0976
Professional Fees—Physical Therapy	0977
Professional Fees—Occupational Therapy	0978
Professional Fees—Speech Pathology	0979

Professional Fees (extension of 096X and 097X)   **098X**

Professional Fees—Emergency Room	0981
Professional Fees—Outpatient Services	0982
Professional Fees—Clinic	0983
Professional Fees—Medical Social Services	0984
Professional Fees—EKG	0985
Professional Fees—EEG	0986
Professional Fees—Hospital Visit	0987
Professional Fees—Consultation	0988
Professional Fees—Private-Duty Nurse	0989

Patient Convenience Items   **099X**

Patient Convenience Items—General	0990
Patient Convenience Items—Cafeteria/Guest Tray	0991
Patient Convenience Items—Private Linen Service	0992
Patient Convenience Items—Telephone/Telegraph	0993
Patient Convenience Items—TV/Radio	0994
Patient Convenience Items—Nonpatient Room Rentals	0995
Patient Convenience Items—Late Discharge Charge	0996
Patient Convenience Items—Admission Kits	0997
Patient Convenience Items—Beauty Shop/Barber	0998
Patient Convenience Items—Other Patient Convenience Items	0999

Appendix 6.2

HCPCS Revenue Code Chart

The following chart reflects HCPCS coding required to be reported under OPPS by hospital outpatient departments. This chart is intended only as a guide to be used by hospitals to assist them in reporting services rendered. Hospitals that are currently utilizing different revenue/ HCPCS reporting may continue to do so. They are not required to change the way they currently report their services to agree with this chart. Note that this chart does not represent all HCPCS coding subjects to OPPS.

Revenue Code	HCPCS Code	Description
*	10040-69990	Surgical Procedure
*	92950-92961	Cardiovascular
*	96570, 96571	Photodynamic Therapy
*	99170, 99185, 99186	Other Services and Procedures
*	99291-99292	Critical Care
*	99440	Newborn Care
*	90782-90799	Therapeutic or Diagnostic Injections
*	D0150, D0240-D0274 D0277, D0460, D0472-D0999, D1510-D1550 D2970, D2999, D3460 D3999, D4260-D4264, D4270-D4273, D4355-D4381, D5911-D5912, D5983-D5985, D5987, D6920, D7110-D7260, D7291, D7940, D9630, D9930, D9940, D9950-D9952	Dental Services
*	92502-92596, 92599	Otorhinolaryngologic Services (ENT)
0278	E0749, E0782, E0783, E0785	Implanted Durable Medical Equipment
0278	E0751, E0753, L8600, L8603, L8610, L8612, L8613, L8614, L8630, L8641, L8642, L8658, L8670, L8699	Implanted Prosthetic Devices

(Continued on next page)

Source: CMS 2006, 27–31.

Revenue Code	HCPCS Code	Description
0302	86485-86586	Immunology
0305	85060-85102, 86077-86079	Hematology
031X	80500-80502	Pathology - Laboratory
0310	88300-88365, 88399	Surgical Pathology
0311	88104-88125, 88160-88199	Cytopathology
032X	70010-76092, 76094-76999	Diagnostic Radiology
0333	77261-77799	Radiation Oncology
034X	78000-79999	Nuclear Medicine
037X	99141-99142	Anesthesia
045X	99281-99285, 99291	Emergency
046X	94010-94799	Pulmonary Function
0480	93600-93790, 93799, G0166	Intraelectrophysiological Procedures and Other Vascular Studies
0481	93501-93572	Cardiac Catheterization
0482	93015-93024	Stress Test
0483	93303-93350	Echocardiography
051X	92002-92499	Ophthalmological Services
051X	99201-99215, 99241-99245, 99271-99275	Clinic Visit
0510, 0517, 0519	95144-95149, 95165, 95170, 95180, 95199	Allergen Immunotherapy
0519	95805-95811	Sleep Testing
0530	98925-98929	Osteopathic Manipulative Procedures
0636	A4642, A9500, A9605	Radionucleides
0636	90476-90665, 90675-90749	Vaccines, Toxoids

Revenue Code	HCPCS Code	Description
0636	90296-90379, 90385, 90389-90396	Immunoglobulins
073X	G0004-G0006, G0015	Event Recording ECG
0730	93005-93009, 93011-93013, 93040-93224, 93278	Electrocardiograms (ECGs)
0731	93225-93272	Holter Monitor
074X	95812-95827, 95950-95962	Electroencephalogram (EEG)
0771	G0008-G0010	Vaccine Administration
088X	90935-90999	Non-ESRD Dialysis
0900	90801, 90802, 90865,90899	Behavioral Health Treatment/Services
0901	90870, 90871	Psychiatry
0903	90910, 90911, 90812-90815, 90823, 90824, 90826-90829	Psychiatry
0909	90880	Psychiatry
0914	90804-90809, 90816-90819, 90821, 90822, 90845, 90862	Psychiatry
0915	90853, 90857	Psychiatry
0916	90846,90847, 90849	Psychiatry
0917	90901-90911	Biofeedback
0918	96100-96117	Central Nervous System Assessments/Tests
092X	95829-95857, 95900-95937, 95970-95999	Miscellaneous Neurological Procedures
0920, 0929	93875-93990	Noninvasive Vascular Diagnosis Studies
0922	95858-95875	Electromyography (EMG)
0924	95004-95078	Allergy Test
0940	96900-96999	Special Dermatological Procedures
0940	98940-98942	Chiropractic Manipulative Treatment
0940	99195	Other Services and Procedures
0943	93797-93798	Cardiac Rehabilitation

*Revenue codes have not been identified for these procedures as they can be performed in a number of revenue centers within a hospital, such as emergency department (0450), operating room (0360), or clinic (0510). Instruct your hospitals to report these HCPCS codes under the revenue center where they were performed.

NOTE: The listing of HCPCS codes contained in the above chart does not ensure coverage of the specific service. Current coverage criteria apply.

Do not install additional edits for the matching of revenue and HCPCS codes.

Appendix 6.3

Sample Job Description for the Chargemaster Coordinator

Job Title: CDM Coordinator (Charge Description Master)

Job Summary

Develops, maintains, and reports on the charge description master (CDM); ensures data and charge integrity between the CDM and the hospital departments; researches coding and revenue reporting requirements and uses strategic pricing applications to maximize reimbursement. This position will assure accurate charge design, build, validation, testing, and quality assurance for all changes to the CDM, electronic and paper charge forms, and charge systems applications.

Essential Functions

1. Maintains the CDM by incorporating new charges/services identified by the departments, third-party changes, CMS regulations, federal and state specific coding updates.

2. Performs a detailed, annual review of the CDM that includes identifying CPT and HCPCS Level II codes that have been deleted, added, or replaced; assigning CPT and HCPCS specific codes when appropriate; identifying description changes; and ensuring the nomenclature reflects the procedures performed.

3. Identifies services that are reimbursable but are not being coded; reviews, assigns, and validates revenue codes.

4. Coordinates annual and biannual meetings with department managers, staff and/or physicians regarding new program and procedure developments, equipment acquisitions and validation of inactive codes.

5. Determines charge and charge attributes for new services and products.

6. Communicates CDM changes to the hospital departments and administration, patient accounting, and others who are impacted by the change.

7. Maintains audit trail of CDM changes.

8. Distributes correspondence of third-party requirements for coding changes to departments for review of the impending changes.

9. Researches and resolves CPT and HCPCS codes, revenue codes, and other issues referred by the Patient Financial Services department.

10. Uses strategic pricing applications.

Sources: The University of Utah 1998; Clarian Health Partners n.d.

11. Uses CMS, third-party payers, and local FI as a technical resource.

12. Establishes and maintains positive working relationships with medical directors, department chairs, and staff.

13. Serves as a resource to hospital departments; for example, assists with the start-up process for new programs and answers implementation questions and regulation questions.

14. Completes and provides management reports as requested.

The preceding essential function statements are not intended to be an exhaustive list of tasks and functions for this position. Other tasks and functions may be assigned as needed to fulfill the mission of the organization.

Qualifications/Knowledge/Skill/Abilities:

- Bachelor's degree in Business Administration or equivalent (required), Master's degree (preferred)

- Five years of experience maintaining price files and record keeping

- Requires knowledge of both clinical and revenue cycle operations

- Requires experience with medical terminology and CPT coding systems

- Requires knowledge of billing and reimbursement processes and methodologies

- Requires computer literacy with experience with Microsoft Office

- Requires excellent written and verbal communication skills with the ability to effectively interact with all levels of internal and external customers

- Requires knowledge regarding CPT-4 and HCPCS coding and UB-92/UB-04 revenue code assignments

- Requires ability to take initiative, effectively use problem-solving skills and adjusts to changes in policy/procedures

- Requires effective organizational skills with attention to detail

- Requires ability to organize and process a high volume of work within established standards

- Requires good interpersonal skills

- Requires ability to work independently

- Requires ability to handle multiple tasks

Appendix 6.4

Sample Packaged Revenue Codes

The following revenue codes when billed under OPPS without HCPCS codes are packaged services for which no separate payment is made. However, the cost of these services is included in the transitional outpatient payment (TOP) and outlier calculations. The revenue codes for packaged services are:

250 Pharmacy
251 Generic
252 Nongeneric
254 Pharmacy Incident to Other Diagnostic
255 Pharmacy Incident to Radiology
257 Nonprescription drugs
258 IV Solutions
259 Other Pharmacy
260 IV Therapy, General Class
262 IV Therapy/Pharmacy Services
263 Supply/Delivery
264 IV Therapy/Supplies
269 Other IV Therapy
270 M&S Supplies
271 Nonsterile Supplies
272 Sterile Supplies
274 Prosthetic/Orthotic Devices
275 Pacemaker Drug
276 Intraocular Lens Source Drug
278 Other Implants
279 Other M&S Supplies
280 Oncology
289 Other Oncology
290 Durable Medical Equipment
343 Diagnostic Radiopharms
344 Therapeutic Radiopharms
370 Anesthesia
371 Anesthesia Incident to Radiology
372 Anesthesia Incident to Other Diagnostic
379 Other Anesthesia
390 Blood Storage and Processing

Source: CMS 2005b; CMS 2006.

399   Other Blood Storage and Processing
560   Medical Social Services
569   Other Medical Social Services
621   Supplies Incident to Radiology
622   Supplies Incident to Other Diagnostic
624   Investigational Device (IDE)
630   Drugs Requiring Specific Identification, General Class
631   Single Source
632   Multiple
633   Restrictive Prescription
681   Trauma Response, Level I
682   Trauma Response, Level II
683   Trauma Response, Level III
684   Trauma Response, Level IV
689   Trauma Response, Other
700   Cast Room
709   Other Cast Room
710   Recovery Room
719   Other Recovery Room
720   Labor Room
721   Labor
762   Observation Room
810   Organ Acquisition
819   Other Organ Acquisition
942   Education/Training

Any other revenue codes that are billable on a hospital outpatient claim must contain a HCPCS code in order to assure payment under OPPS. FIs should return to provider (RTP), claims which contain revenue codes that require HCPCS when no HCPCS is shown on the line.

Part II

Monitoring for Excellence of Service Delivery

Chapter 7

Performance Management and Process Improvement

Anita Orenstein, RHIT, CCS, CCS-P

Effective management of processes in the coding department includes analyzing those processes and improving them to be efficient and adaptable. To be efficient, the coding function must be completed with the lowest possible use of resources. To be adaptable, it must respond to customers' changing requirements. Coding managers should ask themselves the following questions:

- Am I utilizing the coding staff's expertise to the fullest?

- Am I meeting the needs of the facility's customers?

This chapter helps answer those questions and provides the tools necessary to evaluate and improve current coding processes.

Process Improvement: Thinking out of the Box

"Out-of-the-box thinking" is an expression heard frequently in business situations. Often coding managers think that their current processes are the best—or the only—way to perform functions because they are the way things have "always been done." Using out-of-the-box thinking, or changing the paradigm, in relation to those processes may result in a more efficient way of doing things.

Over the years, many changes have occurred in the way health information management (HIM) departments carry out processes. The following examples illustrate some of these changes:

- HIM departments have gone from handwriting **master patient index (MPI)** information on index cards to using computerized MPI systems to using the enterprisewide MPI. The MPI is the link tracking patient, person, or member activity within an organization or enterprise and across patient care settings. The MPI identifies all patients who have been treated in a facility or enterprise and lists the health record or identification number associated with the name.

- The person responsible for reporting daily, monthly, and/or quarterly statistics once maintained those statistics in manual logs and calculated them by applying various formulas. Most facilities currently maintain statistics through automated system logs from which a detailed report of the statistics, along with graphic illustrations, results.

- In the past, coders reviewed the face sheet of a health record and assigned codes based on the final diagnoses and procedures listed on it by the physician. Now, coders analyze the entire health record and assign ICD-9-CM and CPT codes based on physician documentation and the application of official coding guidelines.

Change is all about process improvement: how to complete required tasks more efficiently and with the greatest accuracy possible. The three changes just mentioned, as well as many others, were made because coding professionals changed their paradigms by thinking out of the box.

Change Management

Change can be a difficult concept for some people because they are comfortable in their daily routines. For example, most people have a regular morning routine. It might consist of showering, getting dressed, having breakfast at home, and driving to work. If that routine is interrupted one day because the car is unavailable, the affected individual might have to take the bus to work. To save time, he or she might take a mug of coffee and something to eat on the bus. At first, this change in routine does not feel comfortable. Over time, however, the change becomes a new routine that may even become preferable to the old routine.

Change versus Transition

The terms *change* and *transition* are sometimes used interchangeably, although they have different meanings. Understanding the differences will help those involved in process improvement to move forward with a more positive attitude. Change occurs when something starts or stops, or when something that was done one way is now done in another way. Change can occur all at once or in phases.

Transition, on the other hand, is a psychological process that extends over a period of time. The following three phases take place in any transition process:

- Phase one: Letting go

- Phase two: The neutral zone

- Phase three: A new beginning

Phase One: Letting Go

In phase one, staff members have to let go of the old situation and the old identity that went with it. However, they often have difficulty letting go of responsibilities for which they once took ownership. In phase one, people have several feelings. Table 7.1 illustrates some feelings of loss as well as possible solutions.

Sometimes people seem to be resisting change when, in reality, they are struggling with phase one of the transition. It can help to identify continuities that balance the losses and to reemphasize new connections to new processes. While people are in mourning over the old process, certain behaviors, such as denial, anger, bargaining, grief, and despair, should be expected. Those behaviors usually take place before final acceptance of the change.

Phase Two: The Neutral Zone

Phase two, referred to as the "neutral zone," is considered the heart of transition. This phase is a time of reorientation. Staff still experience feelings of "loss" and may be unclear about

Table 7.1.   Issues of loss and possible solutions

Loss Issue	Possible Solutions
Loss of turf	Emphasize "interest-based" rather than "position-based" status so that staff members feel they are equal.
Loss of attachments	Reattach staff through a process of team building.
Loss of meaning in an issue	Convert this to an information-based issue by confronting the problem rather than simply explaining the solution.
Loss of a competence-based identity	Train staff in new competencies.
Loss of control	Involve staff in creating the new process to compensate for the loss.

the new process. Feelings fluctuate between hopefulness and frustration. Staff sometimes may seem to be just going through the motions of the new process.

The neutral zone can be converted to an opportunity if staff members are given assistance in redefining themselves and their future direction. Coding managers should provide training to enhance staff members' current positions and to provide opportunities for career advancement.

Phase Three: A New Beginning

In phase three, staff may be involved in the following activities:

- Developing new competencies
- Establishing new relationships
- Becoming comfortable with new policies and procedures
- Constructing plans for the future
- Learning to think in new paradigms

Process Analysis: Work Imaging

Before starting a process analysis, coding managers should have a complete understanding of current coding processes. They should ask themselves the following questions:

- Can improvements be made to better utilize the existing staff?
- What noncoding functions does the coding staff complete?
- Is there a way to simplify the process and work "smarter" by eliminating and/or reassigning noncoding functions?

When the process has been defined, coding managers can establish productivity standards. They also can make a true analysis of the coding time required of full-time employees (FTEs) through a work-imaging study. A **work-imaging study** can be described in the following way:

- It is a snapshot of the current process that identifies potential areas for change in the process.

- It quantifies opportunities to improve the healthcare organization's structure.

- It shows where to consolidate functions and responsibilities.

Design and Documentation of a Work-Imaging Study

Designing a work-imaging study need not take a great deal of time or planning. Coding managers simply create a comprehensive list of functions that the current coding staff completes. After they have created the list, they develop a worksheet that documents the "imaging" of each coder's workday. (See table 7.2.)

The coders then complete the worksheet. They document the time they spend each day on functions, as shown in table 7.2. Documentation of functions for 1 to 2 weeks provides a solid foundation for the study.

Analysis of the Work-Imaging Study

When the coders have completed their worksheets, the coding manager calculates the percentage of time spent on each function listed on the worksheets. In the example shown in figure 7.1, only 44 percent of the coders' time was spent on actual coding and abstracting functions. The other functions may be viewed as barriers to the coding process.

The Process Redesign/Improvement Team

The coding team should be involved in process redesign. Because coders have fundamental knowledge of the coding process, they are vital to the success of process redesign activities. It is important to empower staff members to change processes and then to recognize them for their part in the improvements. In addition, staff members accept change much easier when they have been part of the decision-making process for change. By being part of the process

Table 7.2. Work-imaging worksheet

Activity	Monday	Tuesday	Wednesday	Thursday	Friday
Coding and abstracting					
Filing records					
Retrieving records					
Assisting physicians					
Assisting department "walk-ins"					
Locating documentation					
Attending meetings					
Responding to business office questions and issues					
Communicating with physicians					
Attending training					
Performing quality reviews					
Other (specify)					

Figure 7.1. Breakdown of coders time

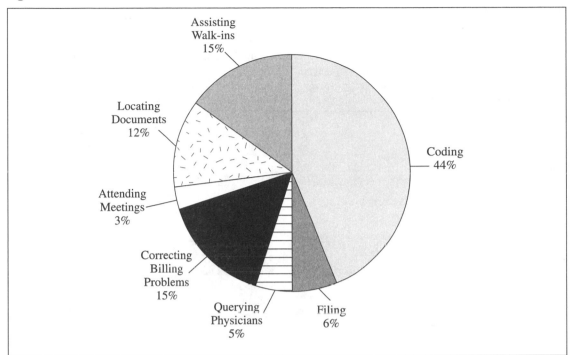

redesign team, the coding staff also will have an easier time going through the early phases of the transition period.

The first step in process improvement is to assemble the team. Table 7.3 lists the members of the **process improvement team** and their respective functions.

The team's success depends on the following seven key elements:

- Establishing ground rules

- Stating the team's purpose/mission

- Identifying customers and their requirements

- Documenting current processes and identifying barriers

- Collecting and analyzing data

- Identifying possible solutions by brainstorming

- Making recommendations for changes in the coding process

Establishing Ground Rules

Ground rules must be agreed on at the very beginning. All members of the team should have input into the ground rules. They should agree to abide by them for the sake of the team's success. Some ground rules that team members should consider are:

- To arrive on time for meetings

- To complete and present the results of assignments from the previous meeting

Table 7.3. The process improvement team

Team Member	Responsibility
Facilitator Does not need the fundamental knowledge of the team members; may be from another department but needs to know performance improvement processes with training and/or experience in facilitating teams in the past	Trains team on performance improvement Remains neutral Is a nonvoting member Makes suggestions Coaches and is a motivator Recognizes team/individual achievements Keeps team on track
Team Leader Is recognized as leader and organizer of the group	Works with facilitator and guides team to plan and coordinate the work of the team • Provides direction • Initiates activities • Encourages members • Contributes ideas • Interprets data • Makes assignments • Schedules meetings • Creates the agenda
Team Members Associated together in their work activity with a fundamental knowledge of the work and process	Identifies current processes and barriers Participates in decision making Identifies opportunities for improvement
Timekeeper	Keeps track of, and calls time remaining on, each agenda item
Recorder	Is responsible for taking minutes

- To respect the opinions of all team members
- To listen to other team members' points of view without criticism
- To abide by decisions made by the team

Stating the Team's Purpose/Mission

The team must answer this question: Why has this team been formed? The team must define its mission in order to create a "map" or plan. For the team in this example, the purpose may be stated as: To meet customers' needs by improving the coding process through better use of the skills, expertise, and time of HIM coders.

Identifying Customers and Their Requirements

The process improvement team must identify the customers associated with the coding process. Such a customer is anyone who uses coded data, for whatever purpose. Customers are both internal (for example, the facility's business office) and external (for example, third-party payers). The process improvement team identifies all these customers and what their requirements are.

Having identified its customers, the team works toward modifying the coding process to meet the customers' requirements. Table 7.4 identifies possible internal and external customers and their requirements that relate to coding functions.

Table 7.4.   Customers of the coding process and their requirements

Internal Customers	Requirements
Business office	Timely and accurate billing
	Timely responses to queries regarding billing issues
Physicians	Availability of chart for completion as soon as possible after discharge, including any necessary coding query forms
	Accurate coded data
External Customers	**Requirements**
Third-party payers	Timely and accurate bills
HIM department	Procedure that will not disrupt the record completion processes
Administration/finance	Discharge to coding within 4 days
	Accurately coded data

Documenting Current Processes and Identifying Barriers

The process improvement team members work together to discuss and document current coding processes. For this step, the team's knowledge is vital because members must answer the following questions:

- What is the current coding process?
- Where are the start and end points of the process?
- What are the barriers to the coding process?

A diagram of a typical coding process with its barriers is shown in figure 7.2.

The team also must consider other functions that affect the coding process. Team members should include the following questions in their evaluation:

- When does the health record arrive in the HIM department after the patient is discharged?
- How is the health record brought to the HIM department?
- What mechanism is in place to ensure that all discharges are sent daily to the HIM department?
- Who in the HIM department is responsible for ensuring that all discharges have been received?
- How soon are health records assembled?
- How soon are they analyzed?
- At what point are health records available to the coders?
- How are the health records made available for the coders?
- When coders have questions for physicians, is there a procedure in place for the health record to be routed back to the coders for completion?
- Who is responsible for locating documentation in the health record that is missing and needed for coding, such as laboratory results and dictation?

Figure 7.2. Typical coding process

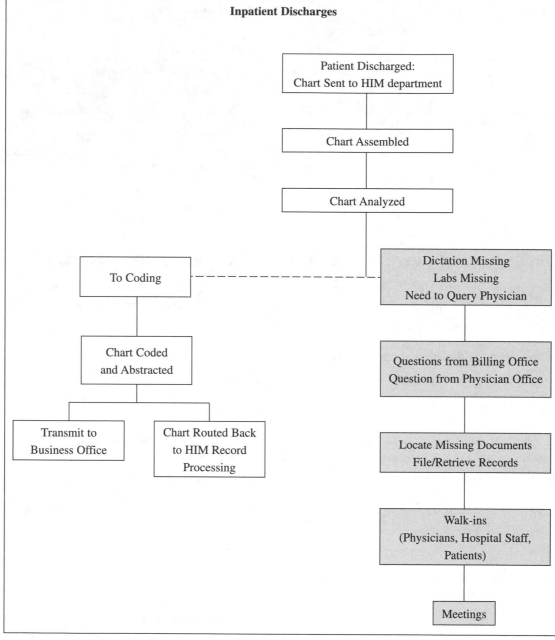

Note: Grey shading incidates barriers to the coding process.

- Do coders have access to the electronic health record?

- What is the turnaround time for transcription?

- Do coders have access to dictation prior to its being transcribed?

- When coding is complete, what is the process for routing the health records back to the HIM department for completion?

- Is concurrent coding performed? If so, what is that process?

Collecting and Analyzing Data

Earlier in this chapter, a sample analysis of the coding process began with collecting data from a work-imaging study. The sample study identified barriers to the coding process. When the barriers are identified and the coding process is changed, data then can be recalculated to show a true picture of how much time will be available to coders for coding. Additional data can be acquired through benchmarking and productivity studies, which are discussed later in this chapter.

The sample work-imaging study indicated that coders spent a significant percentage of time on noncoding functions. The process improvement team should consider assigning those noncoding functions to other HIM department staff. At this point in the process, the team should request that a member of the HIM clerical staff join the team. That person's perspective and knowledge will be helpful in reassigning noncoding functions.

The noncoding functions often can be integrated into the existing clerical functions without the hiring of additional staff. In the event that additional staff is required, a clerical position is easier to fill, is less costly, and requires less training than a coding position.

When noncoding functions are allocated to the clerical staff, the percentage of time that coders spend on coding functions should increase, as illustrated in figure 7.3. The data on the graph in figure 7.3 represent a 33 percent increase in time spent on coding.

Identifying Possible Solutions by Brainstorming

Brainstorming is a useful technique that promotes creative thinking as team members identify possible solutions for process improvement. During brainstorming, the team generates new, potentially useful ideas. Brainstorming requires team members to follow four basic ground rules:

- Welcome all ideas. During brainstorming, no judgments are made about ideas presented—there are no wrong or ridiculous proposals.

Figure 7.3. **Use of coders' time after allocating noncoding functions to clerical staff**

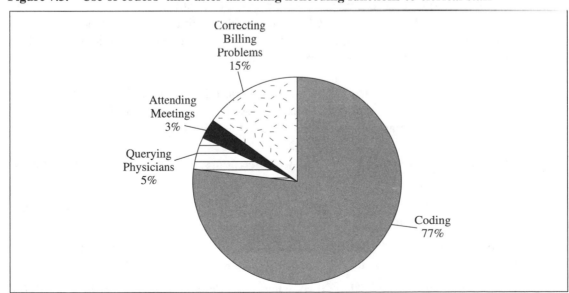

- Be creative in contributions. Think out of the box! Because change involves risk taking, it is important to be open to new ideas. Every person's point of view is valuable. Team members should be encouraged to say whatever occurs to them as a solution, no matter how far-fetched it may seem. Far-fetched ideas may trigger more practical ones and, in some cases, present valid solutions.

- Attempt to contribute a large quantity of ideas in a short amount of time. The more ideas there are, the more likely it is that there will be several useful ones.

- "Piggyback" on one another's ideas. Team members should feel free to combine ideas and to add to or build on the ideas of others to create combinations, improvements, or variations.

Recommendations for Process Change

The process improvement team is responsible for putting the outcome of its work in a report format, along with recommendations for improving the coding process. The recommendations are finalized after all data have been received and analyzed. These data include findings from the benchmarking study (discussed in the next section of this chapter) as well as from productivity measurements. The recommendations should take into account anything that might have an impact on the organization, such as:

- Utilization of staff

- Effect on the budget

- Change in productivity

- Number of days in accounts receivable

- Effects on customer requirements

Benchmarking

The goal of benchmarking is to increase performance by identifying best practices, measuring and comparing a selected work process, and conducting interviews with the benchmark organization or organizations. Opportunities for process improvement can be identified where best practice has been applied in other organizations. A benchmark organization is usually a competitor of similar size.

Before embarking on a benchmarking project, coding managers should determine the criteria or indicators for the benchmark comparison. Areas they should consider and questions they should ask the benchmark organizations include the following:

- How many coder hours, not including overtime hours, does each of the facilities budget for full-time employees?

- What is the average number of health records coded per day per hour by patient type, such as inpatient, outpatient surgical, ancillary, and emergency department?

- What standards does the facility expect coders to meet for both productivity (health records per day) and quality (percentage of accuracy)?

- Is the coding staff credentialed? If so, what type of credentials are represented—RHIT, RHIA, CCA, CCS, CCS-P, CPC, CPC-H, or other?

- Does the organization have a coding incentive plan?

- What is the compensation rate for coding professionals? Are there different compensation levels that depend on experience, mastery-level credential (CCS, CCS-P), and quality and productivity rates?

- Does the organization use contracted services to perform coding?

- Are coders abstracting was well as coding, or are those functions performed separately?

- Who performs quality monitoring? Does the coding supervisor conduct it, or are auditors/quality monitors applied by external reviewers? What are their responsibilities? How frequent are the reviews?

- How many lead coders does the facility have? What are their responsibilities?

- Do coders have clerical support? If so, for what functions?

- What is the facility's case-mix index (CMI)? In benchmarking, knowing the CMI is essential because it is the closest measure for comparing like faculties. CMI is used as a measurement for inpatients. It is the sum of all patient encounters' relative weight, based on DRGs divided by the number of all encounters. The higher the CMI, the more complex the records; therefore, the higher the CMI, the lower the expected productivity. (See chapter 12 for a detailed discussion of the CMI.)

Coding managers can request this information from hospitals of similar size to their own. After the information has been returned, coding managers can compare and analyze the data. Figures 7.4 through 7.9 show graphic representations of example benchmark results. Hospital A, hospital B, and hospital C represent the benchmark organization. The Home Hospital is the facility conducting the study.

Figure 7.4 represents a section of the work-imaging study and displays the percentage of time coders spend on coding and abstracting functions. Figure 7.5 benchmarks the inpatient

Figure 7.4. Work-imaging benchmark

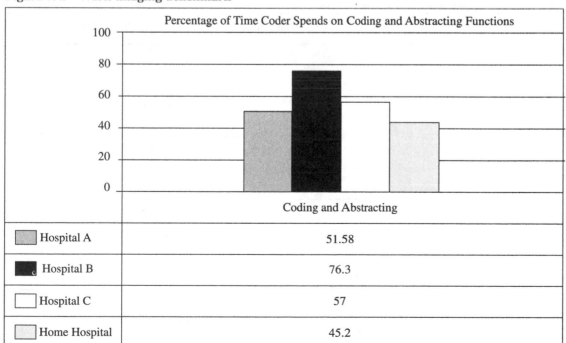

	Coding and Abstracting
Hospital A	51.58
Hospital B	76.3
Hospital C	57
Home Hospital	45.2

coding standards for coders (per day) in each of the facilities. Figure 7.6 graphically illustrates the number of FTE hours for each facility, along with the Medicare CMI. Figure 7.7 displays differences in actual FTE coding hours and budgeted coding hours. The differences may be due to vacant positions or time off due to illness or maternity leave; one of the facilities had a coder called to active duty in the military. The line graph illustrates the average discharged not final billed (DNFB) for that facility. The graph in figure 7.8 shows inpatient coding staffing related to the number of inpatient discharges. Figure 7.9 displays the number of coding supervisors and/or auditors for each facility.

Figure 7.5.   Inpatient coding standard benchmark

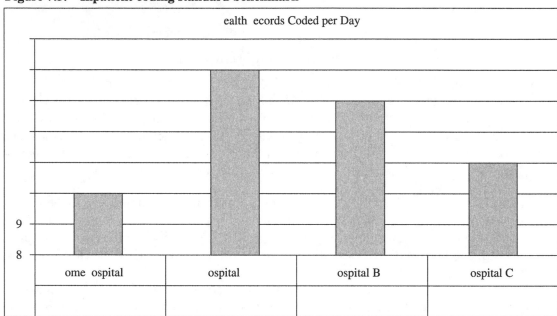

Figure 7.6.   Benchmark: FTE hours and CMI

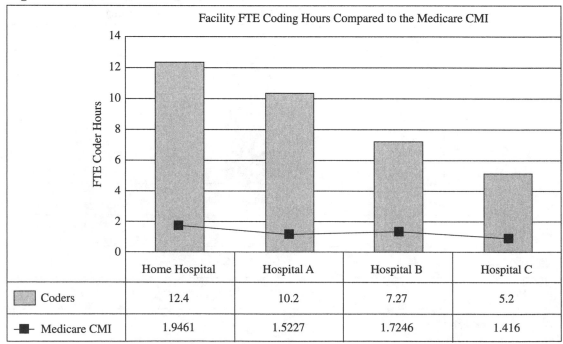

	Home Hospital	Hospital A	Hospital B	Hospital C
Coders	12.4	10.2	7.27	5.2
Medicare CMI	1.9461	1.5227	1.7246	1.416

Analysis of the benchmark data is critical. Now, how can the data be used? An analysis of figures 7.4 through 7.9 results in the following conclusions, each of which is followed by questions the home hospital may want to address with the other facilities:

- Hospital B spends a significantly higher amount of time on the coding and abstracting functions. What steps has hospital B taken to enable coders to spend 76.3 percent of their day on coding and abstracting?

Figure 7.7. Benchmark: Coding hours and DNFB averages

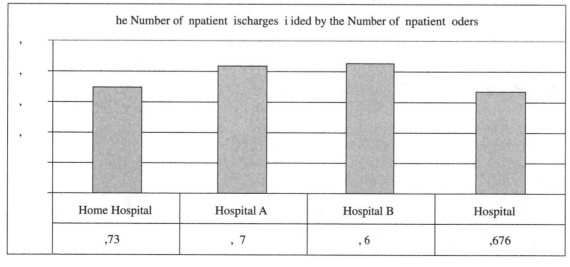

	Home Hospital	Hospital A	Hospital B	Hospital C
Budgeted Coding Hours	68.2	51.4	50.3	38.2
Actual Coding Hours	58.9	51	30.0	27.8
Average DNFB	15.04	14.77	3.52	4.95

Figure 7.8. Benchmark: Coder productivity per discharged inpatient

Home Hospital	Hospital A	Hospital B	Hospital
,73	, 7	, 6	,676

Figure 7.9. Benchmark: Coding supervisors and auditors

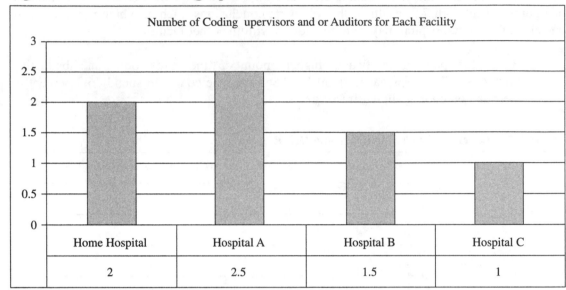

	Home Hospital	Hospital A	Hospital B	Hospital C
	2	2.5	1.5	1

- How were inpatient coding standards developed for each facility? It would be difficult to determine the appropriate standard without that vital information. Was the CMI included in development of the standards?

- Figure 7.6 (p. 202) can be very helpful when analyzing the number of inpatient coders and the relationship to the CMI. It could be assumed that the higher the CMI, the more difficult the charts and the more numerous the coders. However, hospital B has the second highest CMI and yet is staffed with only 7.27 coders. The fact that this hospital's work-imaging study revealed that its coders spent 76.3 percent of their time on coding and abstracting may account for their ability to complete more coding with fewer FTEs.

- Figure 7.7 (p. 203) further demonstrates that hospital B seems to have the best practice in place. Although it is understaffed, it is maintaining low DNFB days at only 3.52 average DNFB days. The analysis of figure 7.8 reveals that hospital B has the second highest ratio of discharges per coder. This may indicate that the coders at hospital B are working more productively.

- Hospital B clearly has been identified as having best practice in the management of its coding functions. The home hospital should consider discussing processes with hospital B so that it can identify and duplicate best practice.

Productivity Standards

When the coding process has been refined, the process improvement team can establish productivity standards. As in the analysis of the coding process, the coding staff's current productivity must be determined. The team can use a productivity measurement worksheet, as shown in table 7.5, to capture the number of health records coded per day.

Each coder should complete a daily worksheet, such as the one in table 7.5, for a specified time period (1 or 2 weeks). After the coders have recorded those data, the team can calculate the average number of health records coded per hour by record type. This calculation provides a baseline of current productivity levels.

Evaluating Coding Staff Productivity

The next step in establishing productivity standards is to evaluate how the productivity of the Home Hospital's coding staff compares with that of other facilities of similar size and case mix. Figure 7.10 illustrates a comparison of standards from the benchmarking study (figure 7.5, p. 202) with the average coding productivity of each of the four hospitals.

Figure 7.11 presents a comparison of the coding productivity standard with the CMI of each hospital. A review of this comparison shows that:

- Hospital A has the lowest CMI with the highest productivity. This makes sense because the lower the case mix, the less complicated the records

- Hospital B does not meet its productivity standard and has the highest CMI in the benchmark study. This may indicate that its standards should be reevaluated.

- Hospital C exceeds its standard; but in relationship to its CMI, the standard may be too low.

Table 7.5. Productivity measurement worksheet

Date:	Number Coded	Time Spent Coding (hours/minutes)
Inpatient records		
Outpatient surgical records		
Emergency department records		
Ancillary records		

Figure 7.10. CMI compared with productivity standard

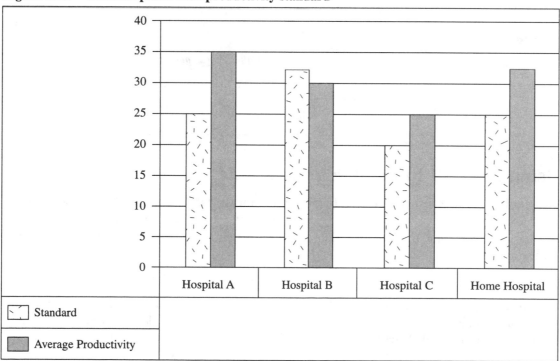

Figure 7.11. Required coding hours per day based on volume

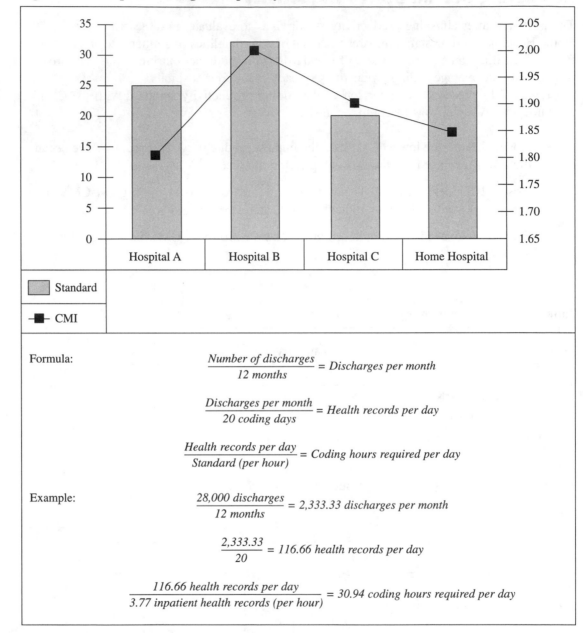

Formula:

$$\frac{Number\ of\ discharges}{12\ months} = Discharges\ per\ month$$

$$\frac{Discharges\ per\ month}{20\ coding\ days} = Health\ records\ per\ day$$

$$\frac{Health\ records\ per\ day}{Standard\ (per\ hour)} = Coding\ hours\ required\ per\ day$$

Example:

$$\frac{28,000\ discharges}{12\ months} = 2,333.33\ discharges\ per\ month$$

$$\frac{2,333.33}{20} = 116.66\ health\ records\ per\ day$$

$$\frac{116.66\ health\ records\ per\ day}{3.77\ inpatient\ health\ records\ (per\ hour)} = 30.94\ coding\ hours\ required\ per\ day$$

Using the CMI to Establish Standards

The coding manager of the Home Hospital now must establish its standards. For purposes of an example, the average productivity for inpatient coders at Home Hospital is 24 health records per day. One method of calculating the productivity standard uses the following formula:

$$CMI \times 12.5 = lower\text{-}limit\ productivity\ rate\ from\ which\ to\ build$$

For example, referring to figure 7.5 (p. 202), the calculation for the health records per hour based on this calculation would be reflected in figure 7.6. This methodology is especially useful in multisystem hospitals because using the CMI formula "levels the playing field."

Using these figures as a base for the standard, the coding manager can create a range for acceptable productivity levels. For example, the range for Home Hospital may be from 23.25 to 26 health records per day. This range is consistent with national studies in which the average standard for inpatient coders is 31 health records per day, with a range of 20 to 60 per day. An average productivity rate greater than 26 health records per day may warrant recognition in the form of an incentive and/or be reflected on the annual performance appraisal.

Considering Factors Other Than CMI

The CMI is not the only factor the coding manager must consider when establishing a productivity standard for coders. For example, if coders do not abstract the health record, the coding manager would have to adjust the formula to allow for that. The same would be true if the facility had an extensive database that required considerable abstracting. In that case, the CMI would be multiplied by a smaller number.

The CMI cannot be utilized for same-day surgical, emergency department, or ancillary records. In those cases, coding managers use the averages from the benchmarking study to compare their own hospital's productivity with that of hospitals of the same size and case mix. In this context, case mix would indicate the probability of similar patient encounters. For example, if the average range for same-day surgical records were 21 to 80 records per day, a coding manager might determine that coders should maintain a range of 40 to 55 records per day.

Coding Volume Analysis

After the analysis of the current coding process has been conducted and its redesign has taken place, the coding manager must ask this question: How many coders does the HIM department need? Coding managers often respond to increases in accounts receivable days by either hiring additional coders or outsourcing work. Either response is an easy way to solve the problem, but neither may be the most cost-effective solution.

Calculating Required Coding Hours

The first step in determining the number of coders needed is to calculate the HIM department's needs based on volume. The formula in figure 7.11 calculates the required coding hours per day for 28,000 inpatient discharges per year when the facility's standard is 3.77 inpatient health records per hour.

The same formula can be applied to each patient type using the number of discharges per year and the number of health records per hour.

Calculating Required Number of Coders

When calculating the number of coders needed to meet the required coding hours per day, the coding manager uses the number of annual budgeted hours per coder minus the number of hours per year that each coder accrues for vacation, sick leave, and training. The coding manager also should use the data gained from the work image during the process redesign.

The data in figure 7.3 showed that after the coding process was redesigned, coders spent an average of 77 percent of their time coding. This equals 6.16 coding hours per day per coder. If the coding manager divides the 23.5 health records per day (figure 7.5) by 6.16 hours, the result is 3.77 health records coded per hour per coder.

Figure 7.12 illustrates a formula for calculating the number of coder hours per day available for coders who spend 77 percent of their time on coding functions. The example is based on five full-time coders, each eligible for 600 hours of vacation/sick leave and 40 hours of training.

Figure 7.11 shows that the required coding hours required per day is 30.94 hours; figure 7.12 shows that 30.8 coder hours are available per day. In this example, the HIM department has an adequate number of coders to meet its coding volume requirements.

How did redesigning the coding process help the department meet its volume requirements? In the work-imaging study, only 44 percent of coder time was spent on coding and abstracting. In figure 7.13, the formula from figure 7.12 is applied to calculate the number of coder hours available at 44 percent productivity. If process improvement had not taken place, the HIM department would have been short by 13.2 hours a day, or more than one full-time coder.

Figure 7.12. Required number of coders per day

Formula: This calculation involves multiplying the annual hours per coder (a) by the number of FTEs (b) in the department to arrive at total annual hours (x) for the staff as a whole. From this number, vacation and sick hours (c) and training hours (d) are subtracted to arrive at the total available hours per year (y). This number is then multiplied by the applicable productivity rate as a percentage (e) to determine the number of productive coding hours for the staff (z), and the calculation is reduced from an annual to a daily figure to arrive at coder hours available per day.

$$a \times b = x$$

$$(x - c) - d = y$$

$$\frac{y \times e}{12 \ months} = z$$

$$\frac{z}{20 \ coding \ days} = Coder \ hours \ available \ per \ day$$

Example:

$$a = 2,080, \ b = 5, \ c = 600, \ d = 200, \ e = 77\%$$

$$2,080 \times 5 = 10,400$$

$$10,400 - 600 - 200 = 9,600$$

$$\frac{9,600 \times 77\%}{12} = 616$$

$$\frac{616}{20} = 30.8 \ coder \ hours \ available \ per \ day$$

Figure 7.13. Coder hours available based on 44 percent of time spent on coding functions

$$a = 2,080, \ b = 5, \ c = 600, \ d = 200, \ e = 44\%$$

$$2,080 \times 5 = 10,400$$

$$10,400 - 600 - 200 = 9,600$$

$$\frac{9,600 \times 44\%}{12} = 352$$

$$\frac{352}{20} = 17.6 \ coder \ hours \ available \ per \ day$$

Staff Development

Staff development means more than just training. True staff development emphasizes personal growth and improvement of employee potential. It maximizes the employees' contributions, improves performance, provides motivation, and improves morale. Training opportunities abound for coding staff. Education is a fundamental element for developing excellent coders. When determining productivity standards and staffing requirements, coding managers should add time for educational opportunities to the equation. Too often, managers believe that training/education takes too much time or is not covered in the budget. Astute HIM managers realize that they cannot afford not to provide continuing training for their coders.

Benefits of Continued Education/Training

A well-trained coding staff helps ensure complete and accurate coding, which is essential for the integrity of the data collected. Precise coding helps ensure compliance with regulatory requirements (discussed in chapter 9) and helps facilitate consistency of coding in the health-care facility.

In addition, coders consider training as an enhancement to their job. Coding professionals take pride in their work and welcome the opportunity to gain knowledge and skill. Organizations that provide continuing education take an additional step in retaining qualified coders.

In-House Training

In-house training programs presented by physicians or clinical department staff on complicated diagnoses, disease processes, and surgical procedures help coders learn to assign the most accurate codes. In addition, the interaction between clinical staff and coders helps cultivate a relationship for better communications. It also affords physicians the opportunity to learn about coding guidelines and regulatory requirements. Additionally, in-house training is an ideal way to communicate to physicians how documentation plays a role in code assignment, the payment process, and compliance issues.

How does a coding manager determine the kind of training to present to the coding staff? Much depends on the findings of quality reviews. (See chapter 8.) Managers can use quality review findings to identify trends and issues that could be addressed in training, such as:

- Complex DRGs
- Disease processes
- Surgical procedures
- Prospective payment systems
- Coding criteria and guidelines
- Laboratory values
- Compliance requirements and regulatory issues

Complex DRGs

Presentations on complex DRGs should include the etiology and manifestations of conditions, along with related complications. For example, a presentation on complex DRGs 575 and 576,

Septicemia, age 18 or older, could include the difference between septicemia, urosepsis, and a urinary tract infection. That presentation also would include the etiology and manifestations for septicemia, abnormal laboratory values, and treatment options.

Moreover, coders must be aware of the coding guidelines related to assigning complex diagnosis codes. An in-house training presentation for the DRGs related to pneumonia could include the following information:

- The etiology, manifestations, and complications of pneumonia, such as respiratory failure

- The diagnosis and treatment of pneumonia

- Official coding guidelines related to pneumonia and complications of pneumonia

- The differences between DRG 089, Simple pneumonia, and DRG 079, Respiratory infections and inflammations, age 18 or older, with CC

- Common errors in assigning DRG 079, including inappropriately assigning "other specified" bacterial pneumonia

Disease Processes

For coders to have a complete understanding of a disease process, reviews should include:

- The etiology, manifestations, and therapeutic and surgical treatments

- Examples of surgical cases for coding

- The ICD-9-CM and CPT coding guidelines for both diagnoses and procedures

Surgical Procedures

Surgical procedures, especially those that are difficult to code, should be reviewed in detail. For example, in coding sinus surgery, a review of the anatomy, physiology, and pathophysiology of the sinuses is valuable in understanding the surgical procedures.

Prospective Payment Systems

How prospective payment systems affect coding is another important topic for in-house training. HIM department coders need a thorough understanding of how DRG results are reported and how they affect the CMI. The accuracy of coding and sequencing absolutely affects DRGs and the CMI, and has a far-reaching impact on healthcare organizations.

Training regarding the CMI should include the following information:

- Finance departments use the CMI for many purposes, such as budgeting for staff and capital expenses, internal and external reporting, planning, clinical programs, and numerous other resources.

- The CMI also can influence coding productivity. That is, an increase in CMI may be indicative of more complicated health records that require more time for complete and accurate coding.

Training for outpatient prospective payment systems (OPPS) could include the following information:

- Ambulatory payment classifications (APCs), the OPPS for Medicare, were implemented in August 2000.

- Outpatient encounters are put into APC groups that, like DRG groupings, are based on the amount of resources they are likely to require.

- Unlike DRGs, multiple APCs can be assigned during a single encounter.

- Comprehensive knowledge of CPT codes, hospital-approved modifiers, and the application of Correct Coding Initiative (CCI) edits are essential for appropriate APC assignment.

Coding Criteria and Guidelines

To ensure consistency of coding, coding managers must make sure that all coders receive up-to-date coding criteria and guidelines. This is especially true for guidelines that are not published in the official coding guidelines or as supplements to the official guidelines but that are requested by payers or other parties.

Physicians also should be involved in the development of criteria for assigning codes to clinical information. In-house training presentations should include demonstrations on the appropriate use of approved physician query forms.

Having skilled coding professionals highly involved in the process of developing and maintaining coding criteria greatly optimizes the opportunity for covering all significant coding areas. If a hospital is part of a multihospital system, the coding manager should organize a committee that develops or reviews such criteria to facilitate consistency among the entities. Both single-hospital and multihospital systems should be sure that all coders receive information consistently so that each coder has the same understanding of how to apply the criteria.

Laboratory Values

Understanding laboratory values helps coders arrive at the most accurate diagnosis code. However, it is inappropriate to code directly from any laboratory report. Instead, an abnormal report may indicate the need to query the physician for clarification or further documentation.

To help coders, in-house training on laboratory values could include the following information:

Quality Standards

A balance must be struck between increasing productivity and maintaining quality results. High output (productivity) is useless without quality data. Although 100 percent code assignment accuracy would be ideal, it is not realistic—many variables are part of the process.

Achieving Minimum Quality Standards

Quality standards should be high enough to validate the data, but achievable with some room for error. Each organization should determine the threshold for its minimum quality standards.

Figure 7.14 illustrates quality standards for inpatient coding compared with the current quality of coding. In this graph, a minimum of 95 percent accuracy is required for each category of coding. The desired accuracy rates vary from category to category. Between the minimum standard and the desired accuracy lies the range of acceptable quality for each category.

Meeting Desired Accuracy

The appropriate assignment of the principal diagnosis code is critical. This is especially true for inpatient coding because the principal diagnosis code usually drives the DRG and, in many cases, the corresponding payment. For this reason, the percentage of accuracy for coding principal diagnoses should be as close to 100 percent as possible. The graph in figure 7.14 shows a desired accuracy of 98 percent for coding principal diagnoses.

Figure 7.14. Current coding quality compared with standards

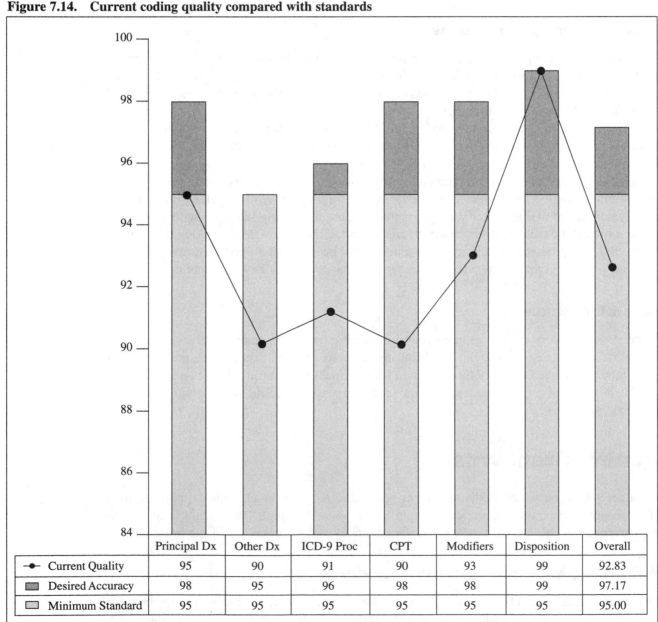

	Principal Dx	Other Dx	ICD-9 Proc	CPT	Modifiers	Disposition	Overall
Current Quality	95	90	91	90	93	99	92.83
Desired Accuracy	98	95	96	98	98	99	97.17
Minimum Standard	95	95	95	95	95	95	95.00

Other diagnosis codes are equally important but do not have the impact on payment or compliance that the principal diagnosis code has. When considering other or secondary diagnoses, coders must realize that the evaluation of CCs is critical, as well as those conditions that do not affect DRG payment. Other diagnoses may be categorized as being "weighted" because some codes are more crucial to capture than others. The quality standard for other diagnoses may therefore be lower than that of the principal diagnosis.

Phase-in Period for Quality Standards

When implementing quality standards, coding managers should phase in the accuracy requirement. They could establish small increments at 30-day intervals until each standard is met. During the phase-in period, coders should receive any training necessary to meet the accuracy requirements.

If the current accuracy rates are significantly lower than the minimum standard, coding managers must allow a long enough phase-in period for coders to meet the requirements. Similar to the program for training new coders, continuous monitoring may be required until coders meet the desired accuracy requirements

Beyond Coding in Managing Coding Services

Coding managers needs to step out of their role as managers of the daily coding workload to examine other factors that influence their ability to manage the coding functions. The coding team is dependent on their clerical counterparts to provide charts in a timely manner. Other considerations include scheduling for coverage and providing coders with workspace that is adequate and quiet enough for concentration on coding. With today's advancing technology, the workforce is demanding options such as telecommuting, and remote coding options can help retain and recruit qualified coders. All of these considerations are included in managing 'beyond' the coding function.

The Clerical Team

Why mention the clerical team in the management of the coding productivity chapter? Because the management of the DNFB is more than just coding! Workflow is a critical component in the management of both the coding and clerical teams. Without efficient chart processing, the coders will not have access to the patient record in a timely manner following discharge. Consider the following scenario of a 600-bed urban hospital.

Example:
The HIM department has coverage for first, second, and third shifts. The clerical staff is responsible for retrieving the health records on the second shift the day of discharge. During their shift, the staff is responsible for coverage of the department, filing of loose miscellaneous reports, and for reviewing the records that have been charted by physicians.

The first shift then assembles and analyzes the records that were retrieved the previous shift. Coders will then have those charts available to them for coding on the third day after discharge.

Figure 7.15 contains a cross-functional flow chart that illustrates the clerical functions and responsibilities for all three clerical shifts.

Figure 7.15. The clerical process

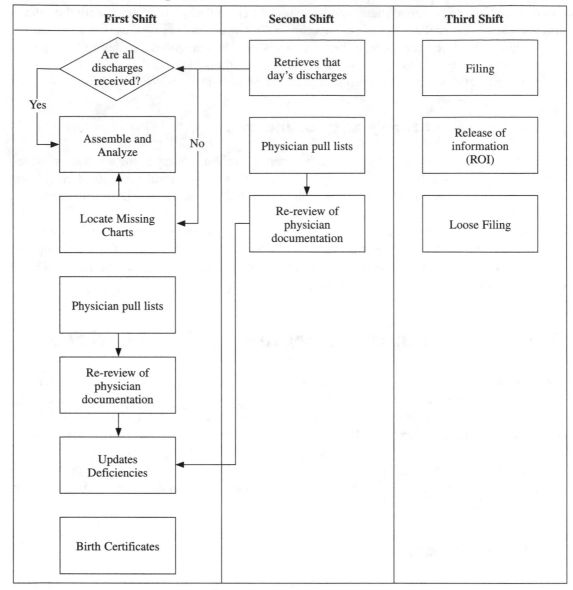

In order to ensure the coders have charts ready for coding the day after the patient's discharge, clerical processes and shift responsibilities must be revised. Figure 7.16 illustrates those changes in responsibilities and ensures that the coders have the health record on the morning following the patient's discharge, reducing the DNFB by 2 days.

Other Departments Affecting HIM Workflow

Other processes outside of HIM can have a dramatic effect on HIM operations and work-flow. It is critical for the coding manager to have an acute awareness of those processes and to collaborate with those other departments to refine processes to meet the needs of everyone involved. The example below shows how the charging processes in a 40-bed rural hospital affects the HIM department's ability to code emergency department (ED) encounters in a timely manner. This small rural facility sees approximately 25 patients daily in the ED.

Figure 7.16. The clerical process, revised

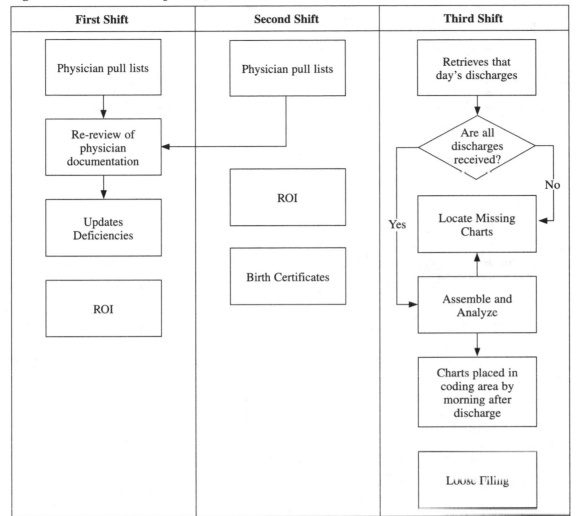

Example:

The HIM department has coverage for the day shift only and has 1.5 FTEs. The problem that this facility experiences involves the processing of ED records. The ED staffs only one nurse, and family practice physicians located within that community provide coverage on a rotating basis. "Borrowing" unit clerks from the nursing floor provides clerical staff when workload is heavy. Because staff is short, it was determined that the charging process would be completed following the patient encounter. As this made sense in terms of providing medical care with a limited staff, it did not necessarily make sense from a business-processing standpoint. Figure 7.17 is a flowchart that illustrates the charging process in this example. The business office is responsible for the charging process, but this passes through many "hands" before it finally arrives in the HIM department for coding up to 5 days following the patient encounter. Because the business office determines the charges based on the medical record documentation, a nurse must perform a quality check prior to coding. The nurse only works in the afternoon, which also slows the process. After process analysis and work redesign, a more efficient process is designed, allowing the HIM department to code for these encounters the day after discharge. Figure 7.18 illustrates that process.

Scheduling for Coverage

Although coders desire flexibility in schedules, a manager needs to keep in mind that coverage for all coding types need to be met. This can be a win-win situation for both the

Figure 7.17. ED charging process

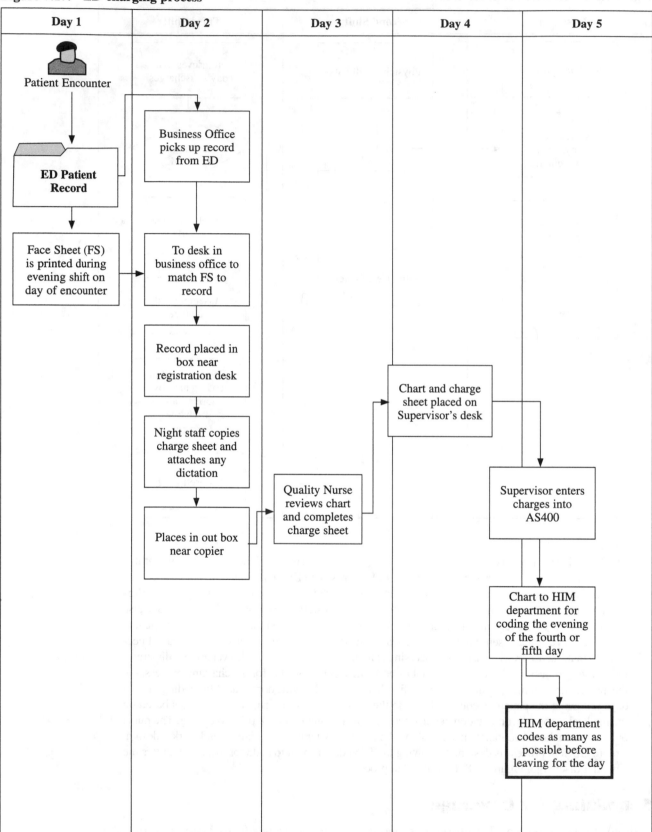

Figure 7.18. ED charging process, revised

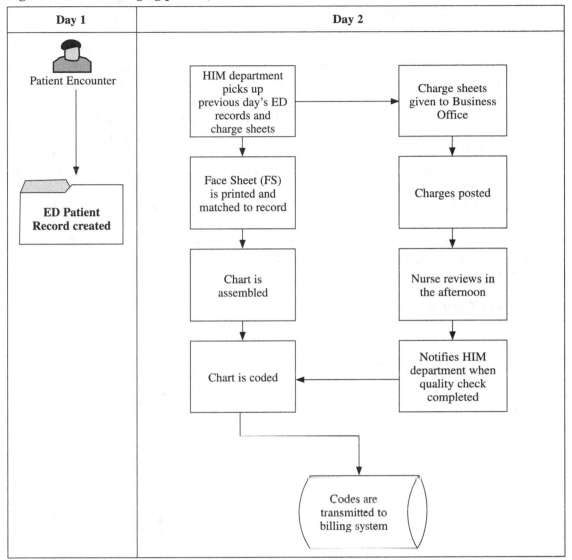

employee and the employer. Because coverage is critical in order to maintain low A/R (accounts receivable) days (or DNFB days), cross training of coders is highly desirable in order to provide coverage in all patient types. Once coders are cross-trained, schedules should be made that will enable the coder to code all patient types on a rotating basis. This allows the coder to maintain proficiency with all patient types and allows the manager to shift work assignments for coverage needs. For example, if there is an increase in outpatient surgery volumes, coding assignments can be made to allow for the volume adjustment without the concern of not having enough outpatient coders. Conversely, when an "inpatient" coder is out on maternity leave, inpatient coding can be assigned to any of the other coders because they are cross-trained.

The Physical Environment

Consider where the coders are located in the HIM department, ergonomic considerations, and flexibility in work schedules and in the work location.

Does it matter where a coder sits? You bet it does! Unlike many of the functions in the HIM department, coders need total concentration and an uninterrupted work area. Once the coder's work is interrupted, they will likely need to reread the chart, losing productivity in the process. When possible, coders should be in a room where they are totally away from the interruptions in the HIM department. With space issues this is not always possible and in those cases, the coding manager should attempt to have as much of a secluded environment as possible.

The example in figure 7.19 shows the office layout of a department with five coders. They are located in an area that is not conducive to interaction with other coders and is in the middle of the clerical work table and copy machine. There is a separate room in that area in which the clerical staff sits. Their responsibilities are the release of information and chart processing. By moving the coders into the clerical space and moving the clerical staff to the coder workstations, better workflow for the clerical team was achieved in addition to the confined workspace for the coders. Clerical staff now has ready access to the copy machine and worktable without interrupting the coding staff. This change is represented in figure 7.20. See chapter 1 for more information on the physical layout of the HIM department.

Figure 7.19. Office layout of a department with five coders

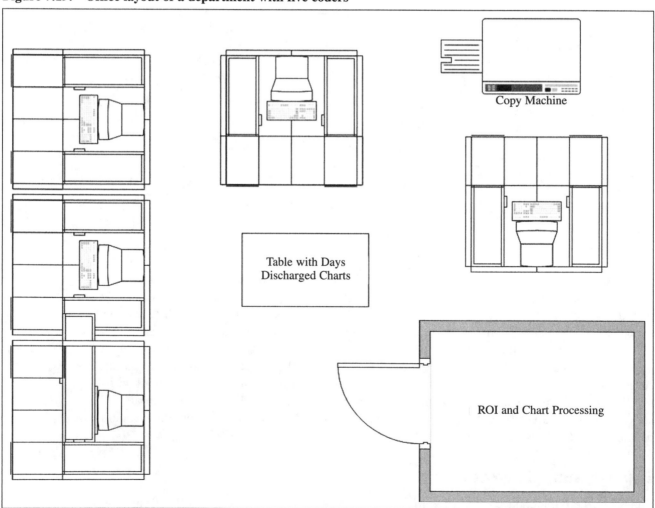

Copy Machine

Table with Days
Discharged Charts

ROI and Chart Processing

Figure 7.20. Office layout of a department with five coders, revised

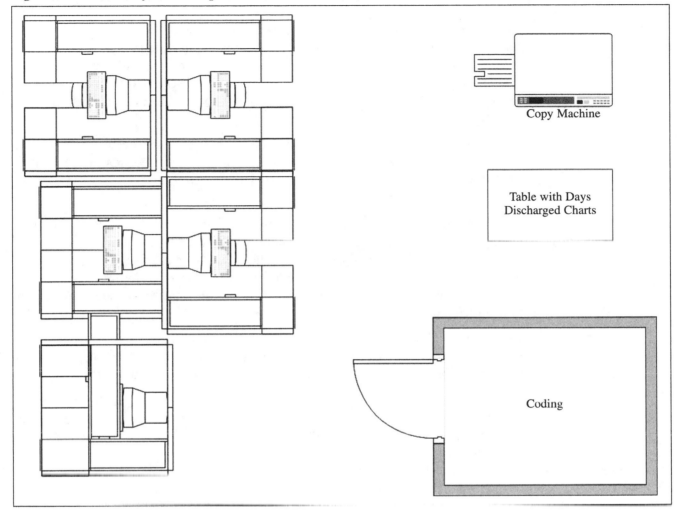

Remote Coding

What about flexibility in work location? Managers have been challenged to find ways to retain coders, utilize existing technology, and provide a more flexible work environment.

There are challenges to managing coding services, including high vacancy rates with 49% projected growth in the profession for the next 4 years. For those experienced coders with the mastery level credentials of CCS and CCS-P, competitive salaries that include sign-on and retention bonuses exist, making it difficult to attract those coders. Implementing a remote coding program is a long-term solution to coder recruitment and retention issues. Shortage of coders results in coding backlogs that result in increased DNFB. This creates the need to utilize outside coding contractors and overtime for coders. Although some coders may be delighted with the opportunity for additional money from the overtime hours, it is not welcome if it is required and for long periods of time. Coder burnout from overtime can result in lower productivity, lower quality, and job dissatisfaction.

Remote coding is an industry trend resulting from a national shortage of qualified clinical coders. It is also a quality of life issue for many qualified coders who would rather spend those additional 2 hours of travel time to and from work with their families.

There are numerous benefits to be realized from implementing a remote coding program:

- Possible increased productivity. This depends on various factors, including the number of additional noncoding activities the coder completed while in the hospital setting. In the case of a coder working from home, those activities cease to exist, allowing more time for coding. Unless the coder is accustomed to coding from an electronic record, there will be a learning curve where productivity is actually lower at first.

- Flexible scheduling. Many facilities have shortages of desk space and are not able to accommodate requests for first shift, and filling vacancies for second or third shift are more difficult. Having a remote coding program can offer flexibility to meet needs of the employees and the facilities.

- Eliminate outsourcing costs. Although outsourcing is an excellent option to provide coverage while experiencing short staffing or coding backlogs, it is much more costly than having the coding completed by the facility. There can also be dissatisfaction among coders when outsourcing services are utilized. Coders are aware of the costs for outsourcing and can sometimes resent the fact that the contracted coders make more money then they do.

- Reduce and maintain DNFB. Remote coding alone won't be able to accomplish this, but it is an important factor in the DNFB process. Provided all other processes are as efficient as possible, not having enough coders will still impact the DNFB.

- Improve coder morale. Everyone wants to feel they have a choice! As mentioned earlier, commute time, time with family, and flexibility in work schedule will all contribute to the coder's morale, which will help to retain those valuable coders and to recruit qualified, experienced coders.

When many hear the term "remote coding" the first thought is that of a home-based coder. This may very well be the case, as in most cases it is, but there are also other forms of remote coding.

Remote coding solutions can help to provide coverage in a variety of ways:

- Coders working from their home. This may include coders currently on staff who want to move to coding at home or it may be a coder hired to work from home who lives in another state.

- Remote coding may be utilized through contracted vendor services.

- Coders in a remote "smart site" or satellite office. An example of this would be a facility that is located in a large urban city where most coders would commute to work daily from the suburb. A smart site could be located in the suburb in which many of the coders live, saving valuable travel time for the coder.

- For multihospital organizations, remote coding may be coders working at their desk, but coding for another hospital—at the other side of town, the opposite end of the state, or in another state all together. Management of the DNFB and coverage for vacations, etc. would be improved with the ability to utilize coders from other hospitals in their system. Additionally, coders would already be familiar with the records, systems, and abstracting requirements.

Considerations

Like any other major initiative, implementing a remote coding project takes a great deal of research, coordination, and planning. Discussion and coordination with the information technology (IT) and human resources (HR) departments are vital in order to meet all the needs of a remote coding program. Some of those considerations are listed below.

Information Technology

- Connectivity: band-width for both uploading and downloading files varies greatly depending on the type of home connection available in the geographic area (DSL, cable, dial-up) and can also be affected by the wiring inside the home.

- Hardware: a decision must be made on who will be responsible for the purchase of the computer and hardware accessories. Will this be the facility or the employee? Will the coder need two monitors? One for viewing the record and a second for the coding and abstracting application?

- Software expenses: Coding and abstracting software costs will also need to be considered. Will these be the responsibility of the facility or the coder? Will there be a web-based application available?

- Technical support: initial set-up and maintenance of remote users is an ongoing concern for the IT department. Will they be responsible for troubleshooting in the remote site? Consider also issues such as inventory control, virus protection, updates, and patches: these are all necessary components for remote PC management.

Operational Management and Workflow

- Getting the information to the coder. How much of the medical record is currently electronic? If there is a paper or hybrid record, will those be scanned for coding? Will those be scanned into the clinical data repository or will a vendor be used for temporary storage while coding? Who will scan the records? How will they be indexed?

- How will work assignments be made and how will productivity be tracked?

- Security of home environment. Remote users will need to have adequate workspace that is safe, free from distraction, properly lighted, ventilated, furnished, and secure from incidental disclosures of protected health information.

- How will the coder attend coding department staff meetings? Will this be a requirement to meet in person or will web or phone conferencing be acceptable?

Human Resources

Working with HR to establish criteria for remote coders is critical prior to implementation to ensure that a fair and equitable program is in place.

Consider the following qualifications in determining policy:

- Productivity: Coders must meet minimum requirements for coding productivity for an established period of time prior to coding from home

- Quality: Coders must meet minimum requirements for coding quality standards for an established period of time prior to coding from home

- Status: Coders must be in good standing. Coders with formal disciplinary action may not be considered.

- Connectivity: Coders must have access to the internet and meet the IT requirements for remote coding

- Downtime: How will downtime be handled? When systems are down, how long will the facility pay the coder without coding productivity? Will the coder need to take personal time off or make up the time later?

- Dependent care: Telecommuting is not a substitute for dependent care (child or adult care). The remote coder should not be the primary caregiver during working hours.

Planning and Implementation

Once a decision has been made to pursue implementation of a remote coding program, a project team should be formed. This team would be responsible for creating and implementing the remote coding program. The team should be composed of the following members:

- Project manager (this individual should have experience with major projects, and have experience in facilitating the project team)

- HIM leadership

- Coding supervisor and/or coder(s)

- Support staff (clerical process)

- IT and HR departments

The process for the design and implementation of the remote coding program will be very similar to that process discussed earlier in this chapter. The project manager would be the facilitator and the team leader would likely be someone from HIM leadership.

Responsibilities of the team would include the following:

- The creation of the team's vision. This should be clear and concise, such as: "Implement remote coding programs as a solution to coder recruitment and retention and DNFB management".

- Establish goals with associated timelines.

- Review and recommend remote coding technology; this will require the evaluation of vendors for scanning and/or web-based applications.

- Assess current status for workflow issues and needs for scanning should that be needed.

- Develop a telecommuting policy

- Identify IT issues

- Determine what work types are to be included in the remote coding project (inpatient, outpatient surgery, emergency department encounters)

- Determine costs and present those to administration for justification of the project

Finally, the team will oversee the implementation and monitoring of the program. It is critical that IT be involved from the very start of the project through implementation. It is also a good idea to create a "virtual" home connection at the facility prior to sending a coder home so that IT may be able to identify connectivity issues. This will also give the coder an opportunity to work with IT troubleshooting before he/she leaves the hospital campus.

Should a healthcare facility determine that remote coding is a solution to the recruitment and retention issues they face, adequate time must be spent in making calculated decisions. Each decision should be based on evaluation, measurement and analysis, and coordination with the entire team. Only then can a successful remote coding program be implemented.

Conclusion

Coding professionals hold a unique position in today's healthcare systems. Healthcare facilities rely on coded data for a variety of statistical uses in addition to reporting codes for payment purposes. A fine balance exists between coding quality and coding productivity. How to maintain this balance has always been a subject of controversy and concern.

Members of a coding staff possess the fundamental knowledge to work together as a team to measure, analyze, and redesign current coding processes. Their involvement helps them appreciate the benefits that process improvement can bring to them as well as to the healthcare organization.

In managing the coding process, it is possible to both maximize coder resources and maintain optimal quality. Coding productivity is an important issue for the efficiency and profitability of a healthcare facility. Establishing quality standards is essential for adequately maintaining a coding staff that meets the needs of the facility's customers.

References and Resources

Bridges, W. 2003. *Managing Transitions: Making the Most of Change,* 2nd ed. Cambridge, MA: Da Capo Press.

Dunn, R. 2001 (April). Developing facility-specific productivity measures. *Journal of American Health Information Management Association* 72(4):73–74.

Dunn, R.T. 2001 (October). Putting productivity plans to work. *Journal of American Health Information Management Association* 72(9):96–100.

Dunn, R.T. 2002 (October). Turning production data into management tools. *Journal of American Health Information Management Association* 73(9):60–68.

Scichilone, R.A. 2006 (September). Coders wanted, experience required. *Journal of American Health Information Management Association* 77(8):46, 48.

Shaw, P.L., C. Elliott, P. Isaacson, and E. Murphy. 2007. *Quality and Performance Improvement: A Tool for Programmed Learning,* 3rd ed. Chicago: AHIMA.

Chapter 8

Quality Control Issues

Donna M. Fletcher, MPA, RHIA

Since implementation of the inpatient and outpatient prospective payment systems (PPSs) and use of data for performance improvement and organization accountability, the need for clinical information in the form of coded data has increased dramatically. The following entities base financial decisions on the information provided by coding professionals:

- Private audit/review organizations
- Third-party administrators
- Employers
- Fiscal intermediaries (FIs) for Medicare and selected other health plans
- Medicare's Hospital Payment Monitoring Program (HPMP)
- Commercial insurance groups

In addition, coded data are driving more and more healthcare industry decision making. This is evidenced by the many initiatives to capture data, such as the:

- Joint Commission on Accreditation of Healthcare Organization's (JCAHO's) ORYX core and non-core measures
- Outcome and Assessment Information Set (OASIS)
- Minimum Data Set (MDS) for long-term care
- National Committee for Quality Assurance's (NCQA) Health Plan Employer Data and Information Set (HEDIS)
- Agency for Healthcare Research and Quality (AHRQ) Patient Safety Indicators

These data are used within facilities to monitor performance improvement efforts and to improve outcomes. In addition, they are used comparatively among facilities as benchmarks and to inform consumers. These data sets have one thing in common: They draw on coded data as raw material for research and comparing patients and institutions with one another.

Consequently, the need for accurate and complete information has resulted in a close examination of the coding process within HIM departments. Practices, policies, staff qualifications, training, and types of quality control programs are critical elements in the data quality review process. In relation to coded data, **data quality reviews** are an examination of health records to determine the level of coding accuracy and to identify areas of coding problems.

As coding professionals face a transition in the reimbursement system of government programs, an accurate database for planning is critical. The data that coding professionals provide today will have a profound impact on future reimbursement. By completely and accurately describing the resources used for patients, coding professionals assure themselves that the database for reimbursement decisions is as detailed as possible. (See appendix 8.1 for an AHIMA practice brief on data quality.)

Additionally, health information professionals must meet the pressures of deadlines and of outside audit/review organizations. In doing so, they realize the critical need for adopting ethical practice standards. Recognizing that responsibility, the AHIMA Board of Directors approved standards of ethical coding in 1991 and revised them in December 1999. (See appendix 8.2 for the current coding standards.)

This chapter discusses the data quality review process and the staff responsibilities in that process. It explains the standard steps that coding supervisors and reviews should take in the review process in terms of both inpatient and outpatient review. The chapter also looks at various types of coding consultants and their use in the review process.

Ensuring Ongoing Data Quality Improvement

Quality, as it applies to coded data, means that the performance of the coding function within a HIM department is accomplished at the highest level of accuracy and efficiency possible. However, ensuring ongoing quality is complex due to factors that impact ICD-9 and CPT/HCPCS code assignment. These factors include the following:

- *Payers and Reimbursement*—Payers may require use of different groupers, such as CMS, state Medicaid, AP-DRGs, payer-specific or another grouper. Sequencing or code assignment in one grouper could result in higher reimbursement or case weight than the same sequencing or code assignment in another grouper. There may also be differences by payer on claims rejected due to selected code assignment.

- *Hospital and Physician Profiling*—Physicians are reluctant to document conditions or situations that have an adverse affect on hospital or physician profiling.

- *Medical Record Documentation*—Documentation factors that affect code assignment are the level of specificity, whether the documentation is that of a physician and whether the complete record is available at the time of coding (CHCA 2006, 3).

These factors further complicate the analysis and reporting of data and interpretation of data used to monitor data quality such as:

- Reimbursement to hospital
- Patient illnesses and related treatments, such as infection rates
- Resources required to treat patients
- JCAHO core and noncore measures

Goals of a Data Quality Improvement Program

The design and implementation of a data quality improvement program begin with setting the following goals:

- To establish an ongoing monitor for identifying problems or opportunities to improve the quality of coded data for inpatient and outpatient cases

- To determine the cause and scope of identified problems

- To set priorities for resolving identified problems

- To implement mechanisms for problem solving through the approval of corrective action plans

- To ensure that corrective action is taken by following up on problems with appropriate monitors

Assessing Data Quality

Coded data quality is the cornerstone of data integrity. Consequently, to direct improvement efforts, basic tenets in data quality management should be assessed to identify coded data issues. (See figure 8.1 for an example of a coded data quality assessment worksheet.) The assessment covers the following data quality management domains:

- Intent: The purpose for which the data are collected

- Collection: The process by which coded data are accumulated

- Warehousing: The processes and systems used to archive coded data

- Analysis: The process of translating coded data into actionable information

When the assessment is completed, a data quality improvement program is implemented to address identified issues.

Methods for Monitoring and Evaluating a Data Quality Improvement Program

The methods for monitoring and evaluation should be clarified in the data quality improvement program. Both internal and external data are important for performance evaluation. External data, such as Medicare inpatient and outpatient claims data, ground the evaluation in measurable industry norms and force hospitals to evaluate performance beyond "local experience." These data establish what is typical and how much variation there is around normal performance. Further, external data encourage hospitals to assess how they differ from the norm and how those differences might affect performance (Price 2005, 26–31).

Numerous documentation and coding areas, both inpatient and outpatient, should be incorporated in the data quality profile, including:

- Key OIG and QIO/HPMP target areas

- CC coding rates (DRGs)

- Medicare case-mix index (DRGs)

- Outpatient Code Editor failure rates

- Outpatient coding into APC levels

- Medicare Discounted Service Index (APCs)

- DRG and APC outlier payment rates (Price 2005, 26–31)

Figure 8.1.   Coded data quality assessment worksheet

Coded data quality is the cornerstone for data analysis and data integrity. To that end, the following checklist outlines basic tenets in data quality management. Use the worksheet to assess overall coded data quality management efforts. Ensure that each item:

• Has been documented clearly.
• Was implemented effectively.
• Is appropriate.
• Is currently in place.

Upon completion of the assessment, direct efforts appropriately to improve coded data quality.

Assessment Items	Considerations include, but are not limited to . . .
Intent—*The purpose for which the data are collected.*	
The purpose/intent/value or the aim for coded data is clear. Coded data are appropriate for the intent.	Confirm the purpose, intent, and value of coded data to validate the hospital's aim for collecting it. Are the data used for: • Comparison • ORYX • Opportunity analyses • Process improvement • Benchmarking • Other How do coded data support these uses?
Coding and classification system conventions are known and communicated.	• Coding conventions are communicated to data users and data analysts.
Coded data are complete.	• What coded data are not collected? • Are coded data collected for all patients? If not, what population of patients is excluded? • Who is responsible for coordinating the ongoing data collection process? • Does a secondary process need to be put in place to ensure collection of the data at a later point? • What percentage of data completion is required?
Values of the coded data are the same across applications and systems.	• Are codes assigned by qualified, credentialed coders? • Who is responsible for coordinating the ongoing coded data collection process? • Who is responsible for monitoring the quality of coded data collection? • Are the data currently collected for another application?
Coded data are available in a timely manner.	• Are processes in place to ensure that coded data are available in a timely manner? • Are documentation time lines met? • Is the record completion process appropriate? • Who is responsible for coordinating the ongoing data collection process? • Are the appropriate people involved in the design of the data collection methodology? • How much time will it take to collect the data? • What impact will data collection have on staffing requirements? • What information is required for coding? • What is the best encoder, grouper, and abstracting system?

Figure 8.1. (Continued)

Assessment Items	Considerations include, but are not limited to . . .
Collection—*The process by which coded data are accumulated*	
Education and training is effective and timely. Communication of coding and classification system conventions are timely and appropriate.	• What training is required for coders? • How will feedback on data quality be provided? • How are implications of poor data quality communicated to those who collect data? • Who is responsible for coordinating the ongoing data collection process? • Who will maintain written coding guidelines? • How are continuing education credits earned? • Are coding conventions communicated to coders, data users, and data analysts?
The most accurate, most timely, and least costly coded data are provided.	• Are codes assigned by qualified, credentialed coders? • How much time will it take to collect the data? • What impact will data collection have on staffing requirements? • How can collection of the data be incorporated into existing work flows? • What is the best encoder, grouper, and abstracting system?
Coded data collection is standardized.	• Who is responsible for coordinating the ongoing data collection process? • Are codes assigned by qualified, credentialed coders? • Who will maintain written coding guidelines? • How can collection of the data be incorporated into existing work flows? • What training is required for coders? • How are continuing education credits earned? • Are the data collected so that they are available for analysis without further manipulation?
Data are collected at the appropriate level of detail or granularity.	• Are codes assigned by qualified, credentialed coders? • Are the data collected so that they are available for analysis without further manipulation?
The data collection instrument is validated.	• Who is responsible for monitoring the quality of data collection? • Who will maintain written coding guidelines? • What is the best encoder, grouper, and abstracting system? • Are the data collected so that they are available for analysis without further manipulation?
Quality (i.e., accuracy) is routinely monitored.	• Who is responsible for monitoring the quality of data collection? • What training is required for those collecting the data? • What percentage of data completion is required? • What process will be used to monitor quality? Are data from comparative databases used to monitor quality? • What incentives can be applied to ensure data quality? • How will feedback on data quality be provided? • What success indicators have been selected? How will they be monitored? • Are audit results available from external organizations (i.e. quality improvement organizations [QIOs]) and consultants?
Warehousing—*Processes and systems used to archive coded data*	
Appropriate edits are in place.	• What edits are appropriate? • How will feedback on data quality be provided?
Data ownership is established.	• Who owns the coded data? • Who ensures that coded data are not altered?
Guidelines for access to coded data and/or systems are in place.	• Who has access to the coded data? • Are coding conventions communicated to coders, data users, and data analysts?

(Continued on next page)

Figure 8.1. **(Continued)**

Assessment Items	Considerations include, but are not limited to . . .
Relationships of data owners, data collectors, and data end users are managed.	• Who is responsible for coordinating the ongoing data management process? • Who is responsible for monitoring the quality of data collection? • Are the appropriate people involved in the design of the data collection methodology? • Are coding conventions communicated to coders, data users, and data analysts?
Data are available on a timely basis.	• Are processes in place to ensure that coded data are available on a timely basis? • Are documentation time lines met? • Is the record completion process appropriate? • Who is responsible for coordinating the ongoing data collection process? • Are the appropriate people involved in the design of the data collection methodology? • How much time will it take to collect the data? • What impact will data collection have on staffing requirements? • What information is required for coding? • What is the best encoder, grouper, and abstracting system?
Analysis—*The process of translating coded data into actionable information*	
Data are collected are in compliance with coding and classification system conventions.	• Are coding conventions communicated to coders, data users, and data analysts? • What training is required to analyze data?
Complete and current coded data are available.	• Are processes in place to ensure that coded data are available in a timely manner? • Are documentation time lines met? • Is the record completion process appropriate? • Who is responsible for coordinating the ongoing data collection process? • Are the appropriate people involved in the design of the data collection methodology? • How much time will it take to collect the data? • What impact will data collection have on staffing requirements? • What information is required for coding? • What is the best encoder, grouper, and abstracting system?
Coded data reflect the treatment of the patient and account for resources expended on the patient's care.	• What documentation is required? • Is the documentation available? • Is documentation available on a timely basis?
Appropriate data comparisons, relationships, and linkages are accessible.	• What documentation is required? • Are codes assigned by qualified, credentialed coders? • Is the documentation available? • Is documentation available on a timely basis?
Data are analyzed at the appropriate level of granularity.	• Are coding conventions communicated to coders, data users, and data analysts? • What training is required to analyze data?

Source: AHIMA Data Quality Management Task Force 1998; Fuller 1998.

Coding managers should share the findings from data quality evaluations and reviews in the following ways:

- Discuss the specific findings from each evaluation and review with the coding staff

- Incorporate specific findings pertinent to individual coders into their employee performance evaluations

- Submit overall findings to the quality improvement committee or its counterpart for further study, if necessary

Staff Responsibilities in the Data Quality Review Process

The HIM department should schedule data quality reviews on a regular and ongoing basis. The review schedule depends on the number of coders and the identified coding problems. If the coding staff consists of several clinical coding specialists, a rotating schedule should be established to review all coders on an annual basis. If the coding staff consists of one or two clinical coding specialists with no supervisor, the HIM department can conduct reviews in one of the following ways:

- Coders review each other's work.

- The HIM department manager reviews the coders' work.

- An external consulting firm is contracted to conduct the review.

The initial review should be conducted using a representative sample of both coding staff and common diagnoses and procedures. This review serves as a baseline for future comparisons. After analyzing the results of the review, the appropriate supervisor identifies problems that relate to coding and abstracting issues.

Coding Managers' Responsibilities in the Data Quality Review Process

Coding managers also play an important part in the data quality review process. They are responsible for:

- Preparing specific coding criteria

- Planning educational sessions for coders

- Evaluating and monitoring education action plans for individual coders

- Monitoring ethical coding practices

- Evaluating and monitoring coding and abstracting quality

- Preparing performance evaluations

Data Quality Reviews and Compliance

The design of any data quality review program should address the compliance initiatives in effect throughout the healthcare organization and within the HIM department. When the analysis of the review is complete, the HIM department should communicate the review's findings to the compliance department. (See chapter 9 for a discussion on how compliance requirements are related to the coding function.)

Review of Inpatient Coding

The HIM department should consider auditing or reviewing health records after coding, but before billing, rather than performing a retrospective audit after claims have been submitted for payment. This issue should be settled with the compliance department during the planning stage of the data quality improvement program.

Selecting the Sample for an Inpatient Review

Health records for inpatient review can be pulled using the inpatient database from the HIM system abstracts. The sample size varies depending on the type of review, the size of the hospital, the number of coders to be included, compliance requirements for sampling, and the number of inpatient discharges. (See chapter 9 for a discussion on sampling for corporate compliance.)

For an initial baseline review, the HIM manager could do sample selection. The best method of sample selection might be to pull a random sample of health records by volume and average charges. For a focused review, the HIM manager might have to develop specific reports. To understand how the codes were reported, code assignment should include the end result, which is generally the UB-92/UB-04 claim form.

Performing Focused Inpatient Reviews

The HIM department can plan focused reviews based on specific problem areas after the initial baseline review has been completed. Some potential problem coding areas for focused reviews include the following:

- Surgical complications

- Obstetrical complications

- DRG 468, 469, 470, 476, and 477 or other DRG code assignments that occur infrequently

- Dehydration as the principal diagnosis

- Medical complications

- Facility top 10 to 15 DRGs by volume and charges

- Areas with significant coding changes in the past year

- Areas with significant changes in coding guidelines in the past year

Topics for focused reviews also may be based on:

- Controversial issues identified in *Coding Clinic*

- Recent data quality issues identified by external review agencies or analysis of comparative data

- Discussions of inpatient coding issues presented in journals

Using published statistical reports for comparisons is another approach to conducting focused reviews. For example, the Office of the Inspector General (OIG) publishes an annual report of focused DRG pairs. The health information manager might be able to use this information to identify other topics for comparisons.

Choosing Forms to be Used in the Inpatient Review

In the inpatient review, forms are used to track cases, identify individual variations, and monitor the type of variations made by individual coders. A form should be completed for each health record included in the sample. Examples of suggested forms are provided in figures 8.2 through 8.5.

Determining How to Review Each Inpatient Health Record

To begin the review, the coding supervisor checks the inpatient health record to ensure that the diagnosis billed as principal meets the official Uniform Hospital Discharge Data Set (UHDDS) definition for principal diagnosis. The **principal diagnosis** must have been present on admission, been a principal reason for admission, and the patient received treatment or evaluation during the stay. When several diagnoses meet all those requirements, any of them could be selected as the principal diagnosis.

If the principal diagnosis was chosen incorrectly, the reviewer must determine the correct diagnosis. If this can be determined using coding conventions and guidelines, the reviewer need not consult the attending physician. If the documentation in the health record is unclear, the reviewer should consult the attending physician. When a physician clarifies the documentation, the clarification should support the code selection and be in the form of an addendum to the health record. If any changes to documentation affect the DRG, the case must be rebilled. Ultimately, the coding supervisor should identify the coding problem and its source and should implement a corrective action to prevent the same errors from recurring.

The following list gives the standard steps in the review process for coding supervisors/reviewers:

1. Review the health record to determine if all secondary diagnoses, CCs, and procedures billed are supported and justified.

2. Review secondary diagnoses to determine if any are supported by the health record, but not reported, and if they affect the DRG assignment.

3. Review the health record to determine that all secondary diagnoses have been completely identified and coded according to guidelines for the addition of secondary diagnoses.

4. For coding procedures, make sure that the entire operative record is available.

5. Review progress notes for bedside procedures to identify any procedures, such as debridements, that might affect DRG assignment.

6. Refer questions to a physician, as needed, and ensure that new information is documented in the health record.

7. Regroup and rebill or resubmit the claim accordingly.

8. Establish the cause of the coding problem.

9. Implement corrective action.

Figure 8.2. Coding compliance review: Inpatient summary

Name: _____ Age: _____ ADM: _____

MR #: _____ Sex: _____ DISCH: _____

ACCT #: _____ MD: _____ Facility: _____

HIC #: _____ LOS: _____ Payer: _____

Original Description and Codes **Revised Description and Codes**

Diagnosis   DRG _____ Diagnosis   DRG _____

1. _____	1. _____	*Variance Type:*
2. _____	2. _____	PrDx Chg /___/
3. _____	3. _____	ReSeq PrDx /___/
4. _____	4. _____	Add 2nd Dx /___/
5. _____	5. _____	Chg 2nd Dx /___/
6. _____	6. _____	PrProc Chg /___/
7. _____	7. _____	Chg 2nd Proc /___/
8. _____	8. _____	Add Proc /___/
9. _____	9. _____	Other /___/
10. _____	10. _____	

Operative Description and Codes **Operative Description and Codes**

1. _____   1. _____

2. _____   2. _____

3. _____   3. _____

4. _____   4. _____

5. _____   5. _____

6. _____   6. _____

Disposition Code: _____ Disposition Code: _____

Summary Findings: _____

_____

_____

Recommendations: _____

_____

_____

_____

Date Reviewed: _____ Date sent to Rebill HIM for: _____

Reviewer: _____ Revised DRG Wt.: _____

Orig. DRG Wt. _____ Pmt.: _____

Pmt: _____ Diff.: _____

Dictation

DxSum (dict): _____ H+P (dict): _____ Oper. (dict): _____

Typed: _____ Typed: _____ Typed: _____

Source: Bowman 2004, CD-ROM.

Figure 8.3. Inpatient review: Variations by coder

Date of Review: _____	
Variation Type	
Inaccurate sequencing or specificity prin Dx, affect DRG	_____
Inaccurate sequencing or specificity prin Dx, no affect DRG	_____
Omission CC, affect DRG	_____
Omission CC, no affect DRG	_____
Inaccurate prin procedure, affect DRG	_____
Omission procedure, affect DRG	_____
More specific coding of Dx or proc, no affect DRG	_____
Inaccurate coding	_____

Source: Bowman 2004, CD-ROM.

Figure 8.4. Rebilling log

Insurance: _____   Patient Type: _____

[Facility or Hospital name]

Date Sent to Business Office: _____

Patient		DRG/ASC Chg		Date of		Received		
Account #	Name	From	To	RA	Rebill	Amount	Date	Comments

(This portion to be completed by Reviewer)   *(This portion to be completed by the Business Office)*

Source: Bowman 2004, CD-ROM.

Figure 8.5. Coding Validation Worksheet: Medicare Coding Compliance—DRG/ICD-9-CM

Patient: _____ Age/Sex: _____ Financial Class: _____ Facility: _____

Health Record No.: _____ Adm. Date: _____

Account No.: _____ Disch. Date: _____

Disposition: _____ LOS: _____ Physician: _____ Date Reviewed: _____

	FACILITY NARRATIVE	FACILITY CODE		REVIEWER NARRATIVE	REVIEWER CODE	TYPE OF CHANGE
1			1			Chg Pdx
2			2			Chg 2d dx
3			3			Add 2d dx
4			4			Chg Pr Proc
5			5			Chg 2d Proc
6			6			Add Proc
7			7			
8			8			
9			9			
1			1			
2			2			
3			3			
4			4			
5			5			
6			6			
7			7			
8			8			
9			9			
10			10			

DRG VARIANCES

Hospital DRG: _____

Relative Weight: _____

Reimbursement: _____   Rationale for Change: _____

Reviewer DRG: _____   _____

Relative Weight: _____   Difference   _____

Reimbursement: _____   [ ]   _____

Dictation: _____ H&P: _____ D/C Summary: _____ Op: _____

Source: Bowman 2004, CD-ROM.

236

Calculating Errors from the Inpatient Review

When all health records in the sample have been reviewed, the results/errors must be summarized for all health records and for individual coders. The two most common methods of calculating errors are the record method and the code method.

The Record Method

The record method of calculating errors considers each health record coded incorrectly as one error. The advantages to the record method are that it allows for benchmarking with other hospitals that frequently use this method, permits reviewers to track errors by case type, and enables reviewers to relate productivity with quality errors on a case-by-case basis.

· The disadvantages to this method are that it oversimplifies the type of health records coded by not identifying the coder's ability to identify codes that must be reported and does not identify the number of secondary diagnoses or procedures missed by the coder.

The Code Method

The code method of calculating errors compares the total number of codes identified by the coder with the total number of possible codes that should have been coded. The advantages to the code method are that it recognizes the coder's ability to identify all codes that require reporting, weighs by code the more resource-intensive cases, and permits better diagnostic results in terms of the kinds of errors the coder is making, such as omission of secondary diagnoses or missed sequencing.

The disadvantages associated with this method are that it is difficult to compare results with benchmarking activities of other organizations that do not use this method and it does not identify the specific coding problems of individual coders or by record type, thus making it difficult to assess educational needs of coders.

It is important that the HIM department compare the accuracy of coders as individuals and as a group, and compare accuracy by type of case and DRG. These comparisons will assist the management team in identifying corrective actions to implement, such as education or training for the coding staff and information for the clinical staff to improve documentation.

Performing a Review of Abstracts and Bills

Abstracts and bills also should be included in the inpatient review when the corresponding health records are being reviewed for coding. The reviewer should print and attach a copy of the abstract to the coding review worksheet, and then should identify and correct abstracting errors.

Completing the Inpatient Review

When the inpatient audit or review has been completed to this point and a final UB-92/UB-04 has been printed, the reviewer should compare all the diagnoses and procedures printed on the bill with the coded information in the health record system. This identifies whether the communication software between the health record system and the billing system is functioning correctly. The HIM department should share the results of this comparison with the patient accounting department.

When the inpatient audit has been completed, the manager of the management team should determine how to share the findings with each coder and with the group of coders. Findings may indicate that documentation issues, coding policy, and procedure changes should be made and that educational programs are needed for the coding staff. Individual audit results by coder should become part of each employee's performance evaluation.

Review of Outpatient Coding

The HIM department should consider reviewing or auditing health records after coding, but before billing, rather than performing a retrospective review after claims have been submitted for payment. This issue should be settled with the compliance department during the planning stage of the data quality improvement program.

Selecting the Sample for an Outpatient Review

When a review or audit is being conducted following the provision of services, coding managers can pull health records for outpatient review by using the outpatient database from the HIM system abstracts. If random sampling is used, the coding manager should request that coders hold all cases for review and selection. If a list of patients is used, the coding manager should pull every fifth case (or some other number).

If an outpatient database is unavailable, the coding manager can develop a sample from a surgery schedule (for a prospective review) or from outpatient remittance advice listings (for a retrospective review). The sample size and its composition, such as ambulatory surgery, endoscopy, clinic visits, or emergency room, should be based on the percentage of business each component represents. For example, if 55 percent of outpatient business is through the ambulatory surgery department, the sample selected should include 55 percent of ambulatory surgery cases.

The sample size also will vary depending on type of review, size of the hospital, number of coders to be included, compliance requirements for the sampling, and number and type of outpatient discharges. (See chapter 9 for a discussion on sampling for corporate compliance.) For an initial baseline review, the HIM manager could do sample selection. The best method of sample selection might be to pull a random sample of cases by volume and average charges. For a focused review, the coding manager might have to develop specific reports. If all outpatient cases are in the abstracting system, the manager may select cases by using a CPT code range or specific groups of CPT codes.

Performing Focused Outpatient Reviews

The HIM department can plan focused outpatient reviews based on specific problem areas after the initial baseline review has been completed. Some potential problem coding areas for focused outpatient reviews include the following:

- Modifier use
- Emergency department use of modifier –25
- Podiatry procedures
- Cardiac catheterizations
- The top 25 APC groups by volume and charges
- Procedure and diagnoses codes by surgery subsection of CPT

Topics for focused reviews also may be based on:

- Problematic coding issues identified in *CPT Assistant*

- Areas of CPT with recent coding changes

- Recent data quality issues identified by external review agencies

- Discussions of outpatient coding issues presented in journals or newsletters

Choosing Forms to Be Used in the Outpatient Review

During the review, forms are used to track outpatient health records, identify individual variations, and monitor the types of variations made by individual coders. A form should be completed for each health record included in the sample. Examples of suggested forms are provided in figures 8.4 (p. 235) and 8.6.

Determining How to Review Each Outpatient Health Record

To begin the review, the reviewer checks each outpatient health record for the types of ICD-9-CM diagnoses and procedures previously described in the subhead Focused Outpatient Reviews. As a reference, the reviewer should use outpatient coding guidelines. For surgical procedures, the reviewer must review the entire operative report to ensure that all appropriate codes are identified and that modifiers are added, as needed.

In addition, the reviewer should run, if available, the most recent version of the Medicare outpatient code editor (OCE) on a sample of the health records. In this way, National Correct Coding Initiative (NCCI) edits, revenue code errors, and modifier errors that may have been overlooked will be identified.

Calculating Errors from the Outpatient Review

When all health records in the sample have been reviewed, the results and errors must be summarized for all health records and for individual coders. As in inpatient reviews, the same two methods of calculating errors—the record method and the code method—are used in outpatient reviews.

It is important that the HIM department compare the accuracy of coders as individuals and as a group, as well as comparing accuracy by type of case and APC. These comparisons will assist the management team in identifying corrective actions, such as implementing education or training programs for coding staff or providing information for the clinical staff to improve documentation.

Performing a Review of Abstracts and Bills

Abstracts and bills also should be included in the outpatient review when the corresponding health records are being reviewed for coding. The reviewer should print and attach a copy of the abstract and the outpatient encounter form, if used, to the coding review worksheet. (See sample worksheets in figures 8.2 through 8.5.) Then, the reviewer should identify and correct abstracting errors.

Figure 8.6. Rebilling summary/coding change

Name: _____ Age: _____ Adm: _____

MR #: _____ Sex: _____ Disch: _____

Acct #: _____ MD: _____ Facility: _____

HIC #: _____ LOS: _____

Disposition: _____

Original Codes: Diagnosis

1. _____
2. _____
3. _____
4. _____
5. _____
6. _____
7. _____
8. _____
9. _____
10. _____

Revised Codes: Diagnosis

1. _____
2. _____
3. _____
4. _____
5. _____
6. _____
7. _____
8. _____
9. _____
10. _____

Operative Codes

1. _____
2. _____
3. _____
4. _____
5. _____
6. _____

Operative Codes

1. _____
2. _____
3. _____
4. _____
5. _____
6. _____

CPT Codes

1. _____
2. _____
3. _____
4. _____
5. _____
6. _____

CPT Codes

1. _____
2. _____
3. _____
4. _____
5. _____
6. _____

The above account/record has been identified to have a coding change. Please rebill with the revised codes as soon as possible. If you have any questions please contact: [enter contact name] @ [enter telephone number and extension].

Date rebilled: _____

Source: Bowman 2004, CD-ROM.

Completing the Outpatient Review

When the outpatient review has been completed to this point and a final UB-92/UB-04 has been printed, the reviewer should compare the diagnoses/procedures printed on the bill with the coded information in the health record system. This identifies whether the communication software between the health record system and the billing system is functioning correctly. The HIM department should share the results of this comparison with the patient accounting department.

When the outpatient audit has been completed, the manager of the team should determine how the findings will be shared individually with each coder and with the group of coders. Findings may indicate that documentation issues, coding policy, and procedure changes should be made and that educational programs are needed for the coding staff. Individual audit results by coder should become part of each employee's performance evaluation.

Performing a Coding Practice Review

As part of the hospital data quality management program, the hospital's coding practices should be compared with those of other hospitals or groups using external databases (for example, Atlas, state databases or databases for selected patient populations, state hospital associations, hospital corporations, or hospital alliances) and make improvements as needed. The procedure is as follows (CHCA 2003b):

1. Determine a patient population to study and obtain comparative data. Select the population based on patient volume, case mix, charges, severity, or a combination of these and other variables.

2. Compare the hospital's coding practices with the comparative data obtained, including factors that impact case mix or severity assignment (that is, principal diagnosis, secondary diagnoses, and principal procedures).

3. Review a sample of records for appropriate code assignment and sequencing and for availability of documentation at time of coding.

4. Analyze the review results.

5. Share the review results with the coding staff.

6. Make improvements as needed.

Conducting a Coding Consistency Review

As part of the hospital's data quality management program and to ensure that all coders assign codes consistently, a coding consistency review should be conducted. The procedure is as follows (CHCA 2003a):

1. Select the patient record(s) to review.

2. Have each coder complete a coding review summary for each of the selected records.

3. Analyze the review findings. Questions may include the following: Are the results the same? Was the same principal diagnosis/procedure selected? If different codes were assigned, why? To direct code assignment, was the key word used in the encoder different?

4. Reach consensus on the appropriate coding practice.

5. Share the review results with the coding staff.

6. Make improvements as needed.

External Coding Consultants Used as Independent Quality Review Resources

The decision to request an external data quality evaluation can be made within the HIM department by either the facility's executives or the finance department. Regardless of the source of the decision, the process of bringing in an external auditor or reviewer can be lengthy. However, using external coding consultants as reviewers can bring a fresh perspective to the facility's coding function.

Types of Coding Consultants

Different types of coding consultants are available to assist with the evaluation of both inpatient and outpatient coding. These consultants can come from:

- Small firms that provide specialized types of reviews

- Larger firms that offer full-service accounts receivable and HIM evaluations

- Certified public accounting firms that work closely with the finance department

The Advantages to Using External Consultants

Using external coding consultants to review inpatient and outpatient coding processes has a number of advantages. For example, external consultants:

- Provide an independent opinion

- Are often more up-to-date on coding regulations and guidelines than internal coding staff because they can devote the necessary time to those activities

- Can verify that the quality of the facility's coded data is as high as possible

- Do not feel the pressure that the coding staff does from the facility's finance department

- Can critically evaluate the coding function and the quality of coded data because they are not involved in the facility's coding operation

Moreover, the facility's coding staff can learn new techniques for evaluating data quality as a result of the external review.

Preparation of a Request for Proposal

When a department in the healthcare facility has made the decision to conduct an external coding evaluation, the department manager must prepare a request for proposal (RFP). The RFP should define the facility's expectations, guide vendors in their responses, and clarify the facility's needs and objectives. An RFP has two major sections: a technical proposal section and a business proposal section.

Technical Section of the RFP

The technical section of the RFP contains the following basic components:

- Cover letter, which introduces the facility, identifies its interest in procuring consulting services, and, in some instances, contains the entire technical proposal section

- Statement of the project's purpose, which identifies the exact nature of the project

- Definition of objectives, which specifically and clearly addresses the nature of the facility's needs

- Scope of work, which delineates the type of review the facility wishes to have completed

- Delivery orders, which include the following information:

  —Profile of requesting facility, which provides a detailed description of the types of services offered by the facility and the details about which services are to be included in the work, volume statistics, and perhaps payor information by volume or percentage of services

  —Functional/technical requirements, including the type of encoder/grouper the facility may require the consultant to use

  —Training requirements needed by consultants to be eligible for consideration

  —Deliverables, or a listing of those products expected at the end of the evaluation

  —Request for references from previous clients with projects similar to the proposal

  —Conditions of bidding, which include how bids will be accepted or conditions that will result in the bid being rejected, a nondiscrimination clause, performance and default clauses, collusive bidding clauses, the implementation team, and the closing date for bids

Business Section of the RFP

The business section of the RFP includes the following components:

- A cost statement

- Limitations

- Contract terms for payment, liability insurance, confidentiality, and so on

Results from Using a Consultant

When the audit has been concluded, the hospital should expect a final report from the consultant or consulting firm that includes:

- The findings, with statistics as appropriate to the type of audit performed

- The identification of specific results of the audit in a table or other organized format with variations shown on a case-by-case basis

- Recommendations for improving both coding and documentation

- The overall impact of the review and its implications for the organization

In addition, the consultants should provide a summary of the coding and documentation issues identified in the audit through educational sessions for the coding and clinical staffs and should present an executive summary of the audit's major findings during an exit conference with the management team.

Confirm the Consultant's Review Results

To ensure that the review is not compromised, select a random sampling of the consultant's work for a second review by a staff member or an outside auditor who is qualified and knowledgeable in the subject matter to scrutinize the original consultant's findings. At a minimum:

- Review all audit documentation

- Evaluate independently the claims/services

- Determine the accuracy of the original audit results

- Assure proper interpretation of relevant policies and guidelines

- Recommend improvements including additional education for the audit staff

- Set a standard process for retaining the second audit's documentation (Derricks 2004)

Conclusion

The increased need for coded data in all areas of healthcare delivery, reimbursement, and accountability has brought about a corresponding need for data quality monitoring and evaluation programs in healthcare organizations. In addition, quality control of coded data is now a mandated effort through which the federal government intends to reduce payment errors and protect Medicare funds. Consequently, auditing and review activities are performed in both inpatient and outpatient settings to ensure the highest levels of coding accuracy and efficiency among coding staff.

Ensuring accuracy of coded data is a shared responsibility among HIM professionals, clinicians, business services staff, and information systems integrity professionals (AHIMA 2003). Maintaining data quality is an ongoing effort that affects many aspects of the current healthcare environment but relies primarily on the commitment and expertise of today's HIM professionals.

References and Resources

AHIMA Coding Products and Services Team. 2003 (July/August). Practice brief: Managing and improving data quality (updated). *Journal of American Health Information Management Association* 74(7): 64A–C.

AHIMA Data Quality Management Task Force. 1998 (March). Practice brief: A checklist to assess data quality management efforts. *Journal of American Health Information Management Association* 69(3):insert following p. 56.

American Health Information Management Association. 2000 (March). Standards of Ethical Coding. *Journal of American Health Information Management Association* 71(3): insert after p. 8.

Bowman, S. *Health Information Management Compliance: A Model Program for Healthcare Organizations,* 3rd ed. Chicago: AHIMA.

Child Health Corporation of America 2006 (March), APR-DRG v20 Severity of Illness Assignment Guidelines.

Child Health Corporation of America. 2003a (August). Coding consistency review procedure.

Child Health Corporation of America. 2003b (August). Coding practice review procedure.

Derricks, J. 2004 (October). Audit the auditors: Are your documentation, coding and billing audit findings valid? 2004 IFHRO Congress, AHIMA Convention Proceedings.

Fuller, S. 1998 (May). Designing a data collection process. *Journal of American Health Information Management Association* 69(5):insert following p. 64.

Price, K., and Farley, D. 2005 (July-August). How does your coding measure up? Analyzing performance data give HIM a boost in managing revenue. *Journal of American Health Information Management Association* 76(7): 26–31.

Appendix 8.1

Practice Brief: Managing and Improving Data Quality (Updated)

Complete and accurate diagnostic and procedural coded data is necessary for research, epidemiology, outcomes and statistical analyses, financial and strategic planning, reimbursement, evaluation of quality of care, and communication to support the patient's treatment.

Consistency of coding has been a major AHIMA initiative in the quest to improve data quality management in healthcare service reporting. The Association has also taken a stand on the quality of healthcare data and information.[1]

Data Quality Mandates

Adherence to industry standards and approved coding principles that generate coded data of the highest quality and consistency remains critical to the healthcare industry and the maintenance of information integrity throughout healthcare systems. HIM professionals must continue to meet the challenges of maintaining an accurate and meaningful database reflective of patient mix and resource use. As long as diagnostic and procedural codes serve as the basis for payment methodologies, the ethics of clinical coders and healthcare organization billing processes will be challenged.

Ensuring accuracy of coded data is a shared responsibility between HIM professionals, clinicians, business services staff, and information systems integrity professionals. The HIM professional has the unique responsibility of administration, oversight, analysis, and/or coding clinical data in all healthcare organizations. Care must be taken in organizational structures to ensure that oversight of the coding and data management process falls within the HIM department's responsibility area so data quality mandates are upheld and appropriate HIM principles are applied to business practices.

Clinical Collaboration

The Joint Commission and the Medicare Conditions of Participation as well as other accreditation agencies require final diagnoses and procedures to be recorded in the medical record and authenticated by the responsible practitioner. State laws also provide guidelines concerning the content of the health record as a legal document.

Clinical documentation primarily created by physicians is the cornerstone of accurate coding, supplemented by appropriate policies and procedures developed by facilities to meet patient care requirements. Coded data originate from the collaboration between clinicians and HIM professionals with clinical terminology, classification system, nomenclature, data analysis, and compliance policy expertise.

Thus, the need for collaboration, cooperation, and communication between clinicians and support personnel continues to grow as information gathering and storage embrace new technology. Movement of the coding process into the business processing side of a healthcare organization must not preclude access to and regular communication with clinicians.

Reprinted from AHIMA Coding Products and Services Team. 2003 (July/August). Practice brief: Managing and improving data quality (updated). *Journal of American Health Information Management Association* 74(7): 64A–C.

Clinical Database Evaluation

Regulatory agencies are beginning to apply data analysis tools to monitor data quality and reliability for reimbursement appropriateness and to identify unusual claims data patterns that may indicate payment errors or health insurance fraud. Examples include the Hospital Payment Monitoring Program tool First Look Analysis Tool for Hospital Outlier Monitoring (FATHOM), used by quality improvement organizations, and the comprehensive error rate testing (CERT) process to be used by Centers for Medicare and Medicaid Services carriers to produce national, contractor, provider type, and benefit category-specific paid claims error rates.

Ongoing evaluation of the clinical database by health information managers facilitates ethical reporting of clinical information and early identification of data accuracy problems for timely and appropriate resolution. Pattern analysis of codes is a useful tool for prevention of compliance problems by identifying and correcting clinical coding errors.

Coding errors have multiple causes, some within the control of HIM processes and others that occur outside the scope of HIM due to inadequacy of the source document or the lack of information integrity resulting from inappropriate computer programming routines or software logic.

Data Quality Management and Improvement Initiatives

The following actions are required in any successful program:

- Evaluation and trending of diagnosis and procedure code selections, the appropriateness of reimbursement group assignment, and other coded data elements such as discharge status are required. This action ensures that clinical concept validity, appropriate code sequencing, specific code use requirements, and clinical pertinence are reflected in the codes reported.

- Reporting data quality review results to organizational leadership, compliance staff, and the medical staff. This stresses accountability for data quality to everyone involved and allows the root causes of inconsistency or lack of reliability of data validity to be addressed. If the source for code assignment is inadequate or invalid, the results may reflect correct coding by the coding professional, but still represent a data quality problem because the code assigned does not reflect the actual concept or event as it occurred.

- Following up on and monitoring identified problems. HIM professionals must resist the temptation to overlook inadequate documentation and report codes without appropriate clinical foundation within the record just to speed up claims processing, meet a business requirement, or obtain additional reimbursement. There is an ethical duty as members of the healthcare team to educate physicians on appropriate documentation practices and maintain high standards for health information practice. Organizational structures must support these efforts by the enforcement of medical staff rules and regulations and continuous monitoring of clinical pertinence of documentation to meet both business and patient care requirements.

HIM clinical data specialists who understand data quality management concepts and the relationship of clinical code assignments to reimbursement and decision support for healthcare will have important roles to play in the healthcare organizations of the future. Continuing education and career boosting specialty advancement programs are expected to be the key to job security and professional growth as automation continues to change healthcare delivery, claims processing, and compliance activities.[2]

Data Quality Recommendations

HIM coding professionals and the organizations that employ them are accountable for data quality that requires the following behaviors.

HIM professionals should:

- Adopt best practices made known in professional resources and follow the code of ethics for the profession or their specific compliance programs.[3] This guidance applies to all settings and all health plans.

- Use the entire health record as part of the coding process in order to assign and report the appropriate clinical codes for the standard transactions and codes sets required for external reporting and meeting internal abstracting requirements.

- Adhere to all official coding guidelines published in the HIPAA standard transactions and code sets regulation. ICD-9-CM guidelines are available for downloading at www.cdc.gov/nchs/data/icd9/icdguide.pdf. Additional official coding advice is published in the quarterly publication *AHA Coding Clinic* for ICD-9-CM. CPT guidelines are located within the CPT code books and additional information and coding advice is provided in the AMA monthly publication CPT Assistant. Modifications to the initial Health Insurance Portability and Accountability Act (HIPAA) standards for electronic transactions or adoption of additional standards are submitted first to the designated standard maintenance organization. For more information, go to http://aspe.osdhhs.gov/admnsimp/final/dsmo.htm and www.hipaa-dsmo.org/faq/.

- Develop appropriate facility or practice-specific guidelines when available coding guidelines do not address interpretation of the source document or guide code selection in specific circumstances. Facility practice guidelines should not conflict with official coding guidelines.

- Maintain a working relationship with clinicians through ongoing communication and documentation improvement programs.

- Report root causes of data quality concerns when identified. Problematic issues that arise from individual physicians or groups of clinicians should be referred to medical staff leadership or the compliance office for investigation and resolution.

- Query when necessary. Best practices and coding guidelines suggest that when coding professionals encounter conflicting or ambiguous documentation in a source document, the physician must be queried to confirm the appropriate code selection.[4]

- Consistently seek out innovative methods to capture pertinent information required for clinical code assignment to minimize unnecessary clinician inquiries. Alternative methods of accessing information necessary for code assignment may prevent the need to wait for completion of the health record, such as electronic access to clinical reports.

- Ensure that clinical code sets reported to outside agencies are fully supported by documentation within the health record and clearly reflected in diagnostic statements and procedure reports provided by a physician.

- Provide the physician the opportunity to review reported diagnoses and procedures on preclaim or postclaim or postbill submission, via mechanisms such as:

  —providing a copy (via mail, fax, or electronic transmission) of the sequenced codes and their narrative descriptions, taking appropriate care to protect patient privacy and security of the information

—placing the diagnostic and procedural listing within the record and bringing it to the physician's attention within the appropriate time frame for correction when warranted

- Create a documentation improvement program or offer educational programs concerning the relationship of health record entries and health record management to data quality, information integrity, patient outcomes, and business success of the organization.

- Conduct a periodic or ongoing review of any automated billing software (chargemasters, service description masters, practice management systems, claims scrubbers, medical necessity software) used to ensure code appropriateness and validity of clinical codes.

- Require a periodic or ongoing review of encounter forms or other resource tools that involve clinical code assignment to ensure validity and appropriateness.

- Complete appropriate continuing education and training to keep abreast of clinical advancements in diagnosis and treatment, billing and compliance issues, regulatory requirements, and coding guideline changes, and to maintain professional credentials.

HIM coding professionals and the organizations that employ them have the responsibility to not engage in, promote, or tolerate the following behaviors that adversely affect data quality. HIM professionals should not:

- Make assumptions requiring clinical judgment concerning the etiology or context of the condition under consideration for code reporting.

- Misrepresent the patient's clinical picture through code assignment for diagnoses/procedures unsupported by the documentation in order to maximize reimbursement, affect insurance policy coverage, or because of other third-party payor requirements. This includes falsification of conditions to meet medical necessity requirements when the patient's condition does not support health plan coverage for the service in question or using a specific code requested by a payor when, according to official coding guidelines, a different code is mandatory.

- Omit the reporting of clinical codes that represent actual clinical conditions or services but negatively affect a facility's data profile, negate health plan coverage, or lower the reimbursement potential.

- Allow changing of clinical code assignments under any circumstances without consultation with the coding professional involved and the clinician whose services are being reported. Changes are allowed only with subsequent validation of the documentation supporting the need for code revision.

- Fail to use the physician query process outlined by professional practice standards or required by quality improvement organizations under contract for federal and state agencies that reimburse for healthcare services.

- Assign codes to an incomplete record without organizational policies in place to ensure the codes are reviewed after the records are complete. Failure to confirm the accuracy and completeness of the codes submitted for a reimbursement claim upon completion of the medical record can increase both data quality and compliance risks.[5]

- Promote or tolerate the falsification of clinical documentation or misrepresentation of clinical conditions or service provided.

Prepared by

AHIMA's Coding Products and Services team:

Kathy Brouch, RHIA, CCS
Susan Hull, MPH, RHIA, CCS
Karen Kostick, RHIT, CCS, CCS-P
Rita Scichilone, MHSA, RHIA, CCS, CCS-P
Mary Stanfill, RHIA, CCS, CCS-P
Ann Zeisset, RHIT, CCS, CCS-P

Acknowledgments

AHIMA Coding (SCC) Community of Practice

AHIMA Coding Policy and Strategy Committee

Sue Prophet-Bowman, RHIA, CCS

Notes

1. For details, see AHIMA's Position Statements on Consistency of Healthcare Diagnostic and Procedural Coding and on the Quality of Healthcare Data and Information at www.ahima.org/dc/positions.

2. For more information on AHIMA's specialty advancement programs, go to http://campus.ahima.org. Institutes for Healthcare Data Analytics and Clinical Data Management are planned for the 2003 AHIMA National Convention. Visit www.ahima.org/convention for more information.

3. AHIMA's Standards of Ethical Coding are available at www.ahima.org/infocenter/guidelines.

4. Prophet, Sue. "Practice Brief: Developing a Physician Query Process." *Journal of AHIMA* 72, no. 9 (2001): 88I–M.

5. More guidelines for HIM policy and procedure development are available in *Health Information Management Compliance: A Model Program for Healthcare Organizations* by Sue Prophet, AHIMA, 2002. Coding from incomplete records is also discussed in the AHIMA Practice Brief "Developing a Coding Compliance Document" in the July/August 2001 *Journal of AHIMA* (vol. 72, no. 7, prepared by AHIMA's Coding Practice Team).

Appendix 8.2

Standards for Ethical Coding

In this era of payment based on diagnostic and procedural coding, the professional ethics of health information coding professionals continue to be challenged. A conscientious goal for coding and maintaining a quality database is accurate clinical and statistical data. The following standards of ethical coding, developed by AHIMA's Coding Policy and Strategy Committee and approved by AHIMA's Board of Directors, are offered to guide coding professionals in this process.

1. Coding professionals are expected to support the importance of accurate, complete, and consistent coding practices for the production of quality healthcare data.

2. Coding professionals in all healthcare settings should adhere to the ICD-9-CM *(International Classification of Diseases, 9th revision, Clinical Modification)* coding conventions, official coding guidelines approved by the Cooperating Parties,* the CPT *(Current Procedural Terminology)* rules established by the American Medical Association, and any other official coding rules and guidelines established for use with mandated standard code sets. Selection and sequencing of diagnoses and procedures must meet the definitions of required data sets for applicable healthcare settings.

3. Coding professionals should use their skills, their knowledge of currently mandated coding and classification systems, and official resources to select the appropriate diagnostic and procedural codes.

4. Coding professionals should only assign and report codes that are clearly and consistently supported by physician documentation in the health record.

5. Coding professionals should consult physicians for clarification and additional documentation prior to code assignment when there is conflicting or ambiguous data in the health record.

6. Coding professionals should not change codes or the narratives of codes on the billing abstract so that meanings are misrepresented. Diagnoses or procedures should not be inappropriately included or excluded because payment or insurance policy coverage requirements will be affected. When individual payer policies conflict with official coding rules and guidelines, these policies should be obtained in writing whenever possible. Reasonable efforts should be made to educate the payer on proper coding practices in order to influence a change in the payer's policy.

7. Coding professionals, as members of the healthcare team, should assist and educate physicians and other clinicians by advocating proper documentation practices,

---

*The Cooperating Parties are the American Health Information Management Association, American Hospital Association, Health Care Financing Administration, and National Center for Health Statistics. All rights reserved. Reprint and quote only with proper reference to AHIMA's authorship.

Reprinted from American Health Information Management Association. 2000 (March). Standards of Ethical Coding. *Journal of American Health Information Management Association* 71(3): insert after p. 8.

further specificity, and resequencing or inclusion of diagnoses or procedures when needed to more accurately reflect the acuity, severity, and the occurrence of events.

8. Coding professionals should participate in the development of institutional coding policies and should ensure that coding policies complement, not conflict with, official coding rules and guidelines.

9. Coding professionals should maintain and continually enhance their coding skills, as they have a professional responsibility to stay abreast of changes in codes, coding guidelines, and regulations.

10. Coding professionals should strive for optimal payment to which the facility is legally entitled, remembering that it is unethical and illegal to maximize payment by means that contradict regulatory guidelines.

Revised 12/99

Chapter 9

Compliance Issues

Cheryl L. Hammen, RHIA

In 1995, the federal government began intensive efforts to identify abusive and fraudulent healthcare claims through various initiatives. As it became evident that healthcare compliance was here to stay, healthcare providers began implementing internal compliance programs with a major focus on coding and billing activities. These programs were developed based on *Compliance Program Guidance* issued by the Office of Inspector General (OIG) of the Department of Health and Human Services (HHS).

Health information managers responsible for coding functions recognized an opportunity to become resources for their facilities. They took the lead in identifying areas of compliance risk that are associated with billing, monitoring these areas and implementing corrective action when necessary. The development of HIM compliance programs to support the facility's compliance program became the norm in hospitals across the country. Steps taken by these innovative leaders are presented in this chapter to provide guidance in ensuring an efficient and effective compliance program.

Healthcare Fraud and Abuse

Healthcare fraud is a deception or misrepresentation by a provider, or by a representative of a provider, that may result in a false or fictitious claim for inappropriate payment by Medicare or other insurers for items or services either not rendered or rendered to a lesser extent than that described in the claim. In other words, healthcare fraud is the submission of a claim for payment of items or services that the person knew—or should have known—were not provided.

Healthcare abuse consists of practices that are inconsistent with generally accepted fiscal, business, or professional practices. Such unacceptable practices result in unnecessary costs to Medicare or to other third-party payers because they are not considered medically necessary or fail to meet recognized medical standards of care.

Optimization of Coding

The term *optimization* generally refers to the procedure or procedures used to make a system or design as effective or functional as possible. When coders "optimize" the coding process, they attempt to make coding for reimbursement as accurate as possible. In this way, the healthcare facility can obtain the highest dollar amount justified within the terms of the government program or the insurance policy involved.

Methods for optimization of coding and subsequent reimbursement began appearing shortly after the implementation of DRGs because hospitals wanted to make sure they obtained the highest possible reimbursement for each inpatient case. Hospitals wanted to ensure that not only all applicable codes, but also the codes providing the best payment appeared on claim forms. A number of optimization tools were developed by hospitals and vendors to meet that objective. These tools included tips on reviewing specific DRGs provided in book form, as well as software programs that "alert" coders to potential optimization opportunities.

Some software programs prompt coding staff or physicians to consider codes that might apply and point out those codes that might pay better. These programs are misused when code selection is based solely on which code pays the most rather than on which code or codes most accurately reflect the services delivered. However, the express intent of most optimization tools is not to cheat insurance plans out of benefits. A valid optimization tool provides the information required to ensure accurate and complete coding. It also provides the user with assistance in selecting the best codes to reflect the clinical circumstances.

Legitimate optimization is achieved through several methods, including:

- Improving documentation or access to documentation for better coding

- Providing educational programs for coders, clinicians, billers, and claims-processing personnel to improve awareness of coding guidelines

- Making use of computer software edits, reminders, and automated assistance

- Reviewing claims to ensure accurate coding for appropriate payments

Clinical coding directly affects the amount of payment a facility receives from a payer (depending on the payer). Individual coders sometimes tend to take an overly conservative approach to coding because they fear allegations of fraudulent or abusive billing practices by the government or others. Sometimes entire organizations have taken this route as a matter of policy. However, neither overly aggressive coding nor overly conservative coding ultimately benefits the organization, from either a financial or compliance perspective.

Government Legislation and Initiatives

Since 1995, several federal initiatives and pieces of legislation related to investigating, identifying, and preventing healthcare fraud and abuse have been passed. The more notable ones are described in the following subheads. They provide background material for understanding the magnitude of fraud and abuse in the mid-1990s and the necessary steps taken to ensure reclamation of inappropriate funds to assist in the continuation of Medicare and Medicaid.

Civil False Claims Act

The Civil False Claims Act was passed during the Civil War. It was an effort to avoid false claims by government contractors for services billed, but not provided, and for items misrepresented in billing. The act was updated in 1986. Later, it was reinforced through passage of the Health Insurance Portability and Accountability Act (HIPAA) of 1996 and the Balanced Budget Act (BBA) of 1997.

Qui tam, or whistle-blowing, legislation has been widely used in the application of the Civil False Claims Act in battling healthcare fraud and abuse. Qui tam legislation refers to a person acting on behalf of the government, although benefiting individually from a successful action. Anyone—a healthcare employee, a competitor, or a patient—may file a lawsuit alleging that there has been a violation of the Civil False Claims Act through the submission of false claims to Medicare, Medicaid, or other federally funded programs.

Successful false claims actions may result in the whistle-blower receiving an award of 15 to 30 percent of the monies recovered. However, seldom does a successful action result in a significant seven-figure award.

Health Insurance Portability and Accountability Act

A major portion of HIPAA focused on identifying healthcare fraud and abuse. Areas such as medically unnecessary services, upcoding, unbundling, and billing for services not provided were targeted.

Upcoding is the practice of using a code that results in a higher payment to the provider than the code that actually reflects the service or item provided. **Unbundling** is the practice of using multiple codes that describe individual steps of a procedure rather than an appropriate single code that describes all steps of the comprehensive procedure performed.

Title II of HIPAA mandated the establishment of fraud and abuse control programs to battle healthcare fraud and abuse. Monies were appropriated to fund those programs, and agencies were identified to participate in the government's efforts. Additionally, the Medicare Integrity Program was established. This program was charged with the following responsibilities, among others:

- Review of provider activities for potential fraudulent activity

- Audit of cost reports

- Payment determinations

- Education of providers and beneficiaries on healthcare fraud and abuse issues

Beneficiary incentive programs were also implemented. Those programs encourage Medicare beneficiaries to review their providers' bills carefully and to report any discrepancies to the secretary of HHS. Beneficiaries also were encouraged to provide suggestions on improving the efficiency of the Medicare program.

HIPAA clarified the application of healthcare fraud and abuse sanctions to include all federal healthcare programs. The act provided guidance on the use of these sanctions, including criteria for modifying or establishing safe harbors and for the issuance of advisory opinions and special fraud alerts. Also included in the act were revisions to previous sanctions related to:

- Mandatory exclusion from Medicare

- Length of exclusion

- Failure to comply with statutory obligations

- Antikickback penalties

- Penalties for disposing of assets in order to gain Medicaid benefits

In response to a HIPAA mandate, data are currently being collected on healthcare providers who have received final adverse actions as the result of fraud and abuse investigation. Data elements to be collected were defined as part of the act. This database continues to be updated on a monthly basis with exclusions and reinstatements.

As a result of this legislation, many agencies began "partnering" to investigate fraud and abuse in the healthcare environment. This included federal, state, and private-sector organizations. Various agencies responsible for investigating and prosecuting healthcare fraud and abuse, such as the Federal Bureau of Investigation (FBI), experienced significant staff increases.

In complying with HIPAA legislation, Congress budgeted $120 million in 1998 to the HHS OIG, CMS, FBI, the Department of Justice (DOJ), and State Medicaid Fraud Control Units. In addition, the Administration on Aging (AOA) provided funding through grants.

Balanced Budget Act of 1997

Title IV, Subtitle D, chapters 1 and 2, of the BBA of 1997 focused on healthcare fraud and abuse issues, especially as they related to penalties. The circumstances under which civil monetary penalties are applied were based on the BBA. Those circumstances include entities that contract with excluded individuals and persons involved with healthcare industry kickbacks.

As a part of the BBA, the following Medicare exclusionary penalties were implemented and are applied to entities that receive monies from federal healthcare programs and are convicted of healthcare-related crimes:

- First offense—5 years

- Second offense—Minimum of 10 years

- Third offense—Permanent exclusion

The right of the Secretary of HHS to refuse to enter into Medicare agreements with those entities convicted of a felony under federal or state law is included in the BBA. Medicare's right to refuse to enter into an agreement with a provider convicted of a felony was extended beyond the individual provider to include family members in control of the entity when ownership or controlling interest was transferred in anticipation of adverse government actions.

Initiatives resulting from mandates in the BBA to improve program integrity included:

- Notifying beneficiaries of their right to request copies of detailed bills for healthcare services received

- Advising beneficiaries to review explanations of benefits and detailed bills for errors and to report these errors to the Secretary of HHS

- Initiating the data collection program, as mandated in HIPAA, to collect information on healthcare fraud and abuse

- Implementing a toll-free fraud and abuse hotline by HHS

Other mandates for improving program integrity included requirements for disclosure of specific information by certain providers wishing to obtain or maintain their participation in the Medicare program.

The use of advisory opinions by HHS to provide information on the prohibition of certain referrals was explained, as was the replacement of reasonable charge methodology with the use of fee schedules for some services.

Requirements for diagnostic information from physicians and nonphysician practitioners to determine medical necessity for certain items and services provided by another entity can be found in Section 4317 (b) (an amendment to Section 1842 (p) of 42 USC 1395u(p) of the BBA), which states:

> In the case of an item or service defined in paragraph (3), (6), (8), or (9) of subsection 1861(s) ordered by a physician or a practitioner specified in subsection (b)(18)(C), but furnished by another entity, if the Secretary (or fiscal agent of the Secretary) requires the entity furnishing the item or service to provide diagnostic or other medical information in order for payment to be made to the entity, the physician or practitioner shall provide that information to the entity at the time that the item or service is ordered by the physician or practitioner.

This is an important amendment because it relates to documentation efforts to obtain diagnoses for outpatient services prior to the performance of those services. This information was clarified by CMS in Transmittal A-01-61, which can be accessed from the CMS Web site at www.cms.hhs.gov.

Operation Restore Trust

Operation Restore Trust began in 1995 as a joint effort of the HHS OIG, CMS, and AOA to target fraud and abuse in healthcare services. The program initially began in five states (California, Illinois, Florida, New York, and Texas), representing one third of the nation's Medicare and Medicaid population.

Interdisciplinary teams of federal, state, and private-sector representatives investigated and audited healthcare providers. These teams identified new approaches for conducting healthcare investigations and audits, including using statistical surveys (statistical surveys are used frequently to determine areas of potential abuse), working with DOJ, and training state organizations to detect and report potential fraud for further investigation.

Eventually, Operation Restore Trust expanded to other states across the country. This program focused on identifying fraud and abuse related to home healthcare services, nursing home services, and the provision of durable medical equipment and supplies. These efforts led to implementation of a national toll-free fraud and abuse hotline, which enabled tipsters to call and report potentially fraudulent activity on the part of healthcare providers. Operation Restore Trust also led to implementation of another initiative—the Voluntary Disclosure Program—and to the use of special fraud alerts based on audit and investigative findings.

In its first 2 years, Operation Restore Trust spent only $7.9 million to identify $188 million in overpayments to providers—a 23-to-1 return on investment. The monies overpaid have been attributed to criminal restitution and fines; civil judgments, settlements and fines; and inappropriately billed or medically unnecessary services.

Medicare Error Rate

From 1996 through 2002, the OIG reported the amount of fee-for-service payments that did not comply with Medicare regulations. In fiscal year 2002, the OIG identified improper Medicare payments totaling $13.3 billion. This should be compared to the $23.2 billion reported in the first OIG error rate audit. This represents a 43 percent improvement since the first audit in 1996.

CMS established the Comprehensive Error Rate Testing (CERT) program and the Hospital Payment Monitoring Program (HPMP) to monitor the accuracy of payments. Each of these programs accounts for approximately 50 percent of the error rate. In order to better understand the cause of the errors, CMS began to calculate additional rates related to the performance of carriers, fiscal intermediaries (FIs), durable medical equipment regional carriers (DMERCs), and quality improvement organizations (QIOs). The CERT program audits the carriers, FIs and DMERCs, whereas the HPMP audits the QIOs. The findings by specific carrier, FI, and so on can be reviewed in the audit reports, located on the Internet by going to the CMS homepage.

In 2004, approximately 160,000 claims were audited. The results by error category from the FY 2004 Improper Medicare Fee-For-Service (FFS) Payment Report Executive Version are broken down as shown in table 9.1.

Table 9.2, from the Improper Medicare FFS Payments Short Report (Web version) for May 2006, shows the amounts of overpayments and underpayments identified since 1996.

The percentage of improper payments has decreased almost every year since the first audit was conducted. This is a tremendous accomplishment, but there is still room for improvement.

Table 9.1. Results of FY 2004 improper fee for service payment audit

Results by Error Category	Percentage
No improper payments	90.7%
Insufficient documentation	4.1%
Nonresponse	2.8%
Medically unnecessary	1.6%
Incorrect coding	0.7%
Other	0.2%

Source: CMS 2004, 8.

Table 9.2. Amounts of overpayments and underpayments identified since 1996

Year	Total Dollars Paid	Overpayments		Underpayments		Overpayments + Underpayments	
		Payment	Rate	Payment	Rate	Improper Payments	Rate
1996	$168.1B	$23.5B	14.0%	$0.3B	0.2%	$23.8B	14.2%
1997	$177.9B	$20.6B	11.6%	$0.3B	0.2%	$20.9B	11.8%
1998	$177.0B	$13.8B	7.8%	$1.2B	0.6%	$14.9B	8.4%
1999	$168.9B	$14.0B	8.3%	$0.5B	0.3%	$14.5B	8.6%
2000	$174.6B	$14.1B	8.1%	$2.3B	1.3%	$16.4B	9.4%
2001	$191.3B	$14.4B	7.5%	$2.4B	1.3%	$16.8B	8.8%
2002	$212.8B	$15.2B	7.1%	$1.9B	0.9%	$17.1B	8.0%
2003	$199.1B	$20.5B	10.3%	$0.9B	0.5%	$12.7B	6.4%
2004	$213.5B	$20.8B	9.7%	$0.9B	0.4%	$21.7B	10.1%
2005	$234.1B	$11.2B	4.8%	$0.9B	0.4%	$12.1B	5.2%
May 2006	$257.4B	$11.9B	4.6%	$1.2B	0.5%	$13.1B	5.1%

Source: CMS 2006a.

OIG Compliance Program Guidance

Over the past several years, the OIG has published several site-of-service documents to help providers develop internal compliance programs that include the seven elements for ensuring compliance as outlined in the U.S. Sentencing Guidelines in 1991:

1. Written policies and procedures

2. Designation of a compliance officer

3. Education and training

4. Communication

5. Auditing and monitoring

6. Disciplinary action

7. Corrective action

In 2004, efforts were underway to update definitions to the U.S. Sentencing Guidelines, with several associations, such as the Health Care Compliance Association, providing comments on draft proposals.

Compliance Program Guidance for Clinical Laboratories

The first OIG site-of-service document, *Compliance Program Guidance for Clinical Laboratories,* addressed clinical laboratories (OIG 1998a). It was first released in February 1997, then again in August 1998 as a revision to reflect CMS policy and the format provided in *Compliance Program Guidance for Hospitals,* which was released in February 1998 (OIG 1998b).

Billing activities in the policies and procedures section of this document are specific to documentation and coding issues. The document instructs clinical laboratories to ensure that codes accurately reflect the services provided. It further instructs them to consider technical expert review to ensure accuracy. Information is provided related to the requirement for accompanying ICD-9-CM diagnosis codes to ensure medical necessity and, therefore, coverage for the procedure performed.

Compliance Program Guidance for Clinical Laboratories instructs clinical laboratories not to do the following:

- *Not* to use diagnostic information from earlier dates of service

- *Not* to use cheat sheets for assigning reimbursable codes

- *Not* to use computer programs that automatically insert diagnosis codes without documentation from the physician

- *Not* to make up diagnostic information for claims

Compliance Program Guidance instructs clinical laboratories to do the following:

- Contact the ordering physician if diagnostic documentation has not been obtained prior to the encounter

- Provide services and diagnostic information for standing orders in connection with an extended course of treatment

- Accurately translate narrative diagnoses into ICD-9-CM codes

It is preferred that physicians provide only a narrative diagnosis with the laboratory ensuring the appropriate diagnostic code assignment.

Compliance Program Guidance for Hospitals

Compliance Program Guidance for Hospitals was released by the OIG in February 1998 (OIG 1998b). Many of the risk areas outlined in this document are related to coding issues, such as:

- Billing for items or services not actually rendered

- Upcoding

- Outpatient services rendered in connection with inpatient stays (72-hour window rule)

- Unbundling

- Billing for discharge instead of transfer

- DRG creep, assigning a code resulting in a DRG with a higher payment rate than that supported by the documentation in the health record

The presence of health record documentation plays a major role in ensuring complete and accurate coding for billing purposes based on the content of this document. The guidance provides for the creation of a mechanism to ensure communication between the coders/billers and the clinical staff to achieve complete and accurate documentation before coding or billing is completed. The Official Coding Guidelines are listed in the guidance as the applicable regulations for coding claims. The document also suggests implementation of random retrospective auditing to test for accuracy. Special training sessions for coders and billers are recommended to ensure ongoing education and skill enhancement.

On January 31, 2005, the OIG published supplemental hospital compliance guidance in the *Federal Register* (OIG 2005). The OIG defined eight areas of increased risk for hospitals:

1. Submission of accurate claims and information

2. The Referral Statutes (physician self-referral and antikickback)

3. Payments to reduce or limit services: gainsharing arrangements

4. Emergency Medical Treatment and Labor Act (EMTALA)

5. Substandard care

6. Relationships with federal healthcare beneficiaries

7. HIPAA privacy and security rules

8. Billing Medicare or Medicaid substantially in excess of usual charges

In regard to coding compliance activities, the submission of accurate claims and information is the focus of concern. There are four main categories related to submission of accurate claims, with individual items specific to each.

- Outpatient Procedure Coding for OPPS

    —Billing as an outpatient for "inpatient only" procedures

    —Submitting claims for medically unnecessary services

    —Submitting duplicate claims and not following the National Correct Coding Initiative (NCCI) edits

    —Submitting incorrect claims due to outdated charge description masters (CDMs)

    —Circumventing the multiple procedure discounting rules

    —Improper evaluation and management (E/M) code selection

    —Improper billing of observation services

- Admissions and Discharges

    —Failure to follow the "same day" rule

    —Abuse of partial hospitalization payments

    —Same-day discharges and readmissions

    —Violation of the postacute care transfer policy (through assignment of incorrect discharge disposition code)

    —Improper churning of patients by long-term care hospitals located within an acute care hospital

- Supplemental Payment Considerations

    —Improper reporting of the costs of "pass-through" items

    —Abuse of DRG outlier payments

    —Improper claims for incorrectly designated "provider-based" entities

    —Improper claims for clinical trials

    —Improper claims for organ acquisition costs

    —Improper claims for cardiac rehabilitation services

    —Failure to follow Medicare rules regarding payment for costs related to educational activities (GME and IME)

- Use of Information Technology

    —Failure to include all billing requirements

    —Failure to include safeguards related to privacy and security rules

Many of these issues are addressed in the 2006 OIG Work Plan and are discussed later in this chapter as they relate to coding compliance activities.

Other Compliance Program Guidance Documents

Many other documents related to *Compliance Program Guidance* have been released since those for clinical laboratories and hospitals. They are all similar in format, using the seven elements for compliance as their main components. The content may differ, however, depending on the site of service. The *Compliance Program Guidance* documents (in addition to those for clinical laboratories and for hospitals) currently available (or in process) include those for:

- Third-party billers

- Hospices

- Durable medical equipment

- Home health agencies

- Medicare+Choice

- Physician practices

- Skilled nursing facilities

- Ambulance industry

- Pharmaceutical manufacturers

- Patients of Public Health Service (PHS) research awards

Copies of the OIG's *Compliance Program Guidance* documents may be obtained at the OIG's Web site at http://www.oig.hhs.gov/fraud/complianceguidance.html.

OIG Work Plans

Annually, the OIG issues its work plan for the following fiscal year. The plan is usually available by October 1 and includes CMS projects; Public Health Service Agency projects; Administrations for Children, Families, and Aging projects; and departmentwide projects within HHS.

The work plan encompasses projects that will be performed under the auspices of the OIG by the Office of Audit Services, the Office of Evaluation and Inspections, the Office of Investigations, and the Office of Counsel to the Inspector General. Each of these agencies assists in the development of the OIG work plan, identifying those areas for which they are responsible. The actions that are performed relate to audit, inspection, investigation, and litigation.

Targets of OIG Work Plans

The major targets of OIG work plans are identified under specific sites or types of service, such as hospitals, nursing homes, or physicians. Areas related to the coding function are frequently found in the work plan. Some coding projects that have appeared in work plans include:

- Pneumonia DRG upcoding project

- Project Bad Bundle

- Physicians at teaching hospitals (PATH)

- Critical care codes

- DRG 14

- Revenue centers without HCPCS codes

- Automated encoding systems for billing

- Home health coding accuracy

In the 2004–006 work plans, coding projects that continue to be assessed include:

- Review of DRGs with aberrant coding patterns

- Coronary artery stent placement for appropriate supporting documentation

- Outpatient prospective payment system (in 2006, this includes unbundling and "inpatient only" billing)

- Evaluation and management coding

- Use of modifier –25

- Overall accuracy in assigning modifiers based on Correct Coding Initiative (CCI) edits

Many targets appear in the work plan multiple years in a row. Given changes in priorities, a major target may move down the list, or it may be that the audit, inspection, or investigation is a lengthy process that requires more than 1 year to complete. The OIG's annual work plan can be obtained from the OIG's Web site at http://www.oig.hhs.gov/publications/workplan.html.

Uses of OIG Work Plans

OIG work plans are important from a coding management perspective because they can be used to:

- Focus monitoring and auditing activities

- Identify problem areas

- Provide education

- Develop policies and procedures

Corporate Compliance and Health Information Management

Because so many compliance issues are related to coding and billing functions, HIM staff has the potential to provide expert advice to senior management, the compliance officer, and other hospital departments. To accomplish this, the health information manager must take the initiative and begin working with staff that is in need of information about compliance-related issues.

Working with the Compliance Committee and Compliance Officer

The HIM department director and the coding manager should have close contact with the facility's compliance committee, the compliance officer, or both. Providing them with current information related to coding and compliance issues establishes the health information manager as a resource for the benefit of the facility as a whole.

In many cases, health information managers rise to the top because they have expertise in the areas of coding, billing, and compliance. The health information manager should be a permanent member of a facility's compliance committee.

Working as a Team

In addition to working with the compliance committee and compliance officer, the HIM department works with other departments as part of a facilitywide team to ensure compliance.

As part of the compliance committee, the health information manager or coding manager works closely with all departments to provide compliance education. However, a team effort is needed in working with certain groups or departments to meet the goals of compliance, appropriate reimbursement, and accurate claims submission.

Working with Medical Staff for Compliance

The health information manager must continuously promote complete, accurate, and timely documentation to ensure appropriate coding, billing, and reimbursement. This requires a close working relationship with the medical staff, perhaps through the use of a physician champion.

Physician champions assist in educating medical staff members on documentation needed for accurate billing. They can demonstrate how improved documentation assists not only with hospital billing and reimbursement, but also with physician office billing and reimbursement. The use of physician champions is not a new concept. They have been used successfully in hospitals across the country. The medical staff is more likely to listen to a peer than to a facility employee, especially when the topic is documentation needed to ensure appropriate reimbursement.

Working with Patient Financial Services for Compliance

The health information manager must also work with patient financial services (PFS) to achieve successes in compliance. Most billers are unaware of the rules that govern coding as described in federal regulations. Health information managers can enhance billers' knowledge of those requirements. In addition, managers can instruct billers on the importance and necessity of contacting the HIM department before changing codes to meet the requirements of certain payers.

Additionally, by developing this relationship, the coding manager can work in concert with PFS on denials from Medicare or other federally funded or private health insurance plans. A process for handling denials should be established that includes:

- Receipt of the denial by the business office

- Notification of the coding manager and case manager by the business office

- Audit of the health record by the HIM department to ensure accurate coding based on existing documentation

- Notification of PFS and case management regarding accuracy of the denial

- Creation of a response to the denial by the coding manager, case manager, and PFS manager

By working as a team, an accurate and timely response to denials can become a routine process. During this process, team members also might identify trends that warrant education for quality improvement purposes.

Working with the Admitting Department for Compliance

The coding manager works closely with the admitting department to ensure the following:

- Accurate patient status

- Receipt of physician documentation with reason for encounter and orders for outpatient services

- Application of advance beneficiary notices (ABNs)

- Education regarding LCDs and NCDs, which outline those diagnoses considered medically necessary for specific procedures

In return, the coding manager provides the admitting department with the expertise needed to ensure compliance in admitting activities related to documentation, coding, and regulations.

Working with Ancillary Departments for Compliance

In most facilities, each ancillary department is responsible for updating its portion of the CDM. Usually, staff members in the ancillary departments do not have the expertise in HCPCS coding to ensure accuracy and timeliness in the updating process. The coding manager should take the lead in providing this expertise to the various ancillary departments. Such action ensures compliance in the facility's charging process using HCPCS codes.

The Health Information Management Coding Compliance Plan

The coding manager faces unique challenges in ensuring coding compliance. Because coding usually determines a facility's reimbursement for services rendered, it is a high-risk area that should be continuously monitored to ensure compliance with all applicable regulations.

In an effort to provide structure and accountability to this important process, HIM departments have implemented coding compliance plans to demonstrate the steps being taken to ensure data quality. The coding compliance plan should be based on the same principles as those of the corporate program. It should include the following elements outlined in OIG compliance guidance documents:

- Code of conduct

- Policies and procedures

- Education and training

- Communication regarding the program

- Auditing

- Corrective action

- Reporting

Numerous benefits can be realized as a result of the coding compliance plan, including the following:

- Improved physician documentation

- Improved coding accuracy

- A decrease in denials

- Relevant physician and coder education

- Proactive research into variations from benchmark data and their underlying causes

- Timely identification, correction, and prevention of potential coding compliance risks

Code of Conduct

The HIM team should demonstrate its commitment and the facility's commitment to ensuring a culture of compliance by developing a code of conduct. Responsibilities related to compliance, the reporting of potential problem areas, and possible disciplinary action should be included in such a code. Use of the corporate compliance hotline should also be included to ensure that employees understand how to report questionable practices without fear of retribution.

To further a culture of compliance, job descriptions for coding functions should include a requirement for adhering to the coding compliance plan. Each employee should be required to sign an acknowledgment indicating awareness of, and agreement with, the plan. The signed acknowledgment should be maintained in the employee's file in case it is needed in the future. If an employee refuses to sign the acknowledgment or to adhere to the plan, the human resources (HR) department should become involved. An employee's refusal to sign the acknowledgment or to adhere to the plan could result in his or her termination for not complying with a term of employment.

Policies and Procedures

Policies and procedures that describe the healthcare facility's coding functions, standards, and practices should be established and documented. Such policies and procedures are needed to demonstrate the efforts being made by the staff to ensure complete and accurate coding and billing for reimbursement.

Health Information Management Coding Compliance Manual

To achieve compliance that mirrors the corporate compliance program, the HIM department should develop a departmental coding compliance manual. Because the HIM department is responsible for the coding function, which is so closely related to many of the facility wide compliance initiatives, this manual should include facility coding policies, procedures, and standards that directly support the corporate compliance program.

Development of Coding Policies and Procedures

In some facilities, the HIM department is required to work with the HR department or another designated department to obtain policy/procedure numbers and to seek organizational approval of proposed coding policies and procedures.

Coding policies should include the following components:

- AHIMA Code of Ethics

- AHIMA Standards of Ethical Coding

- Official Coding Guidelines

- Applicable federal and state regulations

- Internal documentation policies requiring the presence of physician documentation to support all coded diagnosis and procedure code assignments

Procedures related to the actual coding function should include a step-by-step description of the process, thus ensuring maximum accuracy and productivity.

Three Sample Procedures

When documentation is ambiguous or incomplete or when it requires clarification of clinical findings, a procedure should be in place for requesting that the physician provide additional documentation in accordance with procedures for late entries or addenda to the health record.

A second procedure should be developed that provides for a second coding review following the addition of documentation by a physician to the health record. A second review may be needed to ensure complete and accurate coding and billing.

Additionally, a third procedure should be in place to ensure that corrected cases are rebilled following a coding compliance audit. Both increases (if within 60 days of original billing) and decreases to reimbursement should be rebilled. The coding manager should consult patient financial services regarding this procedure. The coding manager and PFS manager should write a policy and procedure to ensure that the process flows smoothly from the HIM department to the business office to the FI or carrier. Follow-up should be included in the procedure to ensure that the rebill actually occurred. (See appendix 9.1 [pp. 293–296] for an AHIMA practice brief on developing a coding compliance policy document.)

Coding Standards

Coding standards should not include numerical goals for case mix, complication and comorbidity (CC) percentage, or any other measurement that encourages payment maximization. However, standards should exist that promote coding accuracy and maximum productivity. The use of benchmarks in determining potential areas of risk or opportunity are considered good business practice, but this should never be confused with attempting to reach a specific numerical goal.

Internal Coding Guidelines

In those instances where no official coding guidelines exist, internal guidelines should be developed to ensure coding consistency and accuracy. These internal guidelines should not conflict with ICD-9-CM, CPT, or HCPCS rules; the Official Coding Guidelines; *Coding Clinic* advice; *CPT Assistant* advice; or federal or state regulations. Coding and sequencing instruction provided in the ICD-9-CM should take precedence over Official Coding Guidelines. However, Official Coding Guidelines should take precedence over facility-specific guidelines.

When clarification of a confusing or new coding issue is necessary, an official source, such as AHA, AHIMA, AMA, CMS, or NCHS, should be contacted. Copies of written requests for guidance and the responses received should be maintained to demonstrate the efforts in place to obtain official guidance in those instances where confusion exists. Until an official response is received, a temporary internal coding guideline should be implemented. A copy of the request for official advice should be attached to the temporary guideline to indicate that a request for official guidance has been made.

Evaluation of Existing Coding Policies, Procedures, Standards, and Internal Guidelines

On an annual basis, coding managers should review and update coding policies, procedures, and standards, as well as internal coding guidelines, to ensure compliance with current regulations. Policies, procedures, and standards for coding should be mandatory regardless of the payment source.

Coder job descriptions should be included in the annual review. This ensures that job descriptions truly reflect the functions currently being performed by coders, the credentials necessary for performing certain coding functions, and the level of education, as well as the number of continuing education hours, required for the coding position.

To ensure that policies are accurate, they should be compared to the release of any official coding guidance or regulations during the past year. Similarly, procedures should be reviewed to determine if any changes have been made that should be incorporated into a procedure's description.

Standards regarding accuracy and productivity levels should be reviewed annually to determine the achievability of the goals and how they compare with standard industry measurements.

Changes made to existing policies, procedures, standards, and internal coding guidelines should include a revision date and follow the facility's procedure for updating these types of documents.

Education and Training

Appropriate and frequent education and training of staff are key factors to ensure ongoing success with the coding compliance program. Potential coding compliance issues may be related to inconsistencies and misinterpretations that arise when coders do not receive ongoing educational opportunities. Coders want to do the right thing; however, without adequate continuing education, accurate coding becomes difficult.

Compliance Education

In conjunction with the corporate compliance officer, the health information manager should provide education and training related to the importance of complete and accurate coding, documentation, and billing on an annual basis. At this time, a review of the facility's corporate compliance plan, the coding compliance plan, fraud and abuse legislation, and the OIG's current work plan should be provided.

Moreover, employees should be provided with acknowledgment forms for the coding compliance plan during compliance education. To ensure compliance, management should designate a time frame for signing and returning the forms to the HR department for placement in the employees' files.

Technical Education

Technical education for coders should be provided monthly (if possible). Such education should include findings associated with data monitoring and ongoing coding audits. Trends identified through those functions should be addressed. A determination should be made prior to the education session as to whether the errors identified in the audit were due to a deficiency in either coding knowledge or clinical knowledge. It may prove useful to have a physician present clinical issues related to specific body systems, diagnoses, or procedures during the session.

Coders should be encouraged to bring difficult cases to the education program. Time should be allotted for coders to present those cases and for the staff to discuss appropriate code assignments.

Areas that should be covered in technical coding education sessions, depending on the type of provider, include:

- OIG focus areas per current work plan

- Clinical information related to problematic body systems, diagnoses, and procedures

- Changes to the PPSs

- Changes to the ICD-9-CM coding and classification system

- Application of the Official Coding Guidelines

- Application of E/M Documentation Guidelines

- *Coding Clinic for ICD-9-CM* to ensure consistent application of published advice

- *CPT Assistant* to ensure consistent application of published advice

Documentation Education

A focused effort should be made to provide documentation education to the medical staff. The coding manager or a physician champion should present documentation issues identified during the audit process, such as incomplete, conflicting, or missing documentation. Many potential compliance issues are the result of inadequate documentation for coding purposes. Improving documentation by the medical staff will ensure coding compliance, as well as the accuracy of the health record.

General areas of concern regarding documentation should also be included. For example, information on inpatient documentation for coding purposes will help ensure that the appropriate documentation is present at the time of discharge. Additionally, education and training related to documentation of the reason for the encounter and of the order for the service should be provided to the physician and/or the physician's office staff. This information will assist in obtaining appropriate documentation and medical necessity at the time of patient registration.

Documentation education should be provided monthly, bimonthly, or quarterly, depending on the severity of the issues. The topics should be related to the underlying cause of errors identified during the audit process.

To improve the overall quality of the health record, ancillary department employees should be included in documentation education. Ancillary departments often benefit from education related to the translation of clinical information into coded data. This is especially useful when this staff is entering charges based on CDM descriptions. When they understand the difficulty associated with that function, the ancillary departments are usually helpful in providing the information needed for accurate coding.

Verbal Communication

Communication between the coding manager and the coding staff is vital to ensure that coding staff are applying policies, procedures, standards, and internal coding guidelines consistently. If the coding manager provides only written copies of new or revised information to the staff with no verbal communication, a high potential exists for individuals to interpret and apply the information inconsistently. By verbally communicating with the staff as a group, the coding manager can ensure that everyone has heard the same message and understands the appropriate application of the information.

The same principle applies when the coding manager passes out copies of new or revised federal and state regulations. Verbal communication ensures that everyone has the same understanding of the intent and application of the regulations.

Additionally, the coding manager should reiterate on a regular basis the steps that coders should take to report potential compliance violations. When he or she repeats the information frequently, coders are less likely to become whistle-blowers and are more likely to understand the action they should take to prompt an internal investigation and resolution—the preferred process.

Auditing

Auditing or reviewing coding and PPS classifications has become an important component in the daily operation of the HIM department. In an effort to ensure compliance, coding managers are spending more time on quality review activities to ensure billing accuracy. This can be a time-consuming process for a manager who is already doing "more with less."

The following sections on internal data monitors, identification of risk areas, considerations in performing an audit, and focus areas for various types of reviews are meant to provide guidance in the manual performance of the auditing function. (Information specific to actually performing the audit or review can be found in chapter 8.)

Internal Data Monitors

Medicare provider analysis and review (MEDPAR) billing data or other national data may be utilized to determine differences between a hospital's billed Medicare inpatient data and a national average of billed Medicare inpatients. Variations identified during this process may indicate fraudulent or abusive coding and billing practices—or there may be a valid explanation for the differences. It is important to note that the existence of a variation does not necessarily mean that there is a compliance issue, but it does indicate that further analysis and an audit should be performed to validate the variations as appropriate for that facility.

DRG monitoring is an excellent method for determining high-risk areas compared with national, regional, or state data. When calculating averages for internal data monitors, the HIM professional must consider whether the calculation will include all payers, only Medicare, or only a specific third-party payer. Also, it is important to use the same period of time in determining both the numerator and the denominator.

Data for the development of national benchmarks for high-risk DRG pairs that are used at your facility can be obtained from Tables 7a and 7b of the proposed and/or final "Changes to the Hospital Inpatient Prospective Payment System" published every year in the *Federal Register* at http://www.gpoaccess.gov/fr/index.html. Data for physician offices and outpatients are available from CMS. Additional sources for obtaining external data for comparison purposes can be found in appendix 9.2 (p. 297).

Areas of External Focus

Data monitors should be established for all areas under investigation by the government or other external reviewers. Those areas may include the following:

- Monitoring of case-mix index

- Percentage of cases that result in the assignment of a DRG with complication or comorbidity

- Audit findings of high-risk DRGs

- Certain problematic diagnoses or procedures

- Variations in length of stay (LOS)

- Variations in charges

Specifics regarding the establishment of data monitors for each of these areas are discussed in the subheads that follow. The HIM professional should remember that many of these areas are "moving targets" that should be evaluated and changed as needed. For example, DRG 14, Intracranial hemorrhage and stroke with infarction; DRG 15, Nonspecific CVA and precerebral occlusion without infarction; and DRG 524, Transient ischemia, might be under investigation one year, but not the next year.

If a facility has significant variations—even after the external focus no longer exists the data monitor should remain in place. However, if no variation exists, the benefit of continued monitoring diminishes.

Tools to use in determining the current external focus include the OIG's annual work plan, identification of its current DRG focus, and knowledge of QIO activities.

Case-Mix Index

Case-mix index (CMI) is the average relative weight for a specified population of inpatients during a specified period of time. In other words, CMI is determined when the DRG relative weights of all discharges in the population for the specified period are added and then divided by the total number of patients in that population for that time period.

Senior management monitors CMI to determine the financial health of an institution. Monitoring should be performed to identify significant, unexplained variations in the CMI. Ongoing analysis should consist of a comparison of the same period of time (for example, a quarter) from one year to the next. A variation in the percentage of change in the CMI from national, regional, or state CMI averages should result in an investigation as to the cause of the variation.

To determine the percentage of change in the CMI, the following formula should be used:

$$\frac{Current\ year's\ CMA\ -\ Last\ year's\ CMI}{Last\ year's\ CMI} \times 100 = Percentage\ of\ change\ in\ CMI$$

The CMI may legitimately vary for any of the following reasons:

- The addition or deletion of services representative of high-weighted DRGs

- Shifts in volumes from low- to high-weighted DRGs or from high- to low-weighted DRGs

- A new local or regional competitor or loss of a competitor

- The addition or loss of specialty physicians to the medical staff

- Changes in coding practices or guidelines

Responsibility for understanding these reasons for CMI variations should fall under the auspices of the health information manager. By analyzing the data proactively, the HIM professional may avoid crisis or reactive measures when called upon to explain the CMI variation. An analysis of the potential causes of a variation may reveal an appropriate explanation. This then should be documented and kept, along with supporting information, for future reference.

Complication and Comorbidity DRG Percentage

Diagnoses that affect certain DRG assignments, when listed as additional diagnoses, are referred to as complications and comorbidities (CCs) in the inpatient PPS. The CC designation indicates that DRGs with CCs have a higher resource intensity, a higher relative weight, and, therefore, a higher reimbursement. Currently (FY 2006), 120 pairs of DRGs split based on the presence or absence of a complicating or comorbid condition. For example, rectal resection splits into two DRGs: DRG 146, Rectal resection with CC, and DRG 147, Rectal resection without CC. DRG 146 has a higher relative weight and reimbursement. There are also seven pairs of DRGs that split based on the presence or absence of a major cardiovascular diagnosis. For instance, DRGs 547 and 548, Coronary bypass with cardiac catheterization, splits based on whether there is a major cardiovascular diagnosis also present.

A CC percentage with a variation significantly higher than the benchmark may be an indicator of overcoding. Using 2005 data, the national average for CC DRG percentage is 80.32 percent. During the mid-1990s in the early days of coding compliance, data indicated that some hospitals consistently showed a CC percentage of 100 percent month after month. Ultimately, many of those hospitals were investigated and settlements were agreed on based on the significant variation initially identified during the government's statistical analysis. (See appendix 9.3 [pp. 298–314] for information related to FY 2005 national averages for CC pairs. Surgical, medical, and total CC pairs are listed separately.)

CC DRG percentages should be monitored on a monthly basis using the following formula (n = number of discharges). Only discharges for those DRGs that split based on the presence or absence of a CC (or an MCV) in the denominator should be monitored.

$$\frac{n(CC\ DRGs)}{n(CC\ DRGs)\ +\ n(no\ CC\ DRGs)} \times 100 = Percentage\ of\ CC\ DRGs$$

An example of this calculation can be seen in the CC/no CC pair, DRG 195/196, Cholecystectomy with common duct exploration. At City Hospital, 187 discharges were assigned to DRG 195 during the period in question. Forty-one cases were assigned to DRG 195 during the same period. The calculation for determining the CC percentage for this pair is as follows:

$$\frac{187}{187\ +\ 41} = \frac{187}{228} = .82017 \times 100 = 82.017\%$$

Of the 228 cases assigned to DRG 195/196 during the period in question, 82 percent were assigned to the higher-weighted DRG 195, reflecting the presence of CCs.

To determine the national average, some hospitals must have a CC percentage greater than the national average and others must have a CC percentage less than the national average. In other words, no "number" is correct for all hospitals. However, when a significant variation from the benchmark number is identified, it should be investigated. When an inappropriate coding practice is identified, a corrective action plan should be instituted.

Audit Findings of High-Risk DRGs

Internal or external coding audits may identify significant areas of variation in DRG assignments. When certain DRGs appear to be problematic for a facility, the HIM professional should establish data monitors. National, regional, or state averages may then be utilized for comparison. Those DRGs may or may not represent the current external investigative focus, but they do represent a high-risk area for the facility. To determine the percentage of a high-risk DRG pair, the following formula (n = number of discharges) should be used:

$$\frac{n(DRG\ X)}{n(DRG\ X)\ +\ n(DRG\ Z)} \times 100 = Percentage\ of\ cases\ in\ DRG\ X$$

For example, in determining the percentage of cases in DRG 475, Respiratory system diagnosis with ventilator support, when the number of cases in DRG 475 and DRG 127, Heart failure and shock, combined represent 100 percent, the following formula should be used (n = number of discharges):

$$\frac{n(DRG\ 475)}{n(DRG\ 475)\ +\ n(DRG\ 127)} \times 100 = Percentage\ of\ cases\ in\ DRG\ 475$$

The following example indicates the percentage of cases that fall into DRG 316, Renal failure, as opposed to DRG 316 and DRG 331/332, Other kidney and urinary tract diagnoses, age >17:

$$\frac{n(DRG\ 316)}{n(DRG\ 316)\ +\ n(DRG\ 331)\ +\ n(DRG\ 332)} \times 100 = Percentage\ of\ cases\ in\ DRG\ 316$$

Appendix 9.4 (pp. 315–316) contains information related to 2005 national averages for high-risk DRG pairs that have been scrutinized by the OIG currently or in the past, or that represent what one might consider a high risk pair due to the nature of the diagnoses or procedures included in the pair (Broussard and Hammen 1999). These high-risk pairs may or may not represent the OIG's current investigative focus.

Twenty Highest-Volume DRGs

By monitoring the 20 highest-volume DRGs at a hospital, the HIM department can determine significant changes that may occur in patient volumes as well as shifts in the volumes.

For example, a high-weighted DRG not previously one of the top 20 in volume begins to appear consistently on the top-20 list month after month. The HIM department should perform additional analysis and audit to determine the underlying cause of the sustained increase. The increase may be legitimately due to the addition of services or specialty physicians. However, the cause must be determined and corrective action taken if the increase was the result of inappropriate coding practices.

Using 2005 national MedPAR data (CMS 2006a), 44 percent—almost half—of all Medicare discharges fell into one of the DRGs shown in appendix 9.3. These DRGs represent the 20 highest-volume Medicare DRGs that occurred nationally in 2005.

Problematic Diagnoses

Data monitors for problematic diagnoses should be instituted when a specific diagnosis is under investigation within a high-risk DRG. At that point, the HIM professional may want to determine the frequency of those diagnoses within the DRG.

For example, DRG 79, Respiratory infections age >17 with CC, represents a significant variation in the percentage of pneumonia cases. Perhaps the assignment of aspiration pneumonia (507.0) as the principal diagnosis was inappropriate. However, by benchmarking and comparing the percentage of cases with aspiration pneumonia as the principal diagnosis versus other principal diagnoses in DRG 79, the need for further audit and investigation may be determined. The calculation would be performed as follows (n = number of discharges):

$$\frac{n(PDX\ 507.0)}{n(DRG\ 79)} \times 100 = Percentage\ of\ cases\ in\ DRG\ 79\ with\ a\ principal\ diagnosis\ of\ 507.0$$

Another example would include monitoring DRG 296 for the percentage of cases with a principal diagnosis of unspecified dehydration (276.51).

$$\frac{n(PDX\ 276.51)}{n(DRG\ 296)} \times 100 = Percentage\ of\ cases\ in\ DRG\ 296\ with\ a\ principal\ diagnosis\ of\ 276.51$$

Problematic Procedures

In monitoring for inpatient compliance, it may prove useful to monitor the occurrence of certain problematic procedures within a category or subcategory of the ICD-9-CM. The difference of one digit in a four-digit procedure code can affect the DRG assignment when it is considered a valid operating room procedure. By monitoring and auditing these high-risk categories, the HIM manager can identify variations from internal benchmarks and institute education and training, where necessary.

Depending on the procedure code assignment from category 38, Incision, excision and occlusion of vessels, the following DRGs may result:

DRG 1/2/3/543	Craniotomy
DRG 7/8	Peripheral, cranial, and other nervous system procedures
DRG 110/111	Major cardiovascular procedure
DRG 119	Vein ligation and stripping
DRG 479/553/554	Other vascular procedures
DRG 528	Intracranial vascular procedure
DRG 533/534	Extracranial procedures

Other DRGs may also apply depending on the principal diagnosis assignment.

The relative weights and thus the reimbursement for these DRGs differ significantly. When one incorrect digit is assigned consistently for a procedure that is frequently performed at a facility, it could result in a pattern of abuse that could capture the attention of external investigators.

For instance, the HIM manager may want to monitor the occurrence of procedure code 38.31, Intracranial vessel resection and anastomosis, as compared to code 38.32, Head and neck vessel resection and anastomosis. The calculation would be performed as follows (n = number of discharges):

$$\frac{n(PX\ 38.31)}{n(PX\ 38.31)\ +\ n(PX\ 38.32)} \times 100 = Percentage\ of\ cases\ assigned\ to\ code\ 38.31$$

The result indicates the percentage of cases assigned to code 38.31 (DRG 1, 2, 3, or 543) rather than to code 38.32 (DRG 533 or 534).

Variations in Length of Stay and in Charges

Variations in length of stay (LOS) should be monitored to determine those cases within a DRG that have a LOS significantly less than the average LOS for other discharges assigned to the same DRG. Potentially, when the LOS is significantly shorter and the patient is discharged to home, there is a chance that DRG creep has occurred.

Variations in charges should be monitored for the same reason. As a benchmark, the charges for each Medicare DRG for the facility are averaged. These averages are used when actual charges are compared to determine variations.

When variations occur in either LOS or charges, those particular cases that fall out should be audited to validate appropriate coding and DRG assignment.

Other Data Monitors

Although inpatient data monitors have been described previously, data monitors may be established for all patient care settings. Some of those not mentioned include:

- The occurrence of component code assignments as a percentage of the comprehensive code assigned to the same encounter

- The 20 highest-volume ambulatory payment classifications (APCs) within the organization for significant changes over time

- A bell curve analysis of E/M code assignments with comparison by physician

- The occurrence of certain modifiers (–59, Distinct procedural services) as a percentage of all outpatient/physician-office encounters

The Next Step

Data monitors should be utilized to determine the next step in the process. If significant variations exist, the coding manager should drill down, or look at a greater level of detail, in the data to identify those specific cases that should be reviewed. The data should be provided in the form of a report representing case-specific information (for example, health record number, account number, diagnosis codes, procedure codes, LOS, and charges).

The coding manager should review the data to determine the cases to be included in the focused audit. Those cases that appear "different" from other cases in the report should be included in the actual audit.

Identification of Risk Areas

Many coding risk areas exist that vary depending on the site of service. Some of these risk areas are discussed in the following sections.

DRG Coding Accuracy

ICD-9-CM coding for Medicare DRG assignment has been a major focus of the OIG's fraud and abuse efforts. Hospitals across the country have been subpoenaed for health records. Those records are then audited to ensure that the coding matches both clinical and physician documentation within the health record.

The criteria for evaluating health records for potentially inappropriate coding or DRG assignments are based on the premise that all coding must be supported by a physician's documentation of the diagnosis or of the procedure in the body of the health record. In addition to blatant violations of coding rules, such as upcoding, it was determined that many violations were caused by poor training or lack of facility-specific coding rules. **Assumption coding**—assigning codes based on clinical signs, symptoms, test findings, or treatment without supporting physician documentation—was also found to be a significant problem.

In addition, appropriate application of the Official Coding and Reporting Guidelines, as well as application of other federal rules and regulations, is reviewed as a requirement of coding accuracy in all care settings.

The initial DRG efforts of the OIG included a comparison of the percentage of cases assigned to DRGs with CCs as opposed to those without CCs, and the DRG pair of complex versus simple pneumonia. In investigating CC percentages, the OIG determined that some hospitals were reporting 100 percent of their cases in DRGs with CCs month after month. At the time those investigations began, the national CC percentage was in the 83 to 85 percent range.

The OIG began its investigation of DRG pairs by comparing the national average for complex versus simple pneumonia to the average for individual hospitals to determine the potential for fraudulent or abusive coding patterns. Since the pneumonia project began in 1998, the OIG has expanded its DRG investigations to include more than 20 pairs of DRGs. It also has employed a more sophisticated statistical methodology for identifying aberrations in hospitals across the country.

As mentioned earlier, when monitoring these averages, health information managers must remember that the existence of a variation does not necessarily mean there is a compliance problem. It does indicate, however, that the variation should be investigated to determine why it exists. In arriving at a national average, some hospitals will have percentages higher than the average and others will have percentages lower than the average.

Variations in CMI

The OIG investigates variations in CMI over time for individual hospitals to determine trends that have occurred and whether such trends were the result of upcoding. Those investigations also include identifying any DRG that significantly influenced national trends in the CMI over time.

Changes in CMI may be attributed to any of the following factors:

- Changes in coding rules
- Changes in medical staff composition
- Changes in services offered
- Local competition
- Referrals

HIM professionals should routinely monitor the CMI and determine the underlying causes of variations as part of their role in coding.

Discharge Status

Hospitals are now reimbursed using a transfer payment methodology when a patient receives postacute care (excluded hospitals, skilled nursing facilities (SNFs), or home healthcare within 3 days of inpatient discharge) for 183 DRGs (see appendix 9.5). CMS is monitoring patients discharged with these DRGs to determine if postacute services are received after discharge. Hospitals stating "home, self-care" as the discharge disposition for those postacute care DRGs may be reviewed by CMS to determine if billing practices are consistent with Medicare policy. In 2004, CMS began comparing acute hospital discharges to their next service provider (for example, home health within 3 days, SNF on day of discharge) through the common working file (CWF) to determine if the appropriate discharge disposition code had been assigned at the acute care site. If the case met criteria for postacute care, monies were being denied until the discharge disposition was corrected to match the postacute care provider setting. The patient status (discharge disposition) codes that indicate a postacute care transfer (and thus affect reimbursement) are:

- A psychiatric hospital or unit (patient status code 65);
- An inpatient rehabilitation hospital or unit (patient status code 62);
- A long term care hospital (patient status code 63);
- A children's hospital (patient status code 05);
- A cancer hospital (patient status code 05);
- A SNF (patient status code 03); or

- A home health agency (patient status code 06) when the patient is provided home health services* under a written plan of care for the provision of home health services from a home health agency and those services begin within 3 days after the date of discharge from the hospital. Title 42 Section 412.4 (c) (3), of the Code of Federal Regulations (CFR) stipulates that a written plan of care is documented and begins within 3 days after the date of discharge.

Other issues related to discharge status have been identified as compliance concerns over the past several years. Cases with a discharge status of "left against medical advice" or "home, self-care" that were found, in fact, to have been transferred to another acute care facility represent compliance issues. Had they been appropriately classified to "transfer to another acute care facility," reimbursement would have been paid at a per diem rate based on LOS rather than at the full DRG rate. Effective FY 2004, hospitals with patients who are discharged as "left against medical advice" will be reimbursed as a qualified transfer if found to be admitted to another hospital on the same day, even though the initial hospital did not transfer the patient. When an inappropriate discharge disposition is coded, there is potential for the occurrence of an honest mistake or for fraudulent or abusive coding. The government looks for *patterns* of abuse to assist in making this determination.

When hospitals merge, another area of potential fraud and abuse in the coding of discharge status occurs. Problems arise when a patient currently listed as an inpatient in hospital A becomes a patient in hospital B upon the merger or acquisition of hospital A with or by hospital B. The correct method of billing this patient is as a single admission under the provider number of the postmerger, or acquiring, hospital for a full DRG payment. However, in certain situations, such a patient might be billed for a transfer at the per diem rate based on LOS under the provider number of hospital A (transferred to hospital B on the date of the merger/acquisition) and for a full DRG payment under the provider number of hospital B (admitted on the date of the merger). Additionally, third-party payers will usually guide the provider in how to handle these situations to fit their particular policies. As with all the examples described in this chapter, the potential for an honest mistake occurring truly depends on the type and amount of training provided to those individuals responsible for ensuring appropriate coding and billing practices.

Services Provided under Arrangement

Services provided under arrangement with another healthcare facility have also been identified as a potential high-risk area for providers. When one facility is in a contractual relationship with another facility to perform services not currently offered at the first facility, the terms of the contractual relationship should be shared with the coding staff at both facilities to ensure complete and accurate coding.

For example, hospital A does not provide cardiac catheterization, but hospital B down the street does. A patient is admitted to inpatient status in hospital A, and the physician determines that a cardiac catheterization procedure is necessary during the current admission. The patient is sent by ambulance to hospital B for the cardiac catheterization and then returned to hospital A after the procedure has been completed.

This example illustrates an appropriate practice. However, the coding staff at the providing facility (hospital B) needs to be aware that the inpatient facility (hospital A) will code the

---

*Home health services provided outside the 3-day window, even if related to the hospital stay, will not be considered a transfer. Also, if care related to the discharge is provided within 3 days but without a written plan of care, then this case *will* be considered a transfer.

procedure and bill Medicare for the cardiac catheterization under the DRG system to avoid duplicate coding and billing. The service provider (hospital B) then will bill the inpatient facility (hospital A) for services provided to the patient.

Medicare rules must be followed in determining certain terms and conditions of the contract. This practice not only affects hospital A's DRG assignment, but also its cost reporting in terms of overhead and administrative costs. It is inappropriate for the billing facility to mark up procedures for these costs when the procedures were not performed at that facility.

72-Hour Window

Medicare issued changes to the 72-hour window rule in the February 11, 1998, *Federal Register*. In summary, the changes included:

- The following services are not subject to the 72-hour window rule and are excluded from the inpatient DRG payment:

  —Hospice, home health, or skilled nursing services covered under Medicare Part A and provided within 72 hours of inpatient admission

  —Ambulance services or maintenance renal dialysis services within 72 hours of admission

  —Nondiagnostic services unrelated to the admission

- The following services are subject to the 72-hour window rule for inclusion in the inpatient DRG payment:

  —All diagnostic services within 72 hours of admission

  —All nondiagnostic services related to the admission

CMS defines nondiagnostic-related services as having the same ICD-9-CM diagnosis code. However, this is not a legal definition, only CMS's interpretation. If coders doubt whether the nondiagnostic service is related to the admission, they should query the physician and obtain supporting documentation.

Through the OIG's 1997 work plan, investigative efforts were begun related to the separate billing of those outpatient services when provided by the admitting hospital, by an entity wholly owned or operated by the admitting hospital, or by another entity under arrangement with the hospital.

Most coding departments are not responsible for determining the presence of outpatient services within 72 hours of inpatient admission. In many instances, this is determined in the business office utilizing commercial software. However, coders should be aware of the intent of the rules to ensure the bundling of outpatient charges, when appropriate.

DRG Payment Window

Per several of the past OIG Work Plans, reviews to investigate the DRG payment window in terms of submitting Medicaid claims for inpatient stay related ancillary services occurring within 3 days of hospital admission. Investigations into the Medicare DRG payment window have resulted in the recoupment of more than $100 million dollars between 1992 and 1996, further investigations may reveal that state Medicaid programs with the same DRG payment window regulations have similar opportunities.

Outpatient Prospective Payment System

The outpatient prospective payment system (OPPS) has become a focus to determine whether payments under OPPS are accurate based on Medicare regulations. Several aspects of the system will be reviewed, including transitional pass-through payments, multiple procedures during one operative episode, and psychotherapy services provided in community health centers. Two areas included in the 2006 OIG Work Plan for investigation under this category include unbundling of hospital outpatient services and "inpatient only" services billed as outpatient services.

Medical Necessity

Medical necessity is a high-risk area in both the hospital and physician-office settings. According to the OIG's *Compliance Program Guidance for Clinical Laboratories* and LCDs, the physician should provide the "reason for the encounter" prior to the performance of the service to ensure medical necessity and Medicare coverage. When the service is not considered medically necessary based on the "reason for the encounter" and the coder is unable to obtain additional, valid diagnoses from the physician, the patient should be provided with a waiver of liability—an advance beneficiary notice (ABN)—indicating that Medicare will not pay and that the patient will be responsible for the entire charge.

A physician or hospital should be able to provide documentation of medical necessity for all outpatient services that are provided and billed to Medicare. When claims submitted to Medicare do not demonstrate medical necessity through documentation, an investigation that identifies a pattern may result in civil penalties.

Evaluation and Management Services

The OIG is investigating the use of E/M codes by physicians with aberrant coding patterns, specifically those with high volumes of high-level codes that provide a higher level of reimbursement to the physician. To be assigned appropriately, these codes must be assigned in accordance with the CPT guidelines surrounding these services and must be based on physician documentation.

Consultation coding is also under investigation with the OIG determining the appropriateness of billing for consultations and the financial impact of inappropriate consultation code assignment.

Other Risk Areas: The CDM and the Superbill

The risk areas already described are by no means all-inclusive. Other risk areas for coding are just as important, depending on the site of service. For example, codes that appear on a hospital's CDM should be audited on an annual basis to ensure that hard coding of certain procedures and services, supplies, drugs, and equipment is accurate. By neglecting to perform this function, a hospital or other provider could be at risk for inappropriate coding, APC assignment, and reimbursement. (The CDM is discussed in detail in chapter 6.)

Another area of concern is the superbill used in the physician office or clinic setting. The superbill also should be audited on an annual basis prior to implementation of updated CPT codes, that is, before January 1 of each year. (Superbills are discussed in chapter 11.)

Coding Compliance Review Considerations

Prior to actually performing coding compliance reviews, the health information manager should consider certain aspects of the review process to ensure consistency and effectiveness. The specific criteria used in the audit process should be included in the HIM department's internal coding compliance plan.

Responsibility for Reviews

Responsibility for coding compliance reviews should be determined prior to implementing the review process in the HIM department. Responsibility for this function, as with any function, should be documented in the department's policy and procedure manual. The policy and procedure should then be included in the coding compliance plan. In most instances, the coding supervisor or the health information manager will be responsible for performing the reviews.

Staff members performing frontline coding should not be responsible for auditing their own work because this could be construed as a conflict of interest. In smaller hospitals or facilities, this may not be practical. In the event the hospital does not have a coding supervisor and the health information manager is not skilled in coding, other options, such as using a local coding consulting company, should be considered for performing the review. When a small hospital is part of a larger chain with other hospitals in the region or with access to corporate resources, HIM could request coding audit assistance from one of the larger facilities in the chain or from its corporate resources.

Internal and External Audits

In a larger hospital, coding compliance reviews may fall under the auspices of an internal audit or compliance department. The coding supervisor or the health information manager then would be responsible only for ensuring the availability of the records prior to the review. The internal auditors would perform the actual review and share the results in accordance with guidelines set through the facilitywide compliance program.

Regardless of whether the coding supervisor, health information manager, or internal auditor reviews health records for compliance, an external review should be performed at least once a year. If problems have been identified in the past, an external audit should be performed twice a year to validate internal findings. Obtaining an objective, third-party review of internal practices ensures that everyone—even those performing ongoing compliance reviews—is compliant with current rules and regulations related to the coding function.

Thus, facilities may choose to do one of the following:

- Outsource coding compliance audit functions to an external auditing company

- Perform all coding compliance audits internally

- Use a combination of internal and external auditing

A combination of the two types of audits provides the best of both worlds; the facility can save money by performing most audits internally, using an external source only once or twice a year.

Prospective and Retrospective Reviews

Another consideration in developing policies and procedures for coding compliance reviews is determining the point in the flow of the health record at which the review will be performed. Should the record be reviewed for coding compliance prior to bill drop (prospective review) or following bill drop (retrospective review)? **Bill drop** indicates that the claim has been released as complete for submission to the insurer for payment.

By reviewing coding prospectively, health information managers can ensure that any errors identified during the review process are corrected and that the DRG is correct prior to bill drop. This reduces the number of rebills that occur over the course of a year and thus reduces the hospital's risk. The drawback of a prospective review is that it cannot be focused on specific types of cases, whether referring to specific inpatient DRGs, specific outpatient APCs, or specific types of physician office visits. When reviewing prospectively, reviewers have limited samples unless they are willing to review a few records every day until the sampling requirements are met.

In performing a retrospective review, the reviewer has the opportunity to focus on certain external or internal high-risk areas. This review also can include a review of the UB-92/UB-04 for the appropriate transfer of codes. Specific numbers of health records per coder or per physician may be selected. However, if DRG inaccuracies are identified, rebilling must be performed, whether or not the correct DRG increases or decreases reimbursement. When a significant number of rebills have occurred, the FI may become interested in why so many claims are being rebilled. This could put the facility at risk for external investigation.

It is probably more prudent (if the audits are performed at the hospital) to conduct prospective reviews as a part of an ongoing internal coding compliance review process. However, either method is appropriate and the selection of methodology must be based on the circumstances that best fit the needs of the hospital.

Frequency of Audits

The coding compliance audit policy should include parameters for the frequency of auditing; daily, weekly, monthly, or quarterly audits may be considered. Establishing the frequency of audits helps ensure that they are performed in a timely manner.

The frequency of coding compliance reviews depends on the individual facility. For example, a supervisor responsible for this function may have only 4 hours per week to devote to coding compliance activities. In such a case, the sampling methodology would have to be determined to accommodate that type of schedule.

In another facility, perhaps the coding supervisor is able to schedule 1 week per quarter for coding compliance reviews. In that case, a much larger sampling can be reviewed during one sitting and can include health records based on facility-specific selection criteria. The frequency of reviews may also depend on whether the reviews are conducted prospectively or retrospectively.

Sampling Methodology

The policy for performing coding compliance audits should include information on selecting the samples for the audit. Various methodologies can be used, including:

- The specific number of health records by type of patient

- A certain percentage of health records by type of patient

- The number/percentage of health records by coder
- A statistically valid sampling formula

The sampling should include:

- Current areas of investigative focus
- Internal high-risk areas
- A random sampling of health records to determine overall accuracy

When established benchmarks are used to monitor coded data, the health information manager should include a review of any areas in which a significant variation from the benchmark has occurred.

Audit Worksheets

A separate audit worksheet is necessary for each type of patient audited because the type of data collected on each will vary to a certain degree. Data elements that should be collected include:

- Type of patient
- Billing number/health record number
- Coder's name
- Physician's name
- Admission/discharge dates
- Length of stay
- Age
- Gender
- Original/audit discharge disposition
- Financial class
- Auditor's name
- Audit date
- Original/audit diagnosis and procedure codes
- Impact on case designation (that is, DRG or APC)
- Impact on reimbursement
- Root cause of error, such as documentation, coding error, Official Coding Guideline, coding convention, *Coding Clinic* advice, and so on
- Documentation present at final coding versus that present during audit
- Rationale for audit recommendations

This information may be collected either on a paper form or electronically. After the audit, the worksheets should be retained as specified in the facility's compliance program. Audit findings and trends identified on the worksheets should be summarized for individual and group education. Accuracy rates should be calculated for individual coders and for the department as a whole, as well as for physicians regarding identified documentation issues.

Coding Compliance Reviews

Using specific criteria, each type of patient should be assessed to determine compliance with applicable regulations and the potential for risk. Current areas of investigative focus should be included in the assessment as well as in those areas in which previous reviews may have revealed problems. (See chapter 8 for techniques about reviewing inpatient and outpatient health records and how to determine errors.)

Reviewing Inpatient Health Records

Complete and accurate coding and DRG assignment of inpatient health records should be assessed to validate that physician and clinical documentation support it. Application of ICD-9-CM coding conventions and Official Coding Guidelines should be utilized in performing the review. The principal diagnosis, all additional diagnoses, and all significant procedures should be reviewed to determine not only upcoding, but also undercoding and total data quality. Timeliness of physician documentation should be reviewed because it can impact coding and billing from a time perspective, as well as from an availability perspective.

The sampling of records to be reviewed should be representative of current areas of investigative focus, including high-risk DRG pairs, CC percentage, and those DRGs with a LOS or charges significantly different from the hospital's average LOS or charges. If a significant variation in case mix exists, the 20 highest-volume DRGs should be reviewed to determine accuracy. Trended variations identified as the result of previous reviews should also be included in the review.

As part of the health record review, the accuracy of discharge status should be determined. For example, if a patient were transferred to another acute care hospital, the transferring hospital would receive only a portion of the DRG reimbursement—a per diem rate—as determined by the actual LOS. That is why the appropriate discharge disposition should be assigned based on health record documentation. If health record documentation provides conflicting information, the hospital should consider instituting a policy and procedure that assigns responsibility for appropriate documentation of discharge disposition to one discipline, such as discharge planning. This improves discharge disposition accuracy for billing purposes. As a part of the review, the discharge disposition should also be reviewed to ensure that it has been transferred appropriately to the UB-92/UB-04.

Inpatient records should also be reviewed to ensure that coding of services provided under arrangement with another facility has been performed appropriately. The appropriate coding depends on whether the facility is a provider or a receiver of services provided under arrangement. In instances in which this is unclear or when the HIM department is unaware of any contractual relationships, the business office director or chief financial officer should be queried.

If preadmission outpatient services provided within 72 hours of inpatient admission are identified during the review, the appropriate area, usually PFS, should be notified so that rebilling can occur. Ensuring compliance with the 72-hour window rule is usually not the responsibility of the HIM department. However, in instances in which errors are identified, they should be addressed.

Ambulatory Surgery and the Emergency Department

The HIM department should validate complete and accurate coding in accordance with ICD-9-CM coding conventions and the Diagnostic Coding and Reporting Guidelines. Additionally, the HIM department should validate CPT coding based on CPT guidelines and include National Correct Coding Initiative (NCCI) edits and outpatient code editor (OCE) edits as part of the review. Each procedure should have a correlating diagnosis to indicate the procedure's medical necessity. Also, appropriate assignment of modifiers should be reviewed because these affect APC assignment and, therefore, outpatient reimbursement.

The coding of the reason for the encounter, all additional diagnoses, and all significant procedures should be reviewed to determine data quality for ambulatory surgery and emergency department coding. Additionally, timeliness of physician documentation should be reviewed because dictation and transcription can affect the timeliness and accuracy of coding.

When the technology is available for reviewing all APC assignments at the point of quality review, APCs should be reviewed to validate appropriate transmission of HCPCS codes to the grouper and to the UB-92/UB-04. If documentation reveals that services or supplies were used, but no charge was generated, the department responsible for the charge entry should receive education on prompt and accurate entry of charges for reimbursement.

E/M codes assigned for emergency department facility charges should be reviewed using hospital-specific criteria to determine the appropriate levels (implementation of facility-standardized criteria is required). Although the coding for the facility charge may not be performed by the HIM coding staff, the codes should be reviewed to ensure accuracy and appropriateness.

When the hospital is also assigning E/M codes for physicians' billing, those codes should be validated based on CMS's E/M Documentation Guidelines.

Referred Outpatients

Only diagnosis codes need to be validated for referred outpatient coding because the procedures should be captured through the facility's CDM. (HIM staff may or may not be called upon to perform an audit of CDM–driven coding.) The HIM department should validate complete and accurate coding in accordance with ICD-9-CM coding conventions and the Diagnostic Coding and Reporting Guidelines. However, the presence of documentation indicating the reason for performing the service and the order for the service should also be verified. If documentation reveals that services or supplies were used, but no charge was generated, the department responsible for the charge entry should receive education on prompt entry of charges for reimbursement.

Physician

E/M codes should be validated based on the presence of documentation to support the level of service provided by the physician and on the appropriate application of E/M Documentation Guidelines. In validating the E/M code assignment, close attention should be paid to E/M for day-of-discharge management services, consultations, critical care services, psychotherapy, and individual psychiatric testing for inpatients. These areas are or have been under investigation, thus warranting a continued close review for compliance with applicable regulations.

The HIM department should validate complete and accurate coding in accordance with ICD-9-CM coding conventions and the Diagnostic Coding and Reporting Guidelines. Additionally, it should validate CPT coding of procedures based on CPT guidelines and include a review for appropriate coding based on NCCI edits. Each procedure should have a correlating diagnosis to indicate the medical necessity of the procedure. Also, appropriate assignment of modifiers should be reviewed because they affect physician reimbursement.

When reviewing records related to physicians at teaching hospitals, the HIM department should validate the existence of documentation to support the presence and supervision of the physician while residents provide services.

Corrective Action

Although corrective action is not the sole responsibility of the coding manager, many of the steps involved in the process fall to the individual in that role. The ultimate goal of corrective action is prevention of the same problem in the future. To reach that point in the corrective action process, many other steps must be performed.

When a compliance problem is identified in the form of a potential coding fraud or abuse issue, the coding manager should work within the guidance provided in the corporate compliance program. Those steps should include notification of the compliance officer. When the compliance officer is involved, the coding manager may or may not be included in the investigation leading to corrective action.

Whether the coding manager is involved or not, the next steps are basically the same. An internal investigation is performed, which usually includes interviews with coding staff, coding management staff, and others who may be involved in the problem. The internal investigation also includes a review of data, policies, and previous educational efforts. This helps to identify the underlying cause of the problem. In other words, is this truly a compliance issue, or was it just an error possibly based on a lack of knowledge?

Senior management, the compliance officer, and legal counsel then work through the details of reporting the issue and providing restitution for overpayments, penalties, and interest. The details of internal disciplinary action depend on the extent of the problem identified through the investigation and include input from the HR department.

Based on the results of the audit, policies and procedures should be updated and/or revised to reflect the appropriate coding practice. Education should then be provided to the coding staff and other staff, as necessary, to ensure a thorough understanding of the appropriate coding practice and future expectations.

At this point, ongoing auditing of the problem area should be instituted to ensure its detection and prevention in the future. Ongoing auditing may be performed either internally or externally, depending on the circumstances surrounding the previously identified problem and on the procedure outlined in the corporate compliance program.

Reporting

All coding compliance activities should be performed, documented, and reported in accordance with direction provided by the corporate compliance program. If no specific guidance is provided, the compliance officer should be able to assist in determining the type of documentation required to demonstrate the compliance efforts of the HIM coding staff.

Usually, the documentation created should include:

- Trends identified

- Financial implications

- Corrective action taken

- Changes made to existing policies and procedures

- Education provided

- Report of findings to the compliance officer

- Dates and statistics for all coding compliance activities

Case-specific findings usually need not be included in the information provided to the compliance department. A summary of the findings, including trends, financial implications, and corrective action, is sufficient in reporting audit activities.

Departmental records of all coding compliance activities should be maintained in the HIM department. Retention of these records depends on the regulations of the state in question and the guidance provided in the corporate compliance plan.

Tools and External Services Used in Coding Compliance

Coding managers make use of a variety of software products for coding, billing, and monitoring functions. Such tools can constitute an important part of the compliance review process.

Software

Encoder and quality review software are valuable tools for ensuring complete and accurate coding for billing purposes. However, inaccuracies and discrepancies in the software may result in compliance risks for the user. Before purchasing software, the HIM manager should be sure that the software vendor provides the following services:

- A hotline for reporting errors and requesting service

- Frequent updates reflecting corrections

- Regular updates to the coding systems and PPSs

- A list of current users for potential buyers to contact regarding their satisfaction with the vendor's software and services

Encoders

Inaccuracies in encoder software may result in a pattern of inappropriate coding that could send up "red flags" for possible investigations. If the ICD-9-CM code books, CPT code book, *Coding Clinic*, or *CPT Assistant* indicate that another code is more appropriate than the code provided through the encoder software, the coding supervisor should notify the vendor about the discrepancy. Corrections made as a result of communication between vendor and user ensures a better product from the vendor in future software updates.

The coding supervisor should keep a log that documents the following information regarding encoder errors:

- The date the error was discovered

- The date the vendor was notified

- The vendor's response to the discrepancy

- The date the software was corrected

The coding staff should be made aware of any encoder discrepancies to avoid assigning incorrect codes. The coding supervisor should stay informed about encoder errors so that, if needed, a study can be conducted of previously coded records to determine the potential financial impact of assigning inappropriate codes over time. If inappropriate codes have been used, rebilling may be necessary. When overpayment to a facility has occurred, the compliance officer should be notified.

Software for Quality Reviews

Software for quality reviews is available from several software companies. Through a series of internal edits, this software identifies accounts that may represent inaccurate or inappropriate coding.

Software for quality reviews can reduce the amount of time needed to perform data-monitoring functions and to determine cases to review for a focused coding compliance audit. Although identification of specific accounts for review is not indicative of errors, it does reduce the amount of time the coding manager must spend in manually reviewing reports to determine those accounts that look "different" from similar accounts.

In the OIG's 1998 report *Using Software to Detect Upcoding of Hospital Bills* (OEI 01-97-00010), optimism was expressed regarding the use of such software. However, state-of-the-art software does not appear to provide the level of accuracy needed to ensure success using only software.

Thus, software for quality reviews still must be coupled with a manual review process to ensure accurate detection of potentially fraudulent or abusive coding practices. In and of itself, no current software package can identify upcoding or undercoding without human intervention in the form of an actual health record review.

Consulting Firms

Time studies may reveal that the coding manager is unable to take on the additional task of conducting coding compliance reviews. As a result, many providers choose to contract with external coding compliance vendors. This is an appropriate solution as long as the vendor can meet certain criteria. External coding compliance companies should meet the following 11 criteria:

1. Follow the Official Coding Guidelines approved by the Cooperating Parties (AMA, AHIMA, CMS, and NCHS). These guidelines are used in coding Medicare, Medicaid, and Tri-Care (Civilian Health and Medical Program of Veterans Administration) claims. These guidelines should also be applied during an audit for a government investigation. The vendor's internal coding guidelines should be reviewed to ensure consistency with the Official Coding Guidelines.

    Additionally, if a quality review of physician coding is being conducted, the vendors should be well versed in the application of E/M Documentation Guidelines that have been approved by CMS in assigning the appropriate level of CPT evaluation and management codes.

2. Identify upcoding, undercoding, and coding quality errors that do not affect the DRG assignment when reporting findings to the client. Total compliance involves ensuring complete and accurate coding reflecting an accurate picture of the patient's care. The provider then can be assured that its billing is accurate and its healthcare statistics provide an accurate view of its case mix for determining future services, managed care contracts, and profiling.

3. Charge a fixed fee rather than a contingency fee. Advice provided by the OIG in its compliance program guidance indicates that compensation for consultants should not provide any financial incentive to upcode claims improperly. By charging the healthcare provider a fixed fee for coding quality reviews rather than a percentage of the money "found," the incentive for upcoding is eliminated.

4. Employ only credentialed coding staff and be willing to provide proof of the credential status of each employee who will be providing services. This includes credentials reflecting RHIA, RHIT, CCS, and CCS-P, which indicate that the individuals have met the competencies set for those particular credentials and have maintained continuing education hours on an ongoing basis.

5. Justify recommendations for changes to coding or prospective payment system assignment through the use of appropriate references. This would include the use of the Official Coding Guidelines, E/M Documentation Guidelines, *Coding Clinic*, or *CPT Assistant*. If the consultant cannot justify a recommended change, the healthcare provider may want to contact an official source, such as the Central Office for ICD-9-CM, for ICD-9-CM questions or the AMA for CPT questions, prior to agreeing with the consultant's recommendation.

6. Educate consulting staff on current areas of investigative focus and on consistent application of guidelines. Vendors should be able to document that they provide at least annual or semiannual educational programs for their consulting staff. This may represent an educational meeting developed and presented by the vendors themselves, or it may represent sending their consulting staff to external programs.

7. Have their own compliance program and provide a copy of it to potential clients. Vendors' coding compliance programs should adhere to the steps outlined in the OIG's compliance program guidance models. The coding philosophy of vendors should reflect that of the client to ensure complete and accurate coding.

8. Educate provider staff as a component of the services. External quality reviews of coding should include education related to upcoding, undercoding, and quality review. It should also provide specific technical or clinical education related to trends identified during the audit process.

9. Have never been convicted of fraudulent practices. In keeping with Sections 4301 and 4302 of the BBA (1997), vendors who have been convicted of fraudulent practices should be avoided. This ensures that the healthcare provider receives high-quality, ethical services.

10. Provide services under attorney–client privilege. When an attorney representing a provider requests auditing services under attorney–client privilege, the vendor works with the attorney designated by the provider. Communication between vendor and healthcare provider is limited to protect the results of the coding compliance audit from future "discovery."

11. Have credible client references. Healthcare providers should not settle for a prepared list of references because it will contain only the names of individuals who will provide positive feedback. Instead, the healthcare provider should request a list of the five clients most recently served by the vendors. When contacting them, the healthcare provider should ensure that these clients were satisfied with the vendors' coding philosophy, fees, and quality of service.

Currently, government investigations are focused on healthcare providers. When a trend has been established between the providers under investigation and use of a particular coding consulting company, increased investigations of vendors and their other clients are likely to occur. Healthcare providers should protect themselves from investigation by ensuring that the company selected for external coding compliance reviews meets the criteria discussed above.

Health Insurance Portability and Accountability Act: Security and Privacy

HIPAA legislation has affected hospital operations and compliance activities nationwide. The impact from a security and privacy aspect as it relates to coding is apparent and should describe practices in place prior to HIPAA. The one aspect that needs consideration is implementation of electronic health records to further secure patient privacy. Coding from an electronic record may have many implications for coders, including the ability to work from home. When that is the reality, policies and procedures need to be established to ensure compliance with HIPAA rules and regulations and maintaining the security of the electronic data in a home office.

Code Sets

In addition to ensuring security and privacy of health information, HIPAA legislation included a provision for the mandatory use of code sets, such as ICD-9-CM, CPT, and HCPCS, in reporting healthcare encounters for reimbursement. This provision also includes the current processes in place for updating the code sets, as well as the use of current guidelines.

The rule includes not only federally funded healthcare programs, but also private third-party payers. In other words, all payers will be required to use the same code sets, follow the same processes for updating the code sets, and—most important—use the same guidelines in applying the code sets. All components of the HIPAA legislation are now in effect (privacy, code sets, and electronic transactions), including that for security.

The mandatory use of code sets offers another opportunity for coding managers to shine. Many of the current payers are unaware of the official guidelines in place for code sets, such as ICD-9-CM. Perhaps coding managers could offer educational sessions regarding the appropriate application of coding guidelines. This would help in the consistent application of code set guidelines in the development of their internal systems and policies.

Protection of Coded Data

External vendors who perform backlog coding activities or audit activities are considered business associates under HIPAA. Those vendors will be performing the coding or auditing function using identifiable health information on behalf of the facility, but they are not internal, permanent employees of the facility. In this situation, the healthcare provider must ensure that the business associate has measures in place to ensure the security and privacy of the information to which it has access. This information must be outlined in the form of a contract between healthcare provider and business associate.

Terms of the contract must include provisions between provider and the business associate that:

- Permit the vendor's use of the identifiable health information

- Prohibit further disclosure of the identifiable health information by the vendor

- Prevent further disclosure of the identifiable health information by the vendor through the use of internal safeguard mechanisms

- Require a report to the provider of any unauthorized disclosure

- Ensure that subcontractors agree to—and follow—the same restrictions as the vendor

- Provide for the return or destruction of identifiable health information in cases in which the vendor provides coding services off-site

When vendors do not adhere to the assurances of security and privacy provided to the healthcare provider, they are considered noncompliant with HIPAA regulations. The coding manager must ensure that all contracts with external vendors or agents performing coding audits are in accordance with the hospital's HIPAA policies and procedures. A business associate's agreement should be signed by hospital management and the vendor.

When in doubt, contracts should be reviewed by legal counsel or the facility's privacy officer to ensure that it safeguards identifiable health information as well as meeting other aspects of the provider–vendor (business associate) relationship.

Conclusion

Although the federal government's efforts to prevent healthcare fraud and abuse have resulted in some hardships for the provider community, they also have resulted in a renewed effort to ensure high-quality services that are coded and billed correctly. Support for coders to attend educational programs has never been better. As a major component of complete and accurate coding to ensure appropriate billing, coders are receiving the education needed to enhance their skills and thus their opportunities for advancement.

A whole new field of opportunity has opened up to health information managers. Many compliance officers across the country have come from an HIM background. By taking the initiative, these leaders have proven that their knowledge in coding, billing, and federal regulations has made them the obvious choice for ensuring compliance throughout their facilities.

The advent of HIPAA legislation for code sets, as well as legislation related to security and privacy, has resulted in other new opportunities for health information coding managers. Many of them are stepping up to the plate and offering their knowledge of code sets, information systems, confidentiality, and federal regulations. As a result, many health information managers have become their facility's security and/or privacy officer.

Now and in the future, health information managers need to recognize when a door to opportunity is opened. By stepping through that door and offering their unique expertise, they will advance the profession and increase the credibility of other HIM professionals.

References

AHIMA Coding Practice Team. 2001 (July–August). Practice brief: Developing a coding compliance policy document. *Journal of American Health Information Management Association* (72)7:88A–C.

Broussard, K., and C. Hammen. 1999. Twenty pairs the OIG may be targeting for investigation. *Journal of Health Care Compliance* 1(3):9–14, 36.

Centers for Medicare and Medicaid Services. 2004 (December). FY 2004 Improper Medicare Fee-For-Service Payment Report Executive Version. Available online from http://coverage.cms.fu.com/certpublic/2004-Medicare-Error-Rate-Short-Report-v9.pdf.

Centers for Medicare and Medicaid Services. 2006a (May 17). Improper Medicare Fee-For-Service Payments Short Report (Web Version) for May 2006.: Findings. Available online from https://www.cms.hhs.gov/apps/er_report/preview_er_report.asp?from=public&which=short&reportID=4&tab=4.

Centers for Medicare and Medicaid Services. 2006b (April 25). Proposed Changes to the Hospital Inpatient Prospective Payment System. *Federal Register* 71(79): 24272–24286 and 24361–24368. Available online from http://www.frwebgate1.access.gpo.gov/cgi-bin/waisgate.cgi?WAISdocID=201896458991+63+0+0&WAISaction=retrieve.

Office of Inspector General. 1998a (Aug. 24). OIG Compliance Program Guidance for Clinical Laboratories. *Federal Register* 63(163): 45078–45087. Available online from http://www.oig.hhs.gov/fraud/complianceguidance.html.

Office of Inspector General. 1998b (Feb. 23). OIG Compliance Program Guidance for Hospitals. *Federal Register* 63(35):8987–98. Available online from http://www.oig.hhs.gov/fraud/complianceguidance.html.

Office of Inspector General. 2005 (Jan. 31). OIG Supplemental Compliance Program Guidance for Hospitals. *Federal Register* 70(19):4858–4876. Available online from http://www.oig.hhs.gov/fraud/complianceguidance.html.

References and Resources

Bryant, G., and C. Hammen. 1999. *Healthcare Fraud and Abuse: Compliance from the HIM Perspective (Program in a box).* Chicago: American Health Information Management Association.

Hammen, C. 1997. Prevention of health care fraud and abuse is top priority for U.S. government. *Advance for Health Information Professionals* 7(8):12–13.

Hammen, C. 1999. Coding compliance consultants must meet compliance criteria. *Journal of Health Care Compliance* 1(6):34.

Hammen, C. 1999. Performing a manual coding audit. *Journal of American Health Information Management Association* 70(6):16–18.

Hammen, C. 1999. Specificity in compliance and medical record documentation. *CodeWrite* 8(4).

Hammen, C. 2001. Alert: the potential impact of an HCFA position on query forms. *CodeWrite* 10(2):9, 12.

Hammen, C. 2001. Using physician profiling to improve documentation. *Journal of American Health Information Management Association* 72(3):19–20.

Hammen, C., and S. Prophet. 1998. Coding compliance: practical strategies for success. *Journal of American Health Information Management Association* 69(2):50–61.

Appendix 9.1

Developing a Coding Compliance Policy Document (AHIMA Practice Brief)

Organizations using diagnosis and procedure codes for reporting healthcare services must have formal policies and corresponding procedures in place that provide instruction on the entire process—from the point of service to the billing statement or claim form. Coding compliance policies serve as a guide to performing coding and billing functions and provide documentation of the organization's intent to correctly report services. The policies should include facility-specific documentation requirements, payer regulations and policies, and contractual arrangements for coding consultants and outsourcing services. This information may be covered in payer/provider contracts or found in Medicare and Medicaid manuals and bulletins.

Following are selected tenets that address the process of code selection and reporting. These tenets may be referred to as coding protocols, a coding compliance program, organizational coding guidelines, or a similar name. These tenets are an important part of any organization's compliance plan and the key to preventing coding errors and resulting reimbursement problems. Examples are taken from both outpatient and inpatient coding processes for illustration purposes only. This document cannot serve as a complete coding compliance plan, but will be useful as a guide for creating a more comprehensive resource to meet individual organizational needs.

A coding compliance plan should include the following components:

- A general policy statement about the commitment of the organization to correctly assign and report codes

  Example: Memorial Medical Center is committed to establishing and maintaining clinical coding and insurance claims processing procedures to ensure that reported codes reflect actual services provided, through accurate information system entries.

- The source of the official coding guidelines used to direct code selection

  Example: ICD-9-CM code selection follows the Official ICD-9-CM Guidelines for Coding and Reporting, developed by the cooperating parties and documented in *Coding Clinic for ICD-9-CM,* published by AHA.

  Example: CPT code selection follows the guidelines set forth in the CPT manual and in *CPT Assistant,* published by AMA.

- The parties responsible for code assignment. The ultimate responsibility for code assignment lies with the physician (provider). However, policies and procedures may document instances where codes may be selected or modified by authorized individuals.

  Example: For inpatient records, medical record analyst I staff are responsible for analysis of records and assignment of the correct ICD-9-CM codes based on documentation by the attending physician.

  Example: Emergency department evaluation and management levels for physician services will be selected by the physician and validated by outpatient record analysts using the HCFA/AMA documentation guidelines. When a variance occurs, the following steps are taken for resolution (the actual document should follow with procedure details).

- The procedure to follow when the clinical information is not clear enough to assign the correct code

Source: Reprinted from AHIMA 2001.

Example: When the documentation used to assign codes is ambiguous or incomplete, the physician must be contacted to clarify the information and complete/amend the record, if necessary. (The actual document should follow with details of how the medical staff would like this to occur, for example, by phone call, by note on the record, etc.). Standard protocols for adding documentation to a record must be followed, in accordance with the applicable laws and regulations.

- Specify the policies and procedures that apply to specific locations and care settings. Official coding guidelines for inpatient reporting and outpatient/physician reporting are different. This means that if a facility-specific coding guideline is being developed for emergency department services, only the coding rules or guidelines that apply in this setting should be designated.

Example: When reporting an injection of a drug provided in the emergency department to a Medicare beneficiary, the appropriate CPT code for the administration of the injection is reported in addition to the evaluation and management service code and drug code. CPT codes are reported whether a physician provides the injection personally or a nurse is carrying out a physician's order. This instruction does not always apply for reporting of professional services in the clinics, because administration of medication is considered bundled with the corresponding evaluation and management service for Medicare patients.

Example: Diagnoses that are documented as "probable," "suspected," "questionable," "rule out," or "working diagnosis" are not to have a code assigned as a confirmed diagnosis. Instead, the code for the condition established at the close of the encounter should be assigned, such as a symptom, sign, abnormal test result, or clinical finding. This guideline applies only to outpatient services.

- Applicable reporting requirements required by specific agencies. The document should include where instructions on payer-specific requirements may be accessed.

Example: For patients with XYZ care plan, report code S0800 for patients having a LASIK procedure rather than an unlisted CPT code.

Example: For Medicare patients receiving a wound closure by tissue adhesive only, report HCPCS Level II code G0168 rather than a CPT code.

Many of these procedures will be put into software databases and would not be written as a specific policy. This is true with most billing software, whether for physician services or through the charge description master used by many hospitals.

- Procedures for correction of inaccurate code assignments in the clinical database and to the agencies where the codes have been reported

Example: When an error in code assignment is discovered after bill release and the claim has already been submitted, this is the process required to update and correct the information system and facilitate claim amendment or correction (the actual document should follow with appropriate details).

- Areas of risk that have been identified through audits or monitoring. Each organization should have a defined audit plan for code accuracy and consistency review and corrective actions should be outlined for problems that are identified.

Example: A hospital might identify that acute respiratory failure is being assigned as the principal diagnosis with congestive heart failure as a secondary diagnosis. The specific reference to *Coding Clinic* could be listed with instructions about correct coding of these conditions and the process to be used to correct the deficiency.

- Identification of essential coding resources available to and used by the coding professionals

Example: Updated ICD-9-CM, CPT, and HCPCS Level II code books are used by all coding professionals. Even if the hospital uses automated encoding software, at least one printed copy of the coding manuals should be available for reference.

Example: Updated encoder software, including the appropriate version of the NCCI edits and DRG and APC grouper software, is available to the appropriate personnel.

Example: Coding Clinic and *CPT Assistant* are available to all coding professionals.

- A process for coding new procedures or unusual diagnoses

Example: When the coding professional encounters an unusual diagnosis, the coding supervisor or the attending physician is consulted. If, after research, a code cannot be identified, the documentation is submitted to AHA for clarification.

- A procedure to identify any optional codes gathered for statistical purposes by the facility and clarification of the appropriate use of E codes

Example: All ICD-9-CM procedure codes in the surgical range (ICD-9-CM Volume III codes 01.01-86.99) shall be reported for inpatients. In addition, codes reported from the non-surgical section include the following (completed document should list the actual codes to be reported).

Example: All appropriate E codes for adverse effects of drugs must be reported. In addition, this facility reports all E codes, including the place of injury for poisonings, all cases of abuse, and all accidents on the initial visit for both inpatient and outpatient services.

- Appropriate methods for resolving coding or documentation disputes with physicians

Example: When the physician disagrees with official coding guidelines, the case is referred to the medical records committee following review by the designated physician liaison from that group.

- A procedure for processing claim rejections

Example: All rejected claims pertaining to diagnosis and procedure codes should be returned to the coding staff for review or correction. Any CDM issues should be forwarded to appropriate departmental staff for corrections. All clinical codes, including modifiers, must never be changed or added without review by coding staff with access to the appropriate documentation.

Example: If a claim is rejected due to the codes provided in the medical record abstract, the billing department notifies the supervisor of coding for a review rather than changing the code to a payable code and resubmitting the claim.

- A statement clarifying that codes will not be assigned, modified, or excluded solely for the purpose of maximizing reimbursement. Clinical codes will not be changed or amended merely due to either physicians' or patients' request to have the service in question covered by insurance. If the initial code assignment did not reflect the actual services, codes may be revised based on supporting documentation. Disputes with either physicians or patients are handled only by the coding supervisor and are appropriately logged for review.

Example: A patient calls the business office saying that her insurance carrier did not pay for her mammogram. After investigating, the HIM coding staff discover that the coding was appropriate for a screening mammogram and that this is a noncovered service with the insurance provider. The code is not changed and the matter is referred back to the business office for explanation to the patient that she should contact her insurance provider with any dispute over coverage of service.

Example: Part of a payment is denied and after review, the supervisor discovers that a modifier should have been appended to the CPT code to denote a separately identifiable service. Modifier –25 is added to the code set and the corrected claim is resubmitted.

Example: A physician approaches the coding supervisor with a request to change the diagnosis codes for his patient because what she currently has is a preexisting condition that is not covered by her current health plan. The coding supervisor must explain to the physician that falsification of insurance claims is illegal. If the physician insists, the physician liaison for the medical record committee is contacted and the matter is turned over to that committee for resolution if necessary.

- The use of and reliance on encoders within the organization. Coding staff cannot rely solely on computerized encoders. Current coding manuals must be readily accessible and the staff must be educated appropriately to detect inappropriate logic or errors in encoding software. When errors in logic or code crosswalks are discovered, they are reported to the vendor immediately by the coding supervisor.

Example: During the coding process, an error is identified in the crosswalk between the ICD-9-CM Volume III code and the CPT code. This error is reported to the software vendor, with proper documentation and notification of all staff using the encoder to not rely on the encoder for code selection.

- Medical records are analyzed and codes selected only with complete and appropriate documentation by the physician available. According to coding guidelines, codes are not assigned without physician documentation. If records are coded without the discharge summary or final diagnostic statements available, processes are in place for review after the summary is added to the record.

Example: When records are coded without a discharge summary, they are flagged in the computer system. When the summaries are added to the record, the record is returned to the coding professional for review of codes. If there are any inconsistencies, appropriate steps are taken for review of the changes.

Additional Elements

A coding compliance document should include a reference to the AHIMA Standards of Ethical Coding, which can be downloaded from AHIMA's Web site at www.ahima.org. Reference to the data quality assessment procedures must be included in a coding compliance plan to establish the mechanism for determining areas of risk. Reviews will identify the need for further education and increased monitoring for those areas where either coding variances or documentation deficiencies are identified.

Specific and detailed coding guidelines that cover the reporting of typical services provided by a facility or organization create tools for data consistency and reliability by ensuring that all coders interpret clinical documentation and apply coding principles in the same manner. The appropriate medical staff committee should give final approval of any coding guidelines that involve clinical criteria to assure appropriateness and physician consensus on the process.

The format is most useful when organized by patient or service type and easily referenced by using a table of contents. If the facility-specific guidelines are maintained electronically, they should be searchable by key terms. Placing the coding guidelines on a facility Intranet or internal computer network is a very efficient way to ensure their use and it also enables timely and efficient updating and distribution. Live links or references should be provided to supporting documents such as Uniform Hospital Discharge Data Sets or other regulatory requirements outlining reporting procedures or code assignments.

Prepared by

AHIMA's Coding Practice Team and reviewed by the Coding Policy and Strategy Committee and the Society for Clinical Coding Data Quality Committee.

Article citation:

AHIMA Coding Practice Team. "Developing a Coding Compliance Policy Document (AHIMA Practice Brief)." *Journal of AHIMA* 72, no. 7 (2001): 88A–C.

Appendix 9.2

Data Sources

Sources for finding external data for data-monitoring comparisons can be found at the following Web sites:

- CMS Web site at http://www.cms.gov. Information by DRG as to the number of Medicare discharges, as well as other information related to charges, LOS, and reimbursement.

- American Hospital Directory Web site at http://www.ahd.com. Specific hospital data can be obtained through this site. General data are free of charge; more specific data can be obtained when a subscription is purchased.

- Data Advantage Web site at http://www.data-advantage.com. Has comparative data products available for inpatients, outpatients, and physician office patients.

- Solucient Web site at http://www.solucient.com or http://www.hcia.com has comparative data and benchmarking products available.

Appendix 9.3

National Averages for CC Pairs

DRG	MDC	Volumes	Type	DRG Title	% with Major Cardiovascular Diagnosis
121	05	150,106	MED	CIRCULATORY DISORDERS W AMI & MAJOR COMP, DISCHARGED ALIVE	73.34%
122	05	54,557	MED	CIRCULATORY DISORDERS W AMI W/O MAJOR COMP, DISCHARGED ALIVE	
547	05	32,613	SURG	CORONARY BYPASS W CARDIAC CATH W MAJOR CV DX	50.37%
548	05	32,131	SURG	CORONARY BYPASS W CARDIAC CATH W/O MAJOR CV DX	
549	05	13,102	SURG	CORONARY BYPASS W/O CARDIAC CATH W MAJOR CV DX	27.54%
550	05	34,474	SURG	CORONARY BYPASS W/O CARDIAC CATH W/O MAJOR CV DX	
551	05	53,809	SURG	PERMANENT CARDIAC PACEMAKER IMPL W MAJ CV DX OR AICD LEAD OR GNRTR	39.64%
552	05	81,920	SURG	OTHER PERMANENT CARDIAC PACEMAKER IMPLANT W/O MAJOR CV DX	
553	05	39,195	SURG	OTHER VASCULAR PROCEDURES W CC W MAJOR CV DX	33.68%
554	05	77,181	SURG	OTHER VASCULAR PROCEDURES W CC W/O MAJOR CV DX	
555	05	37,296	SURG	PERCUTANEOUS CARDIOVASCULAR PROC W MAJOR CV DX	66.29%
556	05	18,962	SURG	PERCUTANEOUS CARDIOVASCULAR PROC W NON-DRUG-ELUTING STENT W/O MAJ CV DX	
557	05	123,883	SURG	PERCUTANEOUS CARDIOVASCULAR PROC W DRUG-ELUTING STENT W MAJOR CV DX	39.17%
558	05	192,407	SURG	PERCUTANEOUS CARDIOVASCULAR PROC W DRUG-ELUTING STENT W/O MAJ CV DX	
		941,636		TOTALS	47.79%

Source: CMS 2006b.

Medical CC-No CC pairs

DRG	MDC	Volumes	Type	DRG Title	CC%
10	01	19,577	MED	NERVOUS SYSTEM NEOPLASMS W CC	86.43%
11	01	3,075	MED	NERVOUS SYSTEM NEOPLASMS W/O CC	
16	01	17,338	MED	NONSPECIFIC CEREBROVASCULAR DISORDERS W CC	85.38%
17	01	2,968	MED	NONSPECIFIC CEREBROVASCULAR DISORDERS W/O CC	
18	01	33,376	MED	CRANIAL & PERIPHERAL NERVE DISORDERS W CC	79.85%
19	01	8,423	MED	CRANIAL & PERIPHERAL NERVE DISORDERS W/O CC	
24	01	63,283	MED	SEIZURE & HEADACHE AGE >17 W CC	69.88%
25	01	27,276	MED	SEIZURE & HEADACHE AGE >17 W/O CC	
28	01	19,839	MED	TRAUMATIC STUPOR & COMA, COMA <1 HR AGE >17 W CC	75.32%
29	01	6,500	MED	TRAUMATIC STUPOR & COMA, COMA <1 HR AGE >17 W/O CC	
31	01	4,967	MED	CONCUSSION AGE >17 W CC	72.79%
32	01	1,857	MED	CONCUSSION AGE >17 W/O CC	
34	01	27,466	MED	OTHER DISORDERS OF NERVOUS SYSTEM W CC	77.82%
35	01	7,830	MED	OTHER DISORDERS OF NERVOUS SYSTEM W/O CC	
46	02	3,942	MED	OTHER DISORDERS OF THE EYE AGE >17 W CC	74.89%
47	02	1,322	MED	OTHER DISORDERS OF THE EYE AGE >17 W/O CC	
68	03	19,066	MED	OTITIS MEDIA & URI AGE >17 W CC	78.57%
69	03	5,201	MED	OTITIS MEDIA & URI AGE >17 W/O CC	
79	04	160,409	MED	RESPIRATORY INFECTIONS & INFLAMMATIONS AGE >17 W CC	95.71%
80	04	7,190	MED	RESPIRATORY INFECTIONS & INFLAMMATIONS AGE >17 W/O CC	
83	04	7,053	MED	MAJOR CHEST TRAUMA W CC	83.65%
84	04	1,379	MED	MAJOR CHEST TRAUMA W/O CC	
85	04	22,193	MED	PLEURAL EFFUSION W CC	92.78%
86	04	1,726	MED	PLEURAL EFFUSION W/O CC	
89	04	555,221	MED	SIMPLE PNEUMONIA & PLEURISY AGE >17 W CC	92.70%
90	04	43,748	MED	SIMPLE PNEUMONIA & PLEURISY AGE >17 W/O CC	
92	04	16,534	MED	INTERSTITIAL LUNG DISEASE W CC	91.96%
93	04	1,446	MED	INTERSTITIAL LUNG DISEASE W/O CC	
94	04	13,561	MED	PNEUMOTHORAX W CC	89.64%
95	04	1,568	MED	PNEUMOTHORAX W/O CC	
96	04	60,151	MED	BRONCHITIS & ASTHMA AGE >17 W CC	69.01%
97	04	27,006	MED	BRONCHITIS & ASTHMA AGE >17 W/O CC	
99	04	21,448	MED	RESPIRATORY SIGNS & SYMPTOMS W CC	76.93%
100	04	6,432	MED	RESPIRATORY SIGNS & SYMPTOMS W/O CC	
101	04	23,374	MED	OTHER RESPIRATORY SYSTEM DIAGNOSES W CC	82.61%
102	04	4,920	MED	OTHER RESPIRATORY SYSTEM DIAGNOSES W/O CC	
130	05	87,632	MED	PERIPHERAL VASCULAR DISORDERS W CC	79.25%
131	05	22,947	MED	PERIPHERAL VASCULAR DISORDERS W/O CC	
132	05	101,483	MED	ATHEROSCLEROSIS W CC	94.52%
133	05	5,883	MED	ATHEROSCLEROSIS W/O CC	

DRG	MDC	Volumes	Type	DRG Title	CC%
135	05	7,172	MED	CARDIAC CONGENITAL & VALVULAR DISORDERS AGE >17 W CC	88.46%
136	05	936	MED	CARDIAC CONGENITAL & VALVULAR DISORDERS AGE >17 W/O CC	
138	05	206,196	MED	CARDIAC ARRHYTHMIA & CONDUCTION DISORDERS W CC	73.57%
139	05	74,082	MED	CARDIAC ARRHYTHMIA & CONDUCTION DISORDERS W/O CC	
141	05	123,475	MED	SYNCOPE & COLLAPSE W CC	71.44%
142	05	49,367	MED	SYNCOPE & COLLAPSE W/O CC	
144	05	104,952	MED	OTHER CIRCULATORY SYSTEM DIAGNOSES W CC	94.82%
145	05	5,728	MED	OTHER CIRCULATORY SYSTEM DIAGNOSES W/O CC	
172	06	33,137	MED	DIGESTIVE MALIGNANCY W CC	93.69%
173	06	2,230	MED	DIGESTIVE MALIGNANCY W/O CC	
174	06	261,063	MED	G.I. HEMORRHAGE W CC	89.72%
175	06	29,906	MED	G.I. HEMORRHAGE W/O CC	
177	06	7,657	MED	UNCOMPLICATED PEPTIC ULCER W CC	75.02%
178	06	2,550	MED	UNCOMPLICATED PEPTIC ULCER W/O CC	
180	06	91,338	MED	G.I. OBSTRUCTION W CC	78.35%
181	06	25,241	MED	G.I. OBSTRUCTION W/O CC	
182	06	297,097	MED	ESOPHAGITIS, GASTROENT & MISC DIGEST DISORDERS AGE >17 W CC	78.40%
183	06	81,861	MED	ESOPHAGITIS, GASTROENT & MISC DIGEST DISORDERS AGE >17 W/O CC	
188	06	93,582	MED	OTHER DIGESTIVE SYSTEM DIAGNOSES AGE >17 W CC	87.67%
189	06	13,160	MED	OTHER DIGESTIVE SYSTEM DIAGNOSES AGE >17 W/O CC	
205	07	32,741	MED	DISORDERS OF LIVER EXCEPT MALIG,CIRR,ALC HEPA W CC	94.13%
206	07	2,042	MED	DISORDERS OF LIVER EXCEPT MALIG,CIRR,ALC HEPA W/O CC	
207	07	38,339	MED	DISORDERS OF THE BILIARY TRACT W CC	80.08%
208	07	9,538	MED	DISORDERS OF THE BILIARY TRACT W/O CC	
240	08	12,903	MED	CONNECTIVE TISSUE DISORDERS W CC	82.00%
241	08	2,833	MED	CONNECTIVE TISSUE DISORDERS W/O CC	
244	08	17,027	MED	BONE DISEASES & SPECIFIC ARTHROPATHIES W CC	74.25%
245	08	5,905	MED	BONE DISEASES & SPECIFIC ARTHROPATHIES W/O CC	
250	08	4,144	MED	FX, SPRN, STRN & DISL OF FOREARM, HAND, FOOT AGE >17 W CC	66.71%
251	08	2,068	MED	FX, SPRN, STRN & DISL OF FOREARM, HAND, FOOT AGE >17 W/O CC	
253	08	24,751	MED	FX, SPRN, STRN & DISL OF UPARM,LOWLEG EX FOOT AGE >17 W CC	71.24%
254	08	9,993	MED	FX, SPRN, STRN & DISL OF UPARM,LOWLEG EX FOOT AGE >17 W/O CC	
272	09	6,079	MED	MAJOR SKIN DISORDERS W CC	82.75%
273	09	1,267	MED	MAJOR SKIN DISORDERS W/O CC	

DRG	MDC	Volumes	Type	DRG Title	CC%
274	09	2,242	MED	MALIGNANT BREAST DISORDERS W CC	92.57%
275	09	180	MED	MALIGNANT BREAST DISORDERS W/O CC	
277	09	119,318	MED	CELLULITIS AGE >17 W CC	77.85%
278	09	33,958	MED	CELLULITIS AGE >17 W/O CC	
280	09	19,321	MED	TRAUMA TO THE SKIN, SUBCUT TISS & BREAST AGE >17 W CC	74.65%
281	09	6,560	MED	TRAUMA TO THE SKIN, SUBCUT TISS & BREAST AGE >17 W/O CC	
283	09	6,782	MED	MINOR SKIN DISORDERS W CC	78.39%
284	09	1,870	MED	MINOR SKIN DISORDERS W/O CC	
296	10	247,607	MED	NUTRITIONAL & MISC METABOLIC DISORDERS AGE >17 W CC	85.29%
297	10	42,717	MED	NUTRITIONAL & MISC METABOLIC DISORDERS AGE >17 W/O CC	
300	10	21,677	MED	ENDOCRINE DISORDERS W CC	84.69%
301	10	3,920	MED	ENDOCRINE DISORDERS W/O CC	
318	11	5,901	MED	KIDNEY & URINARY TRACT NEOPLASMS W CC	93.86%
319	11	386	MED	KIDNEY & URINARY TRACT NEOPLASMS W/O CC	
320	11	225,362	MED	KIDNEY & URINARY TRACT INFECTIONS AGE >17 W CC	87.52%
321	11	32,132	MED	KIDNEY & URINARY TRACT INFECTIONS AGE >17 W/O CC	
323	11	20,435	MED	URINARY STONES W CC, &/OR ESW LITHOTRIPSY	81.54%
324	11	4,625	MED	URINARY STONES W/O CC	
325	11	9,915	MED	KIDNEY & URINARY TRACT SIGNS & SYMPTOMS AGE >17 W CC	79.25%
326	11	2,596	MED	KIDNEY & URINARY TRACT SIGNS & SYMPTOMS AGE >17 W/O CC	
328	11	574	MED	URETHRAL STRICTURE AGE >17 W CC	91.26%
329	11	55	MED	URETHRAL STRICTURE AGE >17 W/O CC	
331	11	56,928	MED	OTHER KIDNEY & URINARY TRACT DIAGNOSES AGE >17 W CC	93.21%
332	11	4,148	MED	OTHER KIDNEY & URINARY TRACT DIAGNOSES AGE >17 W/O CC	
346	12	4,007	MED	MALIGNANCY, MALE REPRODUCTIVE SYSTEM, W CC	94.19%
347	12	247	MED	MALIGNANCY, MALE REPRODUCTIVE SYSTEM, W/O CC	
348	12	4,275	MED	BENIGN PROSTATIC HYPERTROPHY W CC	88.49%
349	12	556	MED	BENIGN PROSTATIC HYPERTROPHY W/O CC	
366	13	4,664	MED	MALIGNANCY, FEMALE REPRODUCTIVE SYSTEM W CC	91.22%
367	13	449	MED	MALIGNANCY, FEMALE REPRODUCTIVE SYSTEM W/O CC	
398	16	18,608	MED	RETICULOENDOTHELIAL & IMMUNITY DISORDERS W CC	91.88%
399	16	1,644	MED	RETICULOENDOTHELIAL & IMMUNITY DISORDERS W/O CC	
403	17	31,520	MED	LYMPHOMA & NONACUTE LEUKEMIA W CC	89.68%
404	17	3,629	MED	LYMPHOMA & NONACUTE LEUKEMIA W/O CC	

DRG	MDC	Volumes	Type	DRG Title	CC%
413	17	5,728	MED	OTHER MYELOPROLIF DIS OR POORLY DIFF NEOPL DIAG W CC	92.25%
414	17	481	MED	OTHER MYELOPROLIF DIS OR POORLY DIFF NEOPL DIAG W/O CC	
419	18	17,739	MED	FEVER OF UNKNOWN ORIGIN AGE >17 W CC	85.31%
420	18	3,054	MED	FEVER OF UNKNOWN ORIGIN AGE >17 W/O CC	
444	21	6,005	MED	TRAUMATIC INJURY AGE >17 W CC	72.65%
445	21	2,261	MED	TRAUMATIC INJURY AGE >17 W/O CC	
449	21	40,821	MED	POISONING & TOXIC EFFECTS OF DRUGS AGE >17 W CC	84.63%
450	21	7,412	MED	POISONING & TOXIC EFFECTS OF DRUGS AGE >17 W/O CC	
452	21	28,666	MED	COMPLICATIONS OF TREATMENT W CC	84.20%
453	21	5,381	MED	COMPLICATIONS OF TREATMENT W/O CC	
454	21	4,755	MED	OTHER INJURY, POISONING & TOXIC EFFECT DIAG W CC	84.31%
455	21	885	MED	OTHER INJURY, POISONING & TOXIC EFFECT DIAG W/O CC	
463	23	32,987	MED	SIGNS & SYMPTOMS W CC	81.11%
464	23	7,681	MED	SIGNS & SYMPTOMS W/O CC	
508	22	663	MED	FULL THICKNESS BURN W/O SKIN GRFT OR INHAL INJ W CC OR SIG TRAUMA	80.85%
509	22	157	MED	FULL THICKNESS BURN W/O SKIN GRFT OR INH INJ W/O CC OR SIG TRAUMA	
510	22	1,798	MED	NONEXTENSIVE BURNS W CC OR SIGNIFICANT TRAUMA	73.87%
511	22	636	MED	NONEXTENSIVE BURNS W/O CC OR SIGNIFICANT TRAUMA	
521	20	32,469	MED	ALCOHOL/DRUG ABUSE OR DEPENDENCE W CC	60.26%
522	20	5,805	MED	ALCOHOL/DRUG ABUSE OR DEPENDENCE W REHABILITATION THERAPY W/O CC	
523	20	15,604	MED	ALCOHOL/DRUG ABUSE OR DEPENDENCE W/O REHABILITATION THERAPY W/O CC	
		4,306,766		TOTAL	83.83%

Surgical CC—No CC pairs

DRG	MDC	Volumes	Type	DRG Title	CC%
1	01	24,336	SURG	CRANIOTOMY AGE >17 W CC	70.30%
2	01	10,279	SURG	CRANIOTOMY AGE >17 W/O CC	
7	01	14,913	SURG	PERIPH & CRANIAL NERVE & OTHER NERV SYST PROC W CC	81.37%
8	01	3,415	SURG	PERIPH & CRANIAL NERVE & OTHER NERV SYST PROC W/O CC	
76	04	47,942	SURG	OTHER RESP SYSTEM O.R. PROCEDURES W CC	95.83%
77	04	2,086	SURG	OTHER RESP SYSTEM O.R. PROCEDURES W/O CC	
110	05	57,543	SURG	MAJOR CARDIOVASCULAR PROCEDURES W CC	84.26%
111	05	10,746	SURG	MAJOR CARDIOVASCULAR PROCEDURES W/O CC	
146	06	10,226	SURG	RECTAL RESECTION W CC	79.68%
147	06	2,608	SURG	RECTAL RESECTION W/O CC	
148	06	132,689	SURG	MAJOR SMALL & LARGE BOWEL PROCEDURES W CC	87.20%
149	06	19,473	SURG	MAJOR SMALL & LARGE BOWEL PROCEDURES W/O CC	
150	06	22,894	SURG	PERITONEAL ADHESIOLYSIS W CC	81.01%
151	06	5,368	SURG	PERITONEAL ADHESIOLYSIS W/O CC	
152	06	5,000	SURG	MINOR SMALL & LARGE BOWEL PROCEDURES W CC	71.97%
153	06	1,947	SURG	MINOR SMALL & LARGE BOWEL PROCEDURES W/O CC	
154	06	26,973	SURG	STOMACH, ESOPHAGEAL & DUODENAL PROCEDURES AGE >17 W CC	81.82%
155	06	5,995	SURG	STOMACH, ESOPHAGEAL & DUODENAL PROCEDURES AGE >17 W/O CC	
157	06	8,294	SURG	ANAL & STOMAL PROCEDURES W CC	69.09%
158	06	3,710	SURG	ANAL & STOMAL PROCEDURES W/O CC	
159	06	19,181	SURG	HERNIA PROCEDURES EXCEPT INGUINAL & FEMORAL AGE >17 W CC	61.66%
160	06	11,929	SURG	HERNIA PROCEDURES EXCEPT INGUINAL & FEMORAL AGE >17 W/O CC	
161	06	10,141	SURG	INGUINAL & FEMORAL HERNIA PROCEDURES AGE >17 W CC	67.18%
162	06	4,954	SURG	INGUINAL & FEMORAL HERNIA PROCEDURES AGE >17 W/O CC	
164	06	5,972	SURG	APPENDECTOMY W COMPLICATED PRINCIPAL DIAG W CC	70.93%
165	06	2,447	SURG	APPENDECTOMY W COMPLICATED PRINCIPAL DIAG W/O CC	
166	06	5,128	SURG	APPENDECTOMY W/O COMPLICATED PRINCIPAL DIAG W CC	51.25%
167	06	4,877	SURG	APPENDECTOMY W/O COMPLICATED PRINCIPAL DIAG W/O CC	
168	03	1,532	SURG	MOUTH PROCEDURES W CC	66.49%
169	03	772	SURG	MOUTH PROCEDURES W/O CC	
170	06	17,895	SURG	OTHER DIGESTIVE SYSTEM O.R. PROCEDURES W CC	92.73%
171	06	1,404	SURG	OTHER DIGESTIVE SYSTEM O.R. PROCEDURES W/O CC	

DRG	MDC	Volumes	Type	DRG Title	CC%
191	07	10,550	SURG	PANCREAS, LIVER & SHUNT PROCEDURES W CC	88.46%
192	07	1,376	SURG	PANCREAS, LIVER & SHUNT PROCEDURES W/O CC	
193	07	4,039	SURG	BILIARY TRACT PROC EXCEPT ONLY CHOLECYST W OR W/O C.D.E. W CC	89.72%
194	07	463	SURG	BILIARY TRACT PROC EXCEPT ONLY CHOLECYST W OR W/O C.D.E. W/O CC	
195	07	2,835	SURG	CHOLECYSTECTOMY W C.D.E. W CC	82.65%
196	07	595	SURG	CHOLECYSTECTOMY W C.D.E. W/O CC	
197	07	16,352	SURG	CHOLECYSTECTOMY EXCEPT BY LAPAROSCOPE W/O C.D.E. W CC	79.91%
198	07	4,110	SURG	CHOLECYSTECTOMY EXCEPT BY LAPAROSCOPE W/O C.D.E. W/O CC	
210	08	126,376	SURG	HIP & FEMUR PROCEDURES EXCEPT MAJOR JOINT AGE >17 W CC	83.09%
211	08	25,712	SURG	HIP & FEMUR PROCEDURES EXCEPT MAJOR JOINT AGE >17 W/O CC	
218	08	29,975	SURG	LOWER EXTREM & HUMER PROC EXCEPT HIP, FOOT, FEMUR AGE >17 W CC	58.74%
219	08	21,059	SURG	LOWER EXTREM & HUMER PROC EXCEPT HIP, FOOT, FEMUR AGE >17 W/O CC	
223	08	12,649	SURG	MAJOR SHOULDER/ELBOW PROC, OR OTHER UPPER EXTREMITY PROC W CC	56.00%
224	08	9,937	SURG	SHOULDER,ELBOW OR FOREARM PROC, EXC MAJOR JOINT PROC, W/O CC	
226	08	6,736	SURG	SOFT TISSUE PROCEDURES W CC	58.05%
227	08	4,868	SURG	SOFT TISSUE PROCEDURES W/O CC	
228	08	2,680	SURG	MAJOR THUMB OR JOINT PROC, OR OTH HAND OR WRIST PROC W CC	70.47%
229	08	1,123	SURG	HAND OR WRIST PROC, EXCEPT MAJOR JOINT PROC, W/O CC	
233	08	18,412	SURG	OTHER MUSCULOSKELET SYS & CONN TISS O.R. PROC W CC	66.99%
234	08	9,074	SURG	OTHER MUSCULOSKELET SYS & CONN TISS O.R. PROC W/O CC	
257	09	13,094	SURG	TOTAL MASTECTOMY FOR MALIGNANCY W CC	53.48%
258	09	11,391	SURG	TOTAL MASTECTOMY FOR MALIGNANCY W/O CC	
259	09	2,658	SURG	SUBTOTAL MASTECTOMY FOR MALIGNANCY W CC	52.22%
260	09	2,432	SURG	SUBTOTAL MASTECTOMY FOR MALIGNANCY W/O CC	
263	09	22,466	SURG	SKIN GRAFT &/OR DEBRID FOR SKN ULCER OR CELLULITIS W CC	85.19%
264	09	3,905	SURG	SKIN GRAFT &/OR DEBRID FOR SKN ULCER OR CELLULITIS W/O CC	
265	09	4,011	SURG	SKIN GRAFT &/OR DEBRID EXCEPT FOR SKIN ULCER OR CELLULITIS W CC	64.36%
266	09	2,221	SURG	SKIN GRAFT &/OR DEBRID EXCEPT FOR SKIN ULCER OR CELLULITIS W/O CC	

DRG	MDC	Volumes	Type	DRG Title	CC%
269	09	11,015	SURG	OTHER SKIN, SUBCUT TISS & BREAST PROC W CC	81.09%
270	09	2,568	SURG	OTHER SKIN, SUBCUT TISS & BREAST PROC W/O CC	
292	10	7,563	SURG	OTHER ENDOCRINE, NUTRIT & METAB O.R. PROC W CC	95.95%
293	10	319	SURG	OTHER ENDOCRINE, NUTRIT & METAB O.R. PROC W/O CC	
304	11	14,043	SURG	KIDNEY,URETER & MAJOR BLADDER PROC FOR NONNEOPL W CC	82.38%
305	11	3,003	SURG	KIDNEY,URETER & MAJOR BLADDER PROC FOR NON-NEOPL W/O CC	
306	11	5,792	SURG	PROSTATECTOMY W CC	74.88%
307	11	1,943	SURG	PROSTATECTOMY W/O CC	
308	11	6,673	SURG	MINOR BLADDER PROCEDURES W CC	67.13%
309	11	3,268	SURG	MINOR BLADDER PROCEDURES W/O CC	
310	11	25,310	SURG	TRANSURETHRAL PROCEDURES W CC	81.17%
311	11	5,873	SURG	TRANSURETHRAL PROCEDURES W/O CC	
312	11	1,322	SURG	URETHRAL PROCEDURES, AGE >17 W CC	72.48%
313	11	502	SURG	URETHRAL PROCEDURES, AGE >17 W/O CC	
334	12	9,483	SURG	MAJOR MALE PELVIC PROCEDURES W CC	43.89%
335	12	12,125	SURG	MAJOR MALE PELVIC PROCEDURES W/O CC	
336	12	28,106	SURG	TRANSURETHRAL PROSTATECTOMY W CC	56.74%
337	12	21,429	SURG	TRANSURETHRAL PROSTATECTOMY W/O CC	
354	13	7,559	SURG	UTERINE, ADNEXA PROC FOR NONOVARIAN/ADNEXAL MALIG W CC	60.21%
355	13	4,995	SURG	UTERINE, ADNEXA PROC FOR NONOVARIAN/ADNEXAL MALIG W/O CC	
358	13	20,877	SURG	UTERINE & ADNEXA PROC FOR NONMALIGNANCY W CC	42.19%
359	13	28,606	SURG	UTERINE & ADNEXA PROC FOR NONMALIGNANCY W/O CC	
370	14	2,212	SURG	CESAREAN SECTION W CC	45.38%
371	14	2,662	SURG	CESAREAN SECTION W/O CC	
401	17	6,443	SURG	LYMPHOMA & NONACUTE LEUKEMIA W OTHER O.R. PROC W CC	82.77%
402	17	1,341	SURG	LYMPHOMA & NONACUTE LEUKEMIA W OTHER O.R. PROC W/O CC	
406	17	2,301	SURG	MYELOPROLIF DISORD OR POORLY DIFF NEOPL W MAJ O.R.PROC W CC	79.10%
407	17	608	SURG	MYELOPROLIF DISORD OR POORLY DIFF NEOPL W MAJ O.R.PROC W/O CC	
442	21	18,533	SURG	OTHER O.R. PROCEDURES FOR INJURIES W CC	83.84%
443	21	3,572	SURG	OTHER O.R. PROCEDURES FOR INJURIES W/O CC	
493	07	60,917	SURG	LAPAROSCOPIC CHOLECYSTECTOMY W/O C.D.E. W CC	71.33%
494	07	24,482	SURG	LAPAROSCOPIC CHOLECYSTECTOMY W/O C.D.E. W/O CC	
497	08	31,247	SURG	SPINAL FUSION EXCEPT CERVICAL W CC	59.34%
498	08	21,409	SURG	SPINAL FUSION EXCEPT CERVICAL W/O CC	
499	08	35,214	SURG	BACK & NECK PROCEDURES EXCEPT SPINAL FUSION W CC	42.99%
500	08	46,705	SURG	BACK & NECK PROCEDURES EXCEPT SPINAL FUSION W/O CC	

DRG	MDC	Volumes	Type	DRG Title	CC%
501	08	3,172	SURG	KNEE PROCEDURES W PDX OF INFECTION W CC	80.75%
502	08	756	SURG	KNEE PROCEDURES W PDX OF INFECTION W/O CC	
506	22	964	SURG	FULL THICKNESS BURN W SKIN GRAFT OR INHAL INJ W CC OR SIG TRAUMA	74.90%
507	22	323	SURG	FULL THICKNESS BURN W SKIN GRFT OR INHAL INJ W/O CC OR SIG TRAUMA	
519	08	12,546	SURG	CERVICAL SPINAL FUSION W CC	43.14%
520	08	16,538	SURG	CERVICAL SPINAL FUSION W/O CC	
529	01	5,110	SURG	VENTRICULAR SHUNT PROCEDURES W CC	60.23%
530	01	3,374	SURG	VENTRICULAR SHUNT PROCEDURES W/O CC	
531	01	4,874	SURG	SPINAL PROCEDURES W CC	63.25%
532	01	2,832	SURG	SPINAL PROCEDURES W/O CC	
533	01	46,528	SURG	EXTRACRANIAL PROCEDURES W CC	52.23%
534	01	42,555	SURG	EXTRACRANIAL PROCEDURES W/O CC	
537	08	8,953	SURG	LOCAL EXCIS & REMOV OF INT FIX DEV EXCEPT HIP & FEMUR W CC	62.13%
538	08	5,456	SURG	LOCAL EXCIS & REMOV OF INT FIX DEV EXCEPT HIP & FEMUR W/O CC	
539	17	4,954	SURG	LYMPHOMA & LEUKEMIA W MAJOR OR PROCEDURE W CC	76.84%
540	17	1,493	SURG	LYMPHOMA & LEUKEMIA W MAJOR OR PROCEDURE W/O CC	
		1,514,216		**TOTAL**	**70.35%**

Total CC—No pairs

DRG	MDC	Volumes	Type	DRG Title	CC%
1	01	24,336	SURG	CRANIOTOMY AGE >17 W CC	70.30%
2	01	10,279	SURG	CRANIOTOMY AGE >17 W/O CC	
7	01	14,913	SURG	PERIPH & CRANIAL NERVE & OTHER NERV SYST PROC W CC	81.37%
8	01	3,415	SURG	PERIPH & CRANIAL NERVE & OTHER NERV SYST PROC W/O CC	
10	01	19,577	MED	NERVOUS SYSTEM NEOPLASMS W CC	86.43%
11	01	3,075	MED	NERVOUS SYSTEM NEOPLASMS W/O CC	
16	01	17,338	MED	NONSPECIFIC CEREBROVASCULAR DISORDERS W CC	85.38%
17	01	2,968	MED	NONSPECIFIC CEREBROVASCULAR DISORDERS W/O CC	
18	01	33,376	MED	CRANIAL & PERIPHERAL NERVE DISORDERS W CC	79.85%
19	01	8,423	MED	CRANIAL & PERIPHERAL NERVE DISORDERS W/O CC	
24	01	63,283	MED	SEIZURE & HEADACHE AGE >17 W CC	69.88%
25	01	27,276	MED	SEIZURE & HEADACHE AGE >17 W/O CC	
28	01	19,839	MED	TRAUMATIC STUPOR & COMA, COMA <1 HR AGE >17 W CC	75.32%
29	01	6,500	MED	TRAUMATIC STUPOR & COMA, COMA <1 HR AGE >17 W/O CC	
31	01	4,967	MED	CONCUSSION AGE >17 W CC	72.79%
32	01	1,857	MED	CONCUSSION AGE >17 W/O CC	
34	01	27,466	MED	OTHER DISORDERS OF NERVOUS SYSTEM W CC	77.82%
35	01	7,830	MED	OTHER DISORDERS OF NERVOUS SYSTEM W/O CC	
46	02	3,942	MED	OTHER DISORDERS OF THE EYE AGE >17 W CC	74.89%
47	02	1,322	MED	OTHER DISORDERS OF THE EYE AGE >17 W/O CC	
68	03	19,066	MED	OTITIS MEDIA & URI AGE >17 W CC	78.57%
69	03	5,201	MED	OTITIS MEDIA & URI AGE >17 W/O CC	
76	04	47,942	SURG	OTHER RESP SYSTEM O.R. PROCEDURES W CC	95.83%
77	04	2,086	SURG	OTHER RESP SYSTEM O.R. PROCEDURES W/O CC	
79	04	160,409	MED	RESPIRATORY INFECTIONS & INFLAMMATIONS AGE >17 W CC	95.71%
80	04	7,190	MED	RESPIRATORY INFECTIONS & INFLAMMATIONS AGE >17 W/O CC	
83	04	7,053	MED	MAJOR CHEST TRAUMA W CC	83.65%
84	04	1,379	MED	MAJOR CHEST TRAUMA W/O CC	
85	04	22,193	MED	PLEURAL EFFUSION W CC	92.78%
86	04	1,726	MED	PLEURAL EFFUSION W/O CC	
89	04	555,221	MED	SIMPLE PNEUMONIA & PLEURISY AGE >17 W CC	92.70%
90	04	43,748	MED	SIMPLE PNEUMONIA & PLEURISY AGE >17 W/O CC	
92	04	16,534	MED	INTERSTITIAL LUNG DISEASE W CC	91.96%
93	04	1,446	MED	INTERSTITIAL LUNG DISEASE W/O CC	
94	04	13,561	MED	PNEUMOTHORAX W CC	89.64%
95	04	1,568	MED	PNEUMOTHORAX W/O CC	

DRG	MDC	Volumes	Type	DRG Title	CC%
96	04	60,151	MED	BRONCHITIS & ASTHMA AGE >17 W CC	69.01%
97	04	27,006	MED	BRONCHITIS & ASTHMA AGE >17 W/O CC	
99	04	21,448	MED	RESPIRATORY SIGNS & SYMPTOMS W CC	76.93%
100	04	6,432	MED	RESPIRATORY SIGNS & SYMPTOMS W/O CC	
101	04	23,374	MED	OTHER RESPIRATORY SYSTEM DIAGNOSES W CC	82.61%
102	04	4,920	MED	OTHER RESPIRATORY SYSTEM DIAGNOSES W/O CC	
110	05	57,543	SURG	MAJOR CARDIOVASCULAR PROCEDURES W CC	84.26%
111	05	10,746	SURG	MAJOR CARDIOVASCULAR PROCEDURES W/O CC	
130	05	87,632	MED	PERIPHERAL VASCULAR DISORDERS W CC	79.25%
131	05	22,947	MED	PERIPHERAL VASCULAR DISORDERS W/O CC	
132	05	101,483	MED	ATHEROSCLEROSIS W CC	94.52%
133	05	5,883	MED	ATHEROSCLEROSIS W/O CC	
135	05	7,172	MED	CARDIAC CONGENITAL & VALVULAR DISORDERS AGE >17 W CC	88.46%
136	05	936	MED	CARDIAC CONGENITAL & VALVULAR DISORDERS AGE >17 W/O CC	
138	05	206,196	MED	CARDIAC ARRHYTHMIA & CONDUCTION DISORDERS W CC	73.57%
139	05	74,082	MED	CARDIAC ARRHYTHMIA & CONDUCTION DISORDERS W/O CC	
141	05	123,475	MED	SYNCOPE & COLLAPSE W CC	71.44%
142	05	49,367	MED	SYNCOPE & COLLAPSE W/O CC	
144	05	104,952	MED	OTHER CIRCULATORY SYSTEM DIAGNOSES W CC	94.82%
145	05	5,728	MED	OTHER CIRCULATORY SYSTEM DIAGNOSES W/O CC	
146	06	10,226	SURG	RECTAL RESECTION W CC	79.68%
147	06	2,608	SURG	RECTAL RESECTION W/O CC	
148	06	132,689	SURG	MAJOR SMALL & LARGE BOWEL PROCEDURES W CC	87.20%
149	06	19,473	SURG	MAJOR SMALL & LARGE BOWEL PROCEDURES W/O CC	
150	06	22,894	SURG	PERITONEAL ADHESIOLYSIS W CC	81.01%
151	06	5,368	SURG	PERITONEAL ADHESIOLYSIS W/O CC	
152	06	5,000	SURG	MINOR SMALL & LARGE BOWEL PROCEDURES W CC	71.97%
153	06	1,947	SURG	MINOR SMALL & LARGE BOWEL PROCEDURES W/O CC	
154	06	26,973	SURG	STOMACH, ESOPHAGEAL & DUODENAL PROCEDURES AGE >17 W CC	81.82%
155	06	5,995	SURG	STOMACH, ESOPHAGEAL & DUODENAL PROCEDURES AGE >17 W/O CC	
157	06	8,294	SURG	ANAL & STOMAL PROCEDURES W CC	69.09%
158	06	3,710	SURG	ANAL & STOMAL PROCEDURES W/O CC	
159	06	19,181	SURG	HERNIA PROCEDURES EXCEPT INGUINAL & FEMORAL AGE >17 W CC	61.66%
160	06	11,929	SURG	HERNIA PROCEDURES EXCEPT INGUINAL & FEMORAL AGE >17 W/O CC	

DRG	MDC	Volumes	Type	DRG Title	CC%
161	06	10,141	SURG	INGUINAL & FEMORAL HERNIA PROCEDURES AGE >17 W CC	67.18%
162	06	4,954	SURG	INGUINAL & FEMORAL HERNIA PROCEDURES AGE >17 W/O CC	
164	06	5,972	SURG	APPENDECTOMY W COMPLICATED PRINCIPAL DIAG W CC	70.93%
165	06	2,447	SURG	APPENDECTOMY W COMPLICATED PRINCIPAL DIAG W/O CC	
166	06	5,128	SURG	APPENDECTOMY W/O COMPLICATED PRINCIPAL DIAG W CC	51.25%
167	06	4,877	SURG	APPENDECTOMY W/O COMPLICATED PRINCIPAL DIAG W/O CC	
168	03	1,532	SURG	MOUTH PROCEDURES W CC	66.49%
169	03	772	SURG	MOUTH PROCEDURES W/O CC	
170	06	17,895	SURG	OTHER DIGESTIVE SYSTEM O.R. PROCEDURES W CC	92.73%
171	06	1,404	SURG	OTHER DIGESTIVE SYSTEM O.R. PROCEDURES W/O CC	
172	06	33,137	MED	DIGESTIVE MALIGNANCY W CC	93.69%
173	06	2,230	MED	DIGESTIVE MALIGNANCY W/O CC	
174	06	261,063	MED	G.I. HEMORRHAGE W CC	89.72%
175	06	29,906	MED	G.I. HEMORRHAGE W/O CC	
177	06	7,657	MED	UNCOMPLICATED PEPTIC ULCER W CC	75.02%
178	06	2,550	MED	UNCOMPLICATED PEPTIC ULCER W/O CC	
180	06	91,338	MED	G.I. OBSTRUCTION W CC	78.35%
181	06	25,241	MED	G.I. OBSTRUCTION W/O CC	
182	06	297,097	MED	ESOPHAGITIS, GASTROENT & MISC DIGEST DISORDERS AGE >17 W CC	78.40%
183	06	81,861	MED	ESOPHAGITIS, GASTROENT & MISC DIGEST DISORDERS AGE >17 W/O CC	
188	06	93,582	MED	OTHER DIGESTIVE SYSTEM DIAGNOSES AGE >17 W CC	87.67%
189	06	13,160	MED	OTHER DIGESTIVE SYSTEM DIAGNOSES AGE >17 W/O CC	
191	07	10,550	SURG	PANCREAS, LIVER & SHUNT PROCEDURES W CC	88.46%
192	07	1,376	SURG	PANCREAS, LIVER & SHUNT PROCEDURES W/O CC	
193	07	4,039	SURG	BILIARY TRACT PROC EXCEPT ONLY CHOLECYST W OR W/O C.D.E. W CC	89.72%
194	07	463	SURG	BILIARY TRACT PROC EXCEPT ONLY CHOLECYST W OR W/O C.D.E. W/O CC	
195	07	2,835	SURG	CHOLECYSTECTOMY W C.D.E. W CC	82.65%
196	07	595	SURG	CHOLECYSTECTOMY W C.D.E. W/O CC	
197	07	16,352	SURG	CHOLECYSTECTOMY EXCEPT BY LAPAROSCOPE W/O C.D.E. W CC	79.91%
198	07	4,110	SURG	CHOLECYSTECTOMY EXCEPT BY LAPAROSCOPE W/O C.D.E. W/O CC	
205	07	32,741	MED	DISORDERS OF LIVER EXCEPT MALIG, CIRR, ALC HEPA W CC	94.13%
206	07	2,042	MED	DISORDERS OF LIVER EXCEPT MALIG, CIRR, ALC HEPA W/O CC	

DRG	MDC	Volumes	Type	DRG Title	CC%
207	07	38,339	MED	DISORDERS OF THE BILIARY TRACT W CC	80.08%
208	07	9,538	MED	DISORDERS OF THE BILIARY TRACT W/O CC	
210	08	126,376	SURG	HIP & FEMUR PROCEDURES EXCEPT MAJOR JOINT AGE >17 W CC	83.09%
211	08	25,712	SURG	HIP & FEMUR PROCEDURES EXCEPT MAJOR JOINT AGE >17 W/O CC	
218	08	29,975	SURG	LOWER EXTREM & HUMER PROC EXCEPT HIP, FOOT, FEMUR AGE >17 W CC	58.74%
219	08	21,059	SURG	LOWER EXTREM & HUMER PROC EXCEPT HIP, FOOT, FEMUR AGE >17 W/O CC	
223	08	12,649	SURG	MAJOR SHOULDER/ELBOW PROC, OR OTHER UPPER EXTREMITY PROC W CC	56.00%
224	08	9,937	SURG	SHOULDER,ELBOW OR FOREARM PROC, EXC MAJOR JOINT PROC, W/O CC	
226	08	6,736	SURG	SOFT TISSUE PROCEDURES W CC	58.05%
227	08	4,868	SURG	SOFT TISSUE PROCEDURES W/O CC	
228	08	2,680	SURG	MAJOR THUMB OR JOINT PROC, OR OTH HAND OR WRIST PROC W CC	70.47%
229	08	1,123	SURG	HAND OR WRIST PROC, EXCEPT MAJOR JOINT PROC, W/O CC	
233	08	18,412	SURG	OTHER MUSCULOSKELET SYS & CONN TISS O.R. PROC W CC	66.99%
234	08	9,074	SURG	OTHER MUSCULOSKELET SYS & CONN TISS O.R. PROC W/O CC	
240	08	12,903	MED	CONNECTIVE TISSUE DISORDERS W CC	82.00%
241	08	2,833	MED	CONNECTIVE TISSUE DISORDERS W/O CC	
244	08	17,027	MED	BONE DISEASES & SPECIFIC ARTHROPATHIES W CC	74.25%
245	08	5,905	MED	BONE DISEASES & SPECIFIC ARTHROPATHIES W/O CC	
250	08	4,144	MED	FX, SPRN, STRN & DISL OF FOREARM, HAND, FOOT AGE >17 W CC	66.71%
251	08	2,068	MED	FX, SPRN, STRN & DISL OF FOREARM, HAND, FOOT AGE >17 W/O CC	
253	08	24,751	MED	FX, SPRN, STRN & DISL OF UPARM, LOWLEG EX FOOT AGE >17 W CC	71.24%
254	08	9,993	MED	FX, SPRN, STRN & DISL OF UPARM, LOWLEG EX FOOT AGE >17 W/O CC	
257	09	13,094	SURG	TOTAL MASTECTOMY FOR MALIGNANCY W CC	53.48%
258	09	11,391	SURG	TOTAL MASTECTOMY FOR MALIGNANCY W/O CC	
259	09	2,658	SURG	SUBTOTAL MASTECTOMY FOR MALIGNANCY W CC	52.22%
260	09	2,432	SURG	SUBTOTAL MASTECTOMY FOR MALIGNANCY W/O CC	
263	09	22,466	SURG	SKIN GRAFT &/OR DEBRID FOR SKN ULCER OR CELLULITIS W CC	85.19%
264	09	3,905	SURG	SKIN GRAFT &/OR DEBRID FOR SKN ULCER OR CELLULITIS W/O CC	

DRG	MDC	Volumes	Type	DRG Title	CC%
265	09	4,011	SURG	SKIN GRAFT &/OR DEBRID EXCEPT FOR SKIN ULCER OR CELLULITIS W CC	64.36%
266	09	2,221	SURG	SKIN GRAFT &/OR DEBRID EXCEPT FOR SKIN ULCER OR CELLULITIS W/O CC	
269	09	11,015	SURG	OTHER SKIN, SUBCUT TISS & BREAST PROC W CC	81.09%
270	09	2,568	SURG	OTHER SKIN, SUBCUT TISS & BREAST PROC W/O CC	
272	09	6,079	MED	MAJOR SKIN DISORDERS W CC	82.75%
273	09	1,267	MED	MAJOR SKIN DISORDERS W/O CC	
274	09	2,242	MED	MALIGNANT BREAST DISORDERS W CC	92.57%
275	09	180	MED	MALIGNANT BREAST DISORDERS W/O CC	
277	09	119,318	MED	CELLULITIS AGE >17 W CC	77.85%
278	09	33,958	MED	CELLULITIS AGE >17 W/O CC	
280	09	19,321	MED	TRAUMA TO THE SKIN, SUBCUT TISS & BREAST AGE >17 W CC	74.65%
281	09	6,560	MED	TRAUMA TO THE SKIN, SUBCUT TISS & BREAST AGE >17 W/O CC	
283	09	6,782	MED	MINOR SKIN DISORDERS W CC	78.39%
284	09	1,870	MED	MINOR SKIN DISORDERS W/O CC	
292	10	7,563	SURG	OTHER ENDOCRINE, NUTRIT & METAB O.R. PROC W CC	95.95%
293	10	319	SURG	OTHER ENDOCRINE, NUTRIT & METAB O.R. PROC W/O CC	
296	10	247,607	MED	NUTRITIONAL & MISC METABOLIC DISORDERS AGE >17 W CC	85.29%
297	10	42,717	MED	NUTRITIONAL & MISC METABOLIC DISORDERS AGE >17 W/O CC	
300	10	21,677	MED	ENDOCRINE DISORDERS W CC	84.69%
301	10	3,920	MED	ENDOCRINE DISORDERS W/O CC	
304	11	14,043	SURG	KIDNEY, URETER & MAJOR BLADDER PROC FOR NON-NEOPL W CC	82.38%
305	11	3,003	SURG	KIDNEY, URETER & MAJOR BLADDER PROC FOR NON-NEOPL W/O CC	
306	11	5,792	SURG	PROSTATECTOMY W CC	74.88%
307	11	1,943	SURG	PROSTATECTOMY W/O CC	
308	11	6,673	SURG	MINOR BLADDER PROCEDURES W CC	67.13%
309	11	3,268	SURG	MINOR BLADDER PROCEDURES W/O CC	
310	11	25,310	SURG	TRANSURETHRAL PROCEDURES W CC	81.17%
311	11	5,873	SURG	TRANSURETHRAL PROCEDURES W/O CC	
312	11	1,322	SURG	URETHRAL PROCEDURES, AGE >17 W CC	72.48%
313	11	502	SURG	URETHRAL PROCEDURES, AGE >17 W/O CC	
318	11	5,901	MED	KIDNEY & URINARY TRACT NEOPLASMS W CC	93.86%
319	11	386	MED	KIDNEY & URINARY TRACT NEOPLASMS W/O CC	
320	11	225,362	MED	KIDNEY & URINARY TRACT INFECTIONS AGE >17 W CC	87.52%
321	11	32,132	MED	KIDNEY & URINARY TRACT INFECTIONS AGE >17 W/O CC	

DRG	MDC	Volumes	Type	DRG Title	CC%
323	11	20,435	MED	URINARY STONES W CC, &/OR ESW LITHOTRIPSY	81.54%
324	11	4,625	MED	URINARY STONES W/O CC	
325	11	9,915	MED	KIDNEY & URINARY TRACT SIGNS & SYMPTOMS AGE >17 W CC	79.25%
326	11	2,596	MED	KIDNEY & URINARY TRACT SIGNS & SYMPTOMS AGE >17 W/O CC	
328	11	574	MED	URETHRAL STRICTURE AGE >17 W CC	91.26%
329	11	55	MED	URETHRAL STRICTURE AGE >17 W/O CC	
331	11	56,928	MED	OTHER KIDNEY & URINARY TRACT DIAGNOSES AGE >17 W CC	93.21%
332	11	4,148	MED	OTHER KIDNEY & URINARY TRACT DIAGNOSES AGE >17 W/O CC	
334	12	9,483	SURG	MAJOR MALE PELVIC PROCEDURES W CC	43.89%
335	12	12,125	SURG	MAJOR MALE PELVIC PROCEDURES W/O CC	
336	12	28,106	SURG	TRANSURETHRAL PROSTATECTOMY W CC	56.74%
337	12	21,429	SURG	TRANSURETHRAL PROSTATECTOMY W/O CC	
346	12	4,007	MED	MALIGNANCY, MALE REPRODUCTIVE SYSTEM, W CC	94.19%
347	12	247	MED	MALIGNANCY, MALE REPRODUCTIVE SYSTEM, W/O CC	
348	12	4,275	MED	BENIGN PROSTATIC HYPERTROPHY W CC	88.49%
349	12	556	MED	BENIGN PROSTATIC HYPERTROPHY W/O CC	
354	13	7,559	SURG	UTERINE, ADNEXA PROC FOR NONOVARIAN/ADNEXAL MALIG W CC	60.21%
355	13	4,995	SURG	UTERINE, ADNEXA PROC FOR NONOVARIAN/ADNEXAL MALIG W/O CC	
358	13	20,877	SURG	UTERINE & ADNEXA PROC FOR NONMALIGNANCY W CC	42.19%
359	13	28,606	SURG	UTERINE & ADNEXA PROC FOR NONMALIGNANCY W/O CC	
366	13	4,664	MED	MALIGNANCY, FEMALE REPRODUCTIVE SYSTEM W CC	91.22%
367	13	449	MED	MALIGNANCY, FEMALE REPRODUCTIVE SYSTEM W/O CC	
370	14	2,212	SURG	CESAREAN SECTION W CC	45.38%
371	14	2,662	SURG	CESAREAN SECTION W/O CC	
398	16	18,608	MED	RETICULOENDOTHELIAL & IMMUNITY DISORDERS W CC	91.88%
399	16	1,644	MED	RETICULOENDOTHELIAL & IMMUNITY DISORDERS W/O CC	
401	17	6,443	SURG	LYMPHOMA & NONACUTE LEUKEMIA W OTHER O.R. PROC W CC	82.77%
402	17	1,341	SURG	LYMPHOMA & NONACUTE LEUKEMIA W OTHER O.R. PROC W/O CC	
403	17	31,520	MED	LYMPHOMA & NONACUTE LEUKEMIA W CC	89.68%
404	17	3,629	MED	LYMPHOMA & NONACUTE LEUKEMIA W/O CC	
406	17	2,301	SURG	MYELOPROLIF DISORD OR POORLY DIFF NEOPL W MAJ O.R.PROC W CC	79.10%
407	17	608	SURG	MYELOPROLIF DISORD OR POORLY DIFF NEOPL W MAJ O.R.PROC W/O CC	

DRG	MDC	Volumes	Type	DRG Title	CC%
413	17	5,728	MED	OTHER MYELOPROLIF DIS OR POORLY DIFF NEOPL DIAG W CC	92.25%
414	17	481	MED	OTHER MYELOPROLIF DIS OR POORLY DIFF NEOPL DIAG W/O CC	
419	18	17,739	MED	FEVER OF UNKNOWN ORIGIN AGE >17 W CC	85.31%
420	18	3,054	MED	FEVER OF UNKNOWN ORIGIN AGE >17 W/O CC	
442	21	18,533	SURG	OTHER O.R. PROCEDURES FOR INJURIES W CC	83.84%
443	21	3,572	SURG	OTHER O.R. PROCEDURES FOR INJURIES W/O CC	
444	21	6,005	MED	TRAUMATIC INJURY AGE >17 W CC	72.65%
445	21	2,261	MED	TRAUMATIC INJURY AGE >17 W/O CC	
449	21	40,821	MED	POISONING & TOXIC EFFECTS OF DRUGS AGE >17 W CC	84.63%
450	21	7,412	MED	POISONING & TOXIC EFFECTS OF DRUGS AGE >17 W/O CC	
452	21	28,666	MED	COMPLICATIONS OF TREATMENT W CC	84.20%
453	21	5,381	MED	COMPLICATIONS OF TREATMENT W/O CC	
454	21	4,755	MED	OTHER INJURY, POISONING & TOXIC EFFECT DIAG W CC	84.31%
455	21	885	MED	OTHER INJURY, POISONING & TOXIC EFFECT DIAG W/O CC	
463	23	32,987	MED	SIGNS & SYMPTOMS W CC	81.11%
464	23	7,681	MED	SIGNS & SYMPTOMS W/O CC	
493	07	60,917	SURG	LAPAROSCOPIC CHOLECYSTECTOMY W/O C.D.E. W CC	71.33%
494	07	24,482	SURG	LAPAROSCOPIC CHOLECYSTECTOMY W/O C.D.E. W/O CC	
497	08	31,247	SURG	SPINAL FUSION EXCEPT CERVICAL W CC	59.34%
498	08	21,409	SURG	SPINAL FUSION EXCEPT CERVICAL W/O CC	
499	08	35,214	SURG	BACK & NECK PROCEDURES EXCEPT SPINAL FUSION W CC	42.99%
500	08	46,705	SURG	BACK & NECK PROCEDURES EXCEPT SPINAL FUSION W/O CC	
501	08	3,172	SURG	KNEE PROCEDURES W PDX OF INFECTION W CC	80.75%
502	08	756	SURG	KNEE PROCEDURES W PDX OF INFECTION W/O CC	
506	22	964	SURG	FULL THICKNESS BURN W SKIN GRAFT OR INHAL INJ W CC OR SIG TRAUMA	74.90%
507	22	323	SURG	FULL THICKNESS BURN W SKIN GRFT OR INHAL INJ W/O CC OR SIG TRAUMA	
508	22	663	MED	FULL THICKNESS BURN W/O SKIN GRFT OR INHAL INJ W CC OR SIG TRAUMA	80.85%
509	22	157	MED	FULL THICKNESS BURN W/O SKIN GRFT OR INH INJ W/O CC OR SIG TRAUMA	
510	22	1,798	MED	NONEXTENSIVE BURNS W CC OR SIGNIFICANT TRAUMA	73.87%
511	22	636	MED	NONEXTENSIVE BURNS W/O CC OR SIGNIFICANT TRAUMA	
519	08	12,546	SURG	CERVICAL SPINAL FUSION W CC	43.14%
520	08	16,538	SURG	CERVICAL SPINAL FUSION W/O CC	

DRG	MDC	Volumes	Type	DRG Title	CC%
521	20	32,469	MED	ALCOHOL/DRUG ABUSE OR DEPENDENCE W CC	60.26%
522	20	5,805	MED	ALCOHOL/DRUG ABUSE OR DEPEND W REHABILITATION THERAPY W/O CC	
523	20	15,604	MED	ALCOHOL/DRUG ABUSE OR DEPEND W/O REHABILITA- TION THERAPY W/O CC	
529	01	5,110	SURG	VENTRICULAR SHUNT PROCEDURES W CC	60.23%
530	01	3,374	SURG	VENTRICULAR SHUNT PROCEDURES W/O CC	
531	01	4,874	SURG	SPINAL PROCEDURES W CC	63.25%
532	01	2,832	SURG	SPINAL PROCEDURES W/O CC	
533	01	46,528	SURG	EXTRACRANIAL PROCEDURES W CC	52.23%
534	01	42,555	SURG	EXTRACRANIAL PROCEDURES W/O CC	
537	08	8,953	SURG	LOCAL EXCIS & REMOV OF INT FIX DEV EXCEPT HIP & FEMUR W CC	62.13%
538	08	5,456	SURG	LOCAL EXCIS & REMOV OF INT FIX DEV EXCEPT HIP & FEMUR W/O CC	
539	17	4,954	SURG	LYMPHOMA & LEUKEMIA W MAJOR OR PROCEDURE W CC	76.84%
540	17	1,493	SURG	LYMPHOMA & LEUKEMIA W MAJOR OR PROCEDURE W/O CC	
		5,820,982		TOTAL	80.32%

Appendix 9.4

2005 National Averages for High-Risk DRG Pairs

DRG	MDC	Volumes	Type	DRG Title	High Risk %
14	01	278,220	MED	INTRACRANIAL HEMORRHAGE OR CEREBRAL INFARCTION	93.28%
15	01	20,045	MED	NONSPECIFIC CVA & PRECEREBRAL OCCLUSION W/O INFARCT	
15	01	20,045	MED	NONSPECIFIC CVA & PRECEREBRAL OCCLUSION W/O INFARCT	15.51%
524	01	109,168	MED	TRANSIENT ISCHEMIA	
79	04	160,409	MED	RESPIRATORY INFECTIONS & INFLAMMATIONS AGE >17 W CC	62.41%
87	04	96,631	MED	PULMONARY EDEMA & RESPIRATORY FAILURE	
79	04	160,409	MED	RESPIRATORY INFECTIONS & INFLAMMATIONS AGE >17 W CC	22.42%
89	04	555,221	MED	SIMPLE PNEUMONIA & PLEURISY AGE >17 W CC	
87	04	96,631	MED	PULMONARY EDEMA & RESPIRATORY FAILURE	18.42%
88	04	427,997	MED	CHRONIC OBSTRUCTIVE PULMONARY DISEASE	
88	04	427,997	MED	CHRONIC OBSTRUCTIVE PULMONARY DISEASE	87.68%
96	04	60,151	MED	BRONCHITIS & ASTHMA AGE >17 W CC	
89	04	555,221	MED	SIMPLE PNEUMONIA & PLEURISY AGE >17 W CC	45.39%
127	05	668,008	MED	HEART FAILURE & SHOCK	
130	05	87,632	MED	PERIPHERAL VASCULAR DISORDERS W CC	95.40%
128	05	4,229	MED	DEEP VEIN THROMBOPHLEBITIS	
132	05	101,483	MED	ATHEROSCLEROSIS W CC	76.29%
140	05	31,544	MED	ANGINA PECTORIS	
132	05	101,483	MED	ATHEROSCLEROSIS W CC	29.86%
143	05	238,376	MED	CHEST PAIN	
138	05	206,196	MED	CARDIAC ARRHYTHMIA & CONDUCTION DISORDERS W CC	62.55%
141	05	123,475	MED	SYNCOPE & COLLAPSE W CC	
174	06	261,063	MED	G.I. HEMORRHAGE W CC	46.77%
182	06	297,097	MED	ESOPHAGITIS, GASTROENT & MISC DIGEST DISORDERS AGE >17 W CC	
182	06	297,097	MED	ESOPHAGITIS, GASTROENT & MISC DIGEST DISORDERS AGE >17 W CC	55.48%
143	05	238,376	MED	CHEST PAIN	
188	06	93,582	MED	OTHER DIGESTIVE SYSTEM DIAGNOSES AGE >17 W CC	50.61%
180	06	91,338	MED	G.I. OBSTRUCTION W CC	
239	08	40,272	MED	PATHOLOGICAL FRACTURES & MUSCULOSKELETAL & CONN TISS MALIGNANCY	28.56%
243	08	100,743	MED	MEDICAL BACK PROBLEMS	

DRG	MDC	Volumes	Type	DRG Title	High Risk %
271	09	21,705	MED	SKIN ULCERS	15.39%
277	09	119,318	MED	CELLULITIS AGE >17 W CC	
296	10	247,607	MED	NUTRITIONAL & MISC METABOLIC DISORDERS AGE >17 W CC	45.46%
182	06	297,097	MED	ESOPHAGITIS, GASTROENT & MISC DIGEST DISORDERS AGE >17 W CC	
316	11	204,595	MED	RENAL FAILURE	45.24%
296	10	247,607	MED	NUTRITIONAL & MISC METABOLIC DISORDERS AGE >17 W CC	
316	11	204,595	MED	RENAL FAILURE	78.23%
331	11	56,928	MED	OTHER KIDNEY & URINARY TRACT DIAGNOSES AGE >17 W CC	
416	18	287,777	MED	SEPTICEMIA AGE >17	64.21%
79	04	160,409	MED	RESPIRATORY INFECTIONS & INFLAMMATIONS AGE >17 W CC	
416	18	287,777	MED	SEPTICEMIA AGE >17	34.14%
89	04	555,221	MED	SIMPLE PNEUMONIA & PLEURISY AGE >17 W CC	
416	18	287,777	MED	SEPTICEMIA AGE >17	56.08%
320	11	225,362	MED	KIDNEY & URINARY TRACT INFECTIONS AGE >17 W CC	
475	04	119,967	MED	RESPIRATORY SYSTEM DIAGNOSIS WITH VENTILATOR SUPPORT	55.39%
87	04	96,631	MED	PULMONARY EDEMA & RESPIRATORY FAILURE	
475	04	119,967	MED	RESPIRATORY SYSTEM DIAGNOSIS WITH VENTILATOR SUPPORT	15.22%
127	05	668,008	MED	HEART FAILURE & SHOCK	
475	04	119,967	MED	RESPIRATORY SYSTEM DIAGNOSIS WITH VENTILATOR SUPPORT	29.42%
416	18	287,777	MED	SEPTICEMIA AGE >17	

Appendix 9.5

2006 Transfer DRGs

DRG	FY06 Final Rule Post-acute Care DRG	FY06 Final Rule Special Pay DRG	MDC	Type	DRG Title	Weights	Geometric Mean LOS	Arithmetic Mean LOS
1	Yes	No	01	SURG	CRANIOTOMY AGE >17 W CC	3.4347	7.6	10.1
2	Yes	No	01	SURG	CRANIOTOMY AGE >17 W/O CC	1.9587	3.5	4.6
7	Yes	Yes	01	SURG	PERIPH & CRANIAL NERVE & OTHER NERV SYST PROC W CC	2.6978	6.7	9.7
8	Yes	Yes	01	SURG	PERIPH & CRANIAL NERVE & OTHER NERV SYST PROC W/O CC	1.5635	2.0	3.0
10	Yes	No	01	MED	NERVOUS SYSTEM NEOPLASMS W CC	1.2222	4.6	6.2
11	Yes	No	01	MED	NERVOUS SYSTEM NEOPLASMS W/O CC	0.8736	2.9	3.8
12	Yes	No	01	MED	DEGENERATIVE NERVOUS SYSTEM DISORDERS	0.8998	4.3	5.5
13	Yes	No	01	MED	MULTIPLE SCLEROSIS & CEREBELLAR ATAXIA	0.8575	4.0	5.0
14	Yes	No	01	MED	INTRACRANIAL HEMORRHAGE OR CEREBRAL INFARCTION	1.2456	4.5	5.8
15	Yes	No	01	MED	NONSPECIFIC CVA & PRECEREBRAL OCCLUSION W/O INFARCT	0.9421	3.7	4.6
16	Yes	No	01	MED	NONSPECIFIC CEREBROVASCULAR DISORDERS W CC	1.3351	5.0	6.5
17	Yes	No	01	MED	NONSPECIFIC CEREBROVASCULAR DISORDERS W/O CC	0.7229	2.5	3.2
18	Yes	No	01	MED	CRANIAL & PERIPHERAL NERVE DISORDERS W CC	0.9903	4.1	5.3
19	Yes	No	01	MED	CRANIAL & PERIPHERAL NERVE DISORDERS W/O CC	0.7077	2.7	3.5
20	Yes	No	01	MED	NERVOUS SYSTEM INFECTION EXCEPT VIRAL MENINGITIS	2.7865	8.0	10.4
24	Yes	No	01	MED	SEIZURE & HEADACHE AGE >17 W CC	0.9970	3.6	4.8
25	Yes	No	01	MED	SEIZURE & HEADACHE AGE >17 W/O CC	0.6180	2.5	3.1
28	Yes	No	01	MED	TRAUMATIC STUPOR & COMA, COMA <1 HR AGE >17 W CC	1.3353	4.4	5.9
29	Yes	No	01	MED	TRAUMATIC STUPOR & COMA, COMA <1 HR AGE >17 W/O CC	0.7212	2.6	3.4
34	Yes	No	01	MED	OTHER DISORDERS OF NERVOUS SYSTEM W CC	1.0062	3.7	4.8
35	Yes	No	01	MED	OTHER DISORDERS OF NERVOUS SYSTEM W/O CC	0.6241	2.4	3.0
73	Yes	No	03	MED	OTHER EAR, NOSE, MOUTH & THROAT DIAGNOSES AGE >17	0.8527	3.3	4.4
75	Yes	No	04	SURG	MAJOR CHEST PROCEDURES	3.0732	7.6	9.9
76	Yes	No	04	SURG	OTHER RESP SYSTEM O.R. PROCEDURES W CC	2.8830	8.4	11.1

Source: Reprinted from CMS 2006b.

DRG	FY06 Final Rule Post-acute Care DRG	FY06 Final Rule Special Pay DRG	MDC	Type	DRG Title	Weights	Geometric Mean LOS	Arithmetic Mean LOS
77	Yes	No	04	SURG	OTHER RESP SYSTEM O.R. PROCEDURES W/O CC	1.1857	3.3	4.7
78	Yes	No	04	MED	PULMONARY EMBOLISM	1.2427	5.4	6.4
79	Yes	No	04	MED	RESPIRATORY INFECTIONS & INFLAMMATIONS AGE >17 W CC	1.6238	6.7	8.5
80	Yes	No	04	MED	RESPIRATORY INFECTIONS & INFLAMMATIONS AGE >17 W/O CC	0.8947	4.4	5.5
82	Yes	No	04	MED	RESPIRATORY NEOPLASMS	1.3936	5.1	6.8
83	Yes	No	04	MED	MAJOR CHEST TRAUMA W CC	0.9828	4.2	5.3
84	Yes	No	04	MED	MAJOR CHEST TRAUMA W/O CC	0.5799	2.6	3.2
85	Yes	No	04	MED	PLEURAL EFFUSION W CC	1.2405	4.8	6.3
86	Yes	No	04	MED	PLEURAL EFFUSION W/O CC	0.6974	2.8	3.6
89	Yes	No	04	MED	SIMPLE PNEUMONIA & PLEURISY AGE >17 W CC	1.0320	4.7	5.7
90	Yes	No	04	MED	SIMPLE PNEUMONIA & PLEURISY AGE >17 W/O CC	0.6104	3.2	3.8
92	Yes	No	04	MED	INTERSTITIAL LUNG DISEASE W CC	1.1853	4.8	6.1
93	Yes	No	04	MED	INTERSTITIAL LUNG DISEASE W/O CC	0.7150	3.1	3.9
101	Yes	No	04	MED	OTHER RESPIRATORY SYSTEM DIAGNOSES W CC	0.8733	3.3	4.3
102	Yes	No	04	MED	OTHER RESPIRATORY SYSTEM DIAGNOSES W/O CC	0.5402	2.0	2.5
104	Yes	No	05	SURG	CARDIAC VALVE & OTH MAJOR CARDIOTHORACIC PROC W CARD CATH	8.2201	12.7	14.9
105	Yes	No	05	SURG	CARDIAC VALVE & OTH MAJOR CARDIOTHORACIC PROC W/O CARD CATH	6.0192	8.4	10.2
108	Yes	No	05	SURG	OTHER CARDIOTHORACIC PROCEDURES	5.8789	8.6	11.0
113	Yes	No	05	SURG	AMPUTATION FOR CIRC SYSTEM DISORDERS EXCEPT UPPER LIMB & TOE	3.1682	10.8	13.7
114	Yes	No	05	SURG	UPPER LIMB & TOE AMPUTATION FOR CIRC SYSTEM DISORDERS	1.7354	6.7	8.9
120	Yes	No	05	SURG	OTHER CIRCULATORY SYSTEM O.R. PROCEDURES	2.3853	5.9	9.2
121	Yes	No	05	MED	CIRCULATORY DISORDERS W AMI & MAJOR COMP, DISCHARGED ALIVE	1.6136	5.3	6.6
126	Yes	No	05	MED	ACUTE & SUBACUTE ENDOCARDITIS	2.7440	9.4	12.0
127	Yes	No	05	MED	HEART FAILURE & SHOCK	1.0345	4.1	5.2
130	Yes	No	05	MED	PERIPHERAL VASCULAR DISORDERS W CC	0.9425	4.4	5.5
131	Yes	No	05	MED	PERIPHERAL VASCULAR DISORDERS W/O CC	0.5566	3.2	3.9
144	Yes	No	05	MED	OTHER CIRCULATORY SYSTEM DIAGNOSES W CC	1.2761	4.1	5.8
145	Yes	No	05	MED	OTHER CIRCULATORY SYSTEM DIAGNOSES W/O CC	0.5835	2.1	2.6
146	Yes	No	06	SURG	RECTAL RESECTION W CC	2.6621	8.6	10.0
147	Yes	No	06	SURG	RECTAL RESECTION W/O CC	1.4781	5.2	5.8
148	Yes	No	06	SURG	MAJOR SMALL & LARGE BOWEL PROCEDURES W CC	3.4479	10.0	12.3

DRG	FY06 Final Rule Post-acute Care DRG	FY06 Final Rule Special Pay DRG	MDC	Type	DRG Title	Weights	Geometric Mean LOS	Arithmetic Mean LOS
149	Yes	No	06	SURG	MAJOR SMALL & LARGE BOWEL PROCEDURES W/O CC	1.4324	5.4	6.0
150	Yes	No	06	SURG	PERITONEAL ADHESIOLYSIS W CC	2.8061	8.9	11.0
151	Yes	No	06	SURG	PERITONEAL ADHESIOLYSIS W/O CC	1.2641	4.0	5.1
154	Yes	No	06	SURG	STOMACH, ESOPHAGEAL & DUODENAL PROCEDURES AGE >17 W CC	4.0399	9.9	13.3
155	Yes	No	06	SURG	STOMACH, ESOPHAGEAL & DUODENAL PROCEDURES AGE >17 W/O CC	1.2889	3.1	4.1
157	Yes	No	06	SURG	ANAL & STOMAL PROCEDURES W CC	1.3356	4.1	5.8
158	Yes	No	06	SURG	ANAL & STOMAL PROCEDURES W/O CC	0.6657	2.1	2.6
170	Yes	No	06	SURG	OTHER DIGESTIVE SYSTEM O.R. PROCEDURES W CC	2.9612	7.8	11.0
171	Yes	No	06	SURG	OTHER DIGESTIVE SYSTEM O.R. PROCEDURES W/O CC	1.1905	3.1	4.1
172	Yes	No	06	MED	DIGESTIVE MALIGNANCY W CC	1.4125	5.1	7.0
173	Yes	No	06	MED	DIGESTIVE MALIGNANCY W/O CC	0.7443	2.7	3.6
176	Yes	No	06	MED	COMPLICATED PEPTIC ULCER	1.1246	4.1	5.2
180	Yes	No	06	MED	G.I. OBSTRUCTION W CC	0.9784	4.2	5.4
181	Yes	No	06	MED	G.I. OBSTRUCTION W/O CC	0.5614	2.8	3.3
188	Yes	No	06	MED	OTHER DIGESTIVE SYSTEM DIAGNOSES AGE >17 W CC	1.1290	4.2	5.6
189	Yes	No	06	MED	OTHER DIGESTIVE SYSTEM DIAGNOSES AGE >17 W/O CC	0.6064	2.4	3.1
191	Yes	No	07	SURG	PANCREAS, LIVER & SHUNT PROCEDURES W CC	3.9680	9.0	12.9
192	Yes	No	07	SURG	PANCREAS, LIVER & SHUNT PROCEDURES W/O CC	1.6793	4.3	5.7
197	Yes	No	07	SURG	CHOLECYSTECTOMY EXCEPT BY LAPAROSCOPE W/O C.D.E. W CC	2.5425	7.5	9.2
198	Yes	No	07	SURG	CHOLECYSTECTOMY EXCEPT BY LAPAROSCOPE W/O C.D.E. W/O CC	1.1604	3.7	4.3
205	Yes	No	07	MED	DISORDERS OF LIVER EXCEPT MALIG, CIRR, ALC HEPA W CC	1.2059	4.4	6.0
206	Yes	No	07	MED	DISORDERS OF LIVER EXCEPT MALIG, CIRR, ALC HEPA W/O CC	0.7292	3.0	3.9
210	Yes	Yes	08	SURG	HIP & FEMUR PROCEDURES EXCEPT MAJOR JOINT AGE >17 W CC	1.9059	6.1	6.9
211	Yes	Yes	08	SURG	HIP & FEMUR PROCEDURES EXCEPT MAJOR JOINT AGE >17 W/O CC	1.2690	4.4	4.7
213	Yes	No	08	SURG	AMPUTATION FOR MUSCULOSKELETAL SYSTEM & CONN TISSUE DISORDERS	2.0428	7.2	9.7
216	Yes	No	08	SURG	BIOPSIES OF MUSCULOSKELETAL SYSTEM & CONNECTIVE TISSUE	1.9131	3.3	5.8
217	Yes	No	08	SURG	WND DEBRID & SKN GRFT EXCEPT HAND, FOR MUSCSKELET & CONN TISS DIS	3.0596	9.3	13.2
218	Yes	No	08	SURG	LOWER EXTREM & HUMER PROC EXCEPT HIP, FOOT, FEMUR AGE >17 W CC	1.6648	4.4	5.6
219	Yes	No	08	SURG	LOWER EXTREM & HUMER PROC EXCEPT HIP, FOOT, FEMUR AGE >17 W/O CC	1.0443	2.6	3.1

DRG	FY06 Final Rule Post-acute Care DRG	FY06 Final Rule Special Pay DRG	MDC	Type	DRG Title	Weights	Geometric Mean LOS	Arithmetic Mean LOS
225	Yes	No	08	SURG	FOOT PROCEDURES	1.2251	3.7	5.2
226	Yes	No	08	SURG	SOFT TISSUE PROCEDURES W CC	1.5884	4.5	6.5
227	Yes	No	08	SURG	SOFT TISSUE PROCEDURES W/O CC	0.8311	2.1	2.6
233	Yes	Yes	08	SURG	OTHER MUSCULOSKELET SYS & CONN TISS O.R. PROC W CC	1.9184	4.6	6.8
234	Yes	Yes	08	SURG	OTHER MUSCULOSKELET SYS & CONN TISS O.R. PROC W/O CC	1.2219	2.0	2.8
235	Yes	No	08	MED	FRACTURES OF FEMUR	0.7768	3.8	4.8
236	Yes	No	08	MED	FRACTURES OF HIP & PELVIS	0.7407	3.8	4.6
238	Yes	No	08	MED	OSTEOMYELITIS	1.4401	6.7	8.7
239	Yes	No	08	MED	PATHOLOGICAL FRACTURES & MUSCULOSKELETAL & CONN TISS MALIGNANCY	1.0767	5.0	6.2
240	Yes	No	08	MED	CONNECTIVE TISSUE DISORDERS W CC	1.4051	5.0	6.7
241	Yes	No	08	MED	CONNECTIVE TISSUE DISORDERS W/O CC	0.6629	3.0	3.7
244	Yes	No	08	MED	BONE DISEASES & SPECIFIC ARTHROPATHIES W CC	0.7200	3.6	4.5
245	Yes	No	08	MED	BONE DISEASES & SPECIFIC ARTHROPATHIES W/O CC	0.4583	2.5	3.1
250	Yes	No	08	MED	FX, SPRN, STRN & DISL OF FOREARM, HAND, FOOT AGE >17 W CC	0.6974	3.2	3.9
251	Yes	No	08	MED	FX, SPRN, STRN & DISL OF FOREARM, HAND, FOOT AGE >17 W/O CC	0.4749	2.3	2.8
253	Yes	No	08	MED	FX, SPRN, STRN & DISL OF UPARM, LOWLEG EX FOOT AGE >17 W CC	0.7747	3.8	4.6
254	Yes	No	08	MED	FX, SPRN, STRN & DISL OF UPARM, LOWLEG EX FOOT AGE >17 W/O CC	0.4588	2.6	3.1
256	Yes	No	08	MED	OTHER MUSCULOSKELETAL SYSTEM & CONNECTIVE TISSUE DIAGNOSES	0.8509	3.9	5.1
263	Yes	No	09	SURG	SKIN GRAFT &/OR DEBRID FOR SKN ULCER OR CELLULITIS W CC	2.1130	8.6	11.4
264	Yes	No	09	SURG	SKIN GRAFT &/OR DEBRID FOR SKN ULCER OR CELLULITIS W/O CC	1.0635	5.0	6.5
265	Yes	No	09	SURG	SKIN GRAFT &/OR DEBRID EXCEPT FOR SKIN ULCER OR CELLULITIS W CC	1.6593	4.4	6.8
266	Yes	No	09	SURG	SKIN GRAFT &/OR DEBRID EXCEPT FOR SKIN ULCER OR CELLULITIS W/O CC	0.8637	2.3	3.2
269	Yes	No	09	SURG	OTHER SKIN, SUBCUT TISS & BREAST PROC W CC	1.8352	6.2	8.6
270	Yes	No	09	SURG	OTHER SKIN, SUBCUT TISS & BREAST PROC W/O CC	0.8313	2.7	3.9
271	Yes	No	09	MED	SKIN ULCERS	1.0195	5.6	7.1
272	Yes	No	09	MED	MAJOR SKIN DISORDERS W CC	0.9860	4.5	5.9
273	Yes	No	09	MED	MAJOR SKIN DISORDERS W/O CC	0.5539	2.9	3.7
277	Yes	No	09	MED	CELLULITIS AGE >17 W CC	0.8676	4.6	5.6
278	Yes	No	09	MED	CELLULITIS AGE >17 W/O CC	0.5391	3.4	4.1
280	Yes	No	09	MED	TRAUMA TO THE SKIN, SUBCUT TISS & BREAST AGE >17 W CC	0.7313	3.2	4.1

DRG	FY06 Final Rule Post-acute Care DRG	FY06 Final Rule Special Pay DRG	MDC	Type	DRG Title	Weights	Geometric Mean LOS	Arithmetic Mean LOS
281	Yes	No	09	MED	TRAUMA TO THE SKIN, SUBCUT TISS & BREAST AGE >17 W/O CC	0.4913	2.3	2.9
283	Yes	No	09	MED	MINOR SKIN DISORDERS W CC	0.7423	3.5	4.6
284	Yes	No	09	MED	MINOR SKIN DISORDERS W/O CC	0.4563	2.4	3.0
285	Yes	No	10	SURG	AMPUTAT OF LOWER LIMB FOR ENDOCRINE, NUTRIT, & METABOL DISORDERS	2.1831	8.2	10.5
287	Yes	No	10	SURG	SKIN GRAFTS & WOUND DEBRID FOR ENDOC, NUTRIT & METAB DISORDERS	1.9470	7.8	10.4
292	Yes	No	10	SURG	OTHER ENDOCRINE, NUTRIT & METAB O.R. PROC W CC	2.6395	7.3	10.3
293	Yes	No	10	SURG	OTHER ENDOCRINE, NUTRIT & METAB O.R. PROC W/O CC	1.3472	3.2	4.5
294	Yes	No	10	MED	DIABETES AGE >35	0.7652	3.3	4.3
296	Yes	No	10	MED	NUTRITIONAL & MISC METABOLIC DISORDERS AGE >17 W CC	0.8187	3.7	4.8
297	Yes	No	10	MED	NUTRITIONAL & MISC METABOLIC DISORDERS AGE >17 W/O CC	0.4879	2.5	3.1
300	Yes	No	10	MED	ENDOCRINE DISORDERS W CC	1.0922	4.6	6.0
301	Yes	No	10	MED	ENDOCRINE DISORDERS W/O CC	0.6118	2.7	3.4
304	Yes	No	11	SURG	KIDNEY, URETER & MAJOR BLADDER PROC FOR NONNEOPL W CC	2.3761	6.1	8.6
305	Yes	No	11	SURG	KIDNEY, URETER & MAJOR BLADDER PROC FOR NONNEOPL W/O CC	1.1595	2.6	3.2
316	Yes	No	11	MED	RENAL FAILURE	1.2692	4.9	6.4
320	Yes	No	11	MED	KIDNEY & URINARY TRACT INFECTIONS AGE >17 W CC	0.8658	4.2	5.2
321	Yes	No	11	MED	KIDNEY & URINARY TRACT INFECTIONS AGE >17 W/O CC	0.5652	3.0	3.6
331	Yes	No	11	MED	OTHER KIDNEY & URINARY TRACT DIAGNOSES AGE >17 W CC	1.0619	4.1	5.5
332	Yes	No	11	MED	OTHER KIDNEY & URINARY TRACT DIAGNOSES AGE >17 W/O CC	0.6160	2.4	3.1
395	Yes	No	16	MED	RED BLOOD CELL DISORDERS AGE >17	0.8328	3.2	4.3
401	Yes	No	17	SURG	LYMPHOMA & NONACUTE LEUKEMIA W OTHER O.R. PROC W CC	2.9678	8.0	11.3
402	Yes	No	17	SURG	LYMPHOMA & NONACUTE LEUKEMIA W OTHER O.R. PROC W/O CC	1.1810	2.8	4.1
403	Yes	No	17	MED	LYMPHOMA & NONACUTE LEUKEMIA W CC	1.8432	5.8	8.1
404	Yes	No	17	MED	LYMPHOMA & NONACUTE LEUKEMIA W/O CC	0.9265	3.0	4.2
415	Yes	No	18	SURG	O.R. PROCEDURE FOR INFECTIOUS & PARASITIC DISEASES	3.9890	11.0	14.8
416	Yes	No	18	MED	SEPTICEMIA AGE >17	1.6774	5.6	7.5
418	Yes	No	18	MED	POSTOPERATIVE & POSTTRAUMATIC INFECTIONS	1.0716	4.8	6.2
423	Yes	No	18	MED	OTHER INFECTIOUS & PARASITIC DISEASES DIAGNOSES	1.9196	6.0	8.4

DRG	FY06 Final Rule Post-acute Care DRG	FY06 Final Rule Special Pay DRG	MDC	Type	DRG Title	Weights	Geometric Mean LOS	Arithmetic Mean LOS
429	Yes	No	19	MED	ORGANIC DISTURBANCES & MENTAL RETARDATION	0.7919	4.3	5.6
430	Yes	No	19	MED	PSYCHOSES	0.6483	5.8	7.9
440	Yes	No	21	SURG	WOUND DEBRIDEMENTS FOR INJURIES	1.9457	5.9	9.2
442	Yes	No	21	SURG	OTHER O.R. PROCEDURES FOR INJURIES W CC	2.5660	6.0	8.9
443	Yes	No	21	SURG	OTHER O.R. PROCEDURES FOR INJURIES W/O CC	0.9943	2.6	3.4
444	Yes	No	21	MED	TRAUMATIC INJURY AGE >17 W CC	0.7556	3.2	4.1
445	Yes	No	21	MED	TRAUMATIC INJURY AGE >17 W/O CC	0.5033	2.2	2.8
462	Yes	No	23	MED	REHABILITATION	0.8700	8.9	10.8
463	Yes	No	23	MED	SIGNS & SYMPTOMS W CC	0.6960	3.1	3.9
464	Yes	No	23	MED	SIGNS & SYMPTOMS W/O CC	0.5055	2.4	2.9
468	Yes	No			EXTENSIVE O.R. PROCEDURE UNRELATED TO PRINCIPAL DIAGNOSIS	4.0031	9.7	13.2
471	Yes	Yes	08	SURG	BILATERAL OR MULTIPLE MAJOR JOINT PROCS OF LOWER EXTREMITY	3.1391	4.5	5.1
475	Yes	No	04	MED	RESPIRATORY SYSTEM DIAGNOSIS WITH VENTILATOR SUPPORT	3.6091	8.1	11.3
477	Yes	No		SURG	NONEXTENSIVE O.R. PROCEDURE UNRELATED TO PRINCIPAL DIAGNOSIS	2.0607	5.8	8.7
478	Yes	No	05	SURG	NO LONGER VALID	0.0000	0.0	0.0
482	Yes	No	PRE	SURG	TRACHEOSTOMY FOR FACE, MOUTH & NECK DIAGNOSES	3.3387	9.6	12.1
485	Yes	No	24	SURG	LIMB REATTACHMENT, HIP AND FEMUR PROC FOR MULTIPLE SIGNIFICANT TRA	3.4952	8.4	10.2
487	Yes	No	24	MED	OTHER MULTIPLE SIGNIFICANT TRAUMA	1.9459	5.3	7.3
497	Yes	Yes	08	SURG	SPINAL FUSION EXCEPT CERVICAL W CC	3.6224	5.0	5.9
498	Yes	Yes	08	SURG	SPINAL FUSION EXCEPT CERVICAL W/O CC	2.7791	3.4	3.8
501	Yes	No	08	SURG	KNEE PROCEDURES W PDX OF INFECTION W CC	2.6462	8.5	10.4
502	Yes	No	08	SURG	KNEE PROCEDURES W PDX OF INFECTION W/O CC	1.4462	4.9	5.9
521	Yes	No	20	MED	ALCOHOL/DRUG ABUSE OR DEPENDENCE W CC	0.6939	4.2	5.6
522	Yes	No	20	MED	ALC/DRUG ABUSE OR DEPEND W REHABILITATION THERAPY W/O CC	0.4794	7.7	9.6
529	Yes	No	01	SURG	VENTRICULAR SHUNT PROCEDURES W CC	2.3160	5.3	8.3
530	Yes	No	01	SURG	VENTRICULAR SHUNT PROCEDURES W/O CC	1.2041	2.4	3.1
531	Yes	No	01	SURG	SPINAL PROCEDURES W CC	3.1279	6.5	9.6
532	Yes	No	01	SURG	SPINAL PROCEDURES W/O CC	1.4195	2.8	3.7
537	Yes	No	08	SURG	LOCAL EXCIS & REMOV OF INT FIX DEV EXCEPT HIP & FEMUR W CC	1.8360	4.8	6.9

DRG	FY06 Final Rule Post-acute Care DRG	FY06 Final Rule Special Pay DRG	MDC	Type	DRG Title	Weights	Geometric Mean LOS	Arithmetic Mean LOS
538	Yes	No	08	SURG	LOCAL EXCIS & REMOV OF INT FIX DEV EXCEPT HIP & FEMUR W/O CC	0.9833	2.1	2.8
541	Yes	No	PRE	SURG	ECMO OR TRACH W MV 96+HRS OR PDX EXC FACE, MOUTH & NECK W MAJ O.R.	19.8038	38.1	45.7
542	Yes	No	PRE	SURG	TRACH W MV 96+HRS OR PDX EXC FACE, MOUTH & NECK W/O MAJ O.R.	12.8719	29.1	35.1
543	Yes	No	01	SURG	CRANIOTOMY W/IMPLANT OF CHEMO AGENT OR ACUTE COMPLX CNS PDX	4.4184	8.5	12.3
544	Yes	Yes	08	SURG	MAJOR JOINT REPLACEMENT OR REATTACHMENT OF LOWER EXTREMITY	1.9643	4.1	4.5
545	Yes	Yes	08	SURG	REVISION OF HIP OR KNEE REPLACEMENT	2.4827	4.5	5.2
547	Yes	No	05	SURG	CORONARY BYPASS W CARDIAC CATH W MAJOR CV DX	6.1948	10.8	12.3
548	Yes	No	05	SURG	CORONARY BYPASS W CARDIAC CATH W/O MAJOR CV DX	4.7198	8.2	9.0
549	Yes	Yes	05	SURG	CORONARY BYPASS W/O CARDIAC CATH W MAJOR CV DX	5.0980	8.7	10.3
550	Yes	Yes	05	SURG	CORONARY BYPASS W/O CARDIAC CATH W/O MAJOR CV DX	3.6151	6.2	6.9
553	Yes	No	05	SURG	OTHER VASCULAR PROCEDURES W CC W MAJOR CV DX	3.0957	6.6	9.7
554	Yes	No	05	SURG	OTHER VASCULAR PROCEDURES W CC W/O MAJOR CV DX	2.0721	4.0	5.9

Chapter 10

Reporting Issues

Desla R. Mancilla, MPA, RHIA

With the evolution of automated systems, coded data are no longer available only in the form of standard reports from the health information management (HIM) department. They now can be customized and used in a variety of ways. HIM department staff or users anywhere in the facility can design and run reports. More important, reports can be used to integrate and summarize data collected and stored in many disparate systems. In addition to internal facility users of reports based on diagnostic and procedure codes, there are many external demands for these reports as well.

The term **information** implies the transformation of raw data into a usable format. Data collected by healthcare facilities are voluminous. The resulting information must be manageable, yet comprehensive enough to accurately depict the overall process and results of patient care.

In the realm of healthcare information, data sources are numerous. Traditionally, paper records were created and analyzed as required data elements were abstracted to a paper document. Subsequently, the paper documents were accumulated and sent to companies to generate reports. Those reports were eventually returned to the originating facility for assessment and interpretation.

Today, with the ever-advancing capabilities provided by automated collection and analysis systems, information is at the fingertips of the user within moments of data collection. However, unformatted data are difficult to understand. Therefore, reports are created, formatted, and distributed to users throughout the healthcare enterprise for a multitude of purposes.

Healthcare facilities everywhere and of every kind—rural, urban, large, small, private, for profit, nonprofit, long-term care, ambulatory care, and others—devote significant resources, both financial and human, to the processes associated with collecting, analyzing, maintaining, reporting, and distributing information vital to the organization's success.

This chapter defines the sources of data as they relate to the coding process, identifies the type of information needed to create reports based on coded data, and describes where and how various users inside and outside the healthcare facility need and use coded information.

Sources of Data

The sources of data must be understood, particularly when the data are converted into diagnostic and procedural codes. Such codes are one step in the process of making data more usable. Coding professionals are charged with the task of analyzing raw data and assigning codes that represent the significant conditions and resources expended on the care of a patient.

Codes, both diagnostic and procedural, are **aggregate data**—a mass or body of data that is treated as a unit. A code represents the sum of the coder's analysis of extensive documentation.

The documentation that coders analyze may be in the form of handwritten notes or reports from healthcare providers. Often it consists of computer-generated information from one of many ancillary-, nursing-, or physician-based analysis or treatment systems. For example, an echocardiography result may appear as:

- An interpretation handwritten by a physician

- An interpretation dictated by a physician and transcribed into a report by a transcriptionist

- A computer-generated result

The computer-generated result represents the capabilities of knowledge-based systems that require little or no human intervention in the analysis process.

Traditionally, one of the major delays in the coding process has resulted from the time spent waiting for all pertinent test results and transcribed reports to reach the coding department. In an effort to speed up the process, and subsequently to reduce billing delays, some facilities have developed great efficiencies in the coding process. They allow coders to access the required information before it is available in its final form. For example, some facilities have developed mechanisms that allow coders to dial into the dictation system to hear a healthcare provider's dictation before it has been transcribed.

In other facilities, interfaces from feeder systems to the hospital information system allow coders to see the test results online and in real time. They do not have to wait for the results to be printed, distributed, and "charted" on the paper record. A **feeder system** is an automated data system that feeds results into a comprehensive database, such as the echocardiography system discussed above. A **hospital information system (HIS)** is the comprehensive database that contains all the clinical, administrative, financial, and demographic information about each patient served by a hospital.

All of those factors are important in the life cycle of report creation, generation, and distribution. Reports based on coded information are instrumental in promoting managerial efficiency in all aspects of the healthcare facility's operation. Planning, assessment, and development of services, as well as countless financial decisions, are based on reports detailing individual and aggregate coded information.

Abstracting

Abstracting is the process of extracting elements of data from a source document (a paper record, for example) and entering them into an automated system. The purpose of this endeavor is to make those data elements available for later use. After a data element has been captured in electronic form, it generally can be searched for, and reported on, as a discrete entity. In addition, it can be aggregated into a group of data elements to provide information needed by the user.

Paper versus Electronic Record Systems

Abstracting is not done in the same way when patient records and source documents are electronic rather than paper. With electronic record systems, the data elements do not have to be abstracted because they already are available in electronic form. However, all electronic data are not searchable. Therefore, data elements intended for inclusion in a required report should be stored in indexed data fields that allow for search and retrieval of the required information.

The distinction between the abstracting process in paper and electronic forms must be further detailed to distinguish between a true electronic patient record system and an **optical image–based system.** In a totally electronic record system, all parts of the record are created initially in electronic form. In an optical image–based system, the information is created initially in paper form and then scanned into a system for storage and retrieval. The abstraction process varies depending on the types of electronic systems used within the organization.

Cycle of Capturing Data

To understand how data are captured in an automated system, it is important to understand the flow cycle from the point of registration to the point of discharge. In an acute care facility, it is common for a patient to register for the service being provided. The patient gives patient access department personnel pertinent demographic information that is entered into the registration system. Insurance, emergency contact, and physician data also are generally collected at the point of registration. Throughout the patient's stay, a wide variety of other information is generated, some in paper form and some in electronic form.

In the traditional paper-based facility, the healthcare provider, or some other party authorized to take verbal orders, writes an order for a test in the health record. The order then is generally entered into the HIS. After the order is entered into this system, the responsible ancillary department performs the test. The test is often performed using biomedical or clinical equipment that is itself another type of automated system.

The test result then can be processed in one of the following ways:

- It can be printed and "charted," which is time-consuming and resource intensive.

- It can be sent from the biomedical system to the HIS through an interface or some other direct-access mechanism, which allows nursing, ancillary, and medical staff members to access the result as soon as it is available.

If no automated mechanism is in place to transfer the results to the HIS, the responsible ancillary department typically contacts the physician and the nursing unit with abnormal test results for prompt attention.

Many departments have automated data systems, also called feeder systems, such as those just described. For example, the emergency department may have a system to assist in triage and in tracking patients seen in the department. Respiratory therapy may have a system that not only assists in the interpretation of clinical testing, but also serves as a documentation system for the therapists. In that type of automated data system, therapists no longer write care notes by hand. Instead, they use the system to create and maintain the history of their treatment services. After the results of all the feeder systems, or automated data systems, are in the HIS, they are integrated with the patient's demographic and financial information, thus creating a comprehensive history of all aspects of care.

Departments that do not have automated data systems create and maintain their information in paper form. The paper records are sent to the HIM department for integration with all other parts of the patient record. In some facilities, these paper documents are scanned into an optical imaging system. The entire record then can be stored in, and retrieved from, an automated system when needed at some point after patient discharge.

The problem for the coder becomes one of timing. He or she must understand where data are stored and how to access them for use in the coding process. Procedurally, coders abide by the guidelines of their organization and of the agencies that direct what information is to be used when determining the appropriate codes to be assigned.

Types of Data Elements

The types of data elements that are abstracted, or defined as indexed fields in an automated system, vary from facility to facility. Generally, however, any data elements that are needed for selecting cases for reports must be abstracted or indexed. Typical data fields that can be searched for the purpose of case finding and reporting include:

- Patient name

- Zip code

- Health record number

- Patient account number

- Guarantor number

- Financial class

- Insurance company and plan number

- Attending physician

- ICD-9-CM diagnosis codes

- ICD-9-CM procedure codes

- DRG number

- APC number

- CPT code

Some of these fields are abstracted; others are present in the system from the point of patient registration onward.

Patient Name Data Field

Patient name data fields are searchable for the obvious reason of finding a specific case. A discrete field is generally used to collect both the first and last names of the patient. Specific individual records are needed for every imaginable reason—from patient care, to assessment of services, to continuation of medical care.

Zip Code Data Field

Many facilities use the practice of zip code aggregation and analysis to determine populations to which they should market their services. In that way, certain populations can be targeted based on demographics known to be associated with a specific zip code. For example, in communities with young populations, marketing of sports medicine and obstetrical services is commonplace. Conversely, zip codes associated with a largely geriatric population are likely candidates for targeted marketing of long-term and other types of residential care.

Health Record Number Data Field

The health record number is used to identify all occasions of service for a specific patient within a given facility. Moreover, it can be used throughout the entire healthcare enterprise to track a variety of services within an integrated healthcare delivery network. Health record numbers are used in reports to identify specific cases meeting selection criteria. In addition, the presence of a health record number on a report assists in the process of finding the record, in either paper or electronic form.

Patient Account Number Data Field

The patient account number is used to separate charges and related services for a specific patient with multiple visits. For example, a patient might have three inpatient visits within a month. In each of those visits, a chest x-ray may have been performed. The account number denotes which x-ray was taken during a specific time frame, essentially allowing for classification of services and charges by date.

An account number is critical for finding specific occasions of service for a particular patient or for identifying groups of related events. For example, a user may need to find all records in which a left heart catheterization was performed. He or she would create a report to search for such cases by procedure code number and would direct the report to print the account number for each case found in the search process. The specific records corresponding to the account numbers listed on the report then would be used in the data analysis project.

Guarantor Number Data Field

The guarantor number identifies all of the patient accounts that a specific party is responsible for paying. In the traditional nuclear family, a married male is the guarantor for his spouse and children, even though his spouse may work and have her own insurance coverage. The guarantor number allows for efficiency in the billing process by grouping active account information together during a billing cycle. In this way, a single statement including all account activity can be sent to the guarantor, or his insurer, instead of multiple statements.

Financial Class Data Field

The financial class is a highly significant data element because it represents the payer, or insurer, of the account. Managed care contracts identify specific criteria that are covered and limitations of coverage. If an organization wants to know which accounts fall out of the specified criteria, a report is often created based on financial class.

In another scenario, a facility that needs to know how many Medicare days of service it has provided over a given time can query its system by financial class code. The query will be designed further to count the days of service for each individual account in order to report a total number of days of service provided within each managed care contract group.

Insurance Company and Plan Number Data Field

The insurance company and the plan number also are collected and used in the reporting process because a broad spectrum of insurers may fall into a single financial class. A financial class representing commercial insurance is one possible example. Users needing to run a report for a specific insurance company would be unable to do so based on the financial class data field. Instead, they would have to request further details in the form of the insurance company and plan number.

Attending Physician Number Data Field

Information about the attending physician is extremely important in the reporting process. Many departments within the facility need information based on physician services. The physician is often identified in the system based on a number. Subsequently, reports are run for individual physicians, physicians by service, or even by physicians grouped by medical service department. The concept of physician profiling appears later in this chapter, but it is important to note at this point that the attending physician number is usually held in a separate field from the number fields for the other physicians involved with a case.

The physician numbers of other types of physicians are abstracted for later use in reporting. Numbers for all secondary, consulting, and admitting physicians, as well as surgeons, surgical assistants, and covering physicians, are generally input as part of the data abstraction process. This is necessary to identify all cases in which a physician may have been involved.

The finance department in healthcare facilities also is interested in information trends regarding physicians and patient admissions. For example, an analysis of zip codes can determine that individuals from certain geographic areas in the community are more likely to be admitted through the emergency department than by a general medicine or family practice physician. In such a situation, the healthcare facility may want to develop a facility-sponsored family medicine practice in that geographic area to augment business from that part of the community. Services supported by specialty physicians such as cardiologists, nephrologists, neurologists, and neurosurgeons are generally known to increase reimbursement to the facility. On the other hand, less resource-intensive general practice services create less revenue. Nevertheless, general medical practitioners must be located within the community to ensure initial placement in the facility of patients who then can be referred to specialists as necessary.

ICD-9-CM Diagnosis Codes Data Fields

The ICD-9-CM principal diagnosis code is critical in the process of generating reports. Clinical users select cases based on a specific medical condition, and the principal diagnosis most succinctly describes the clinical assessment and treatment of the patient.

However, the principal diagnosis alone does not fully describe the care provided to a patient. ICD-9-CM secondary diagnosis codes also are important. They provide detailed evidence of the patient's overall condition.

Automated data systems allow for storage of many diagnosis codes. Typically, the principal diagnosis field is listed first and stored as a separate index from the secondary codes. However, there is usually great flexibility in designing reports based on combinations of principal and secondary diagnoses.

ICD-9-CM Procedure Codes Data Fields

The ICD-9-CM primary procedure code and secondary procedure codes are similar to their diagnostic counterparts. When these codes are applied, they generally are associated with detailed information about the physician or caregiver who performed the procedure, along with the date and time of service. Many facilities also choose to associate an anesthesia type with the procedure for future reference.

DRG Number Data Field

The DRG number is of primary significance in reporting because it is the single element that combines clinical care with the resources required to provide it. The DRG is calculated based on a combination of codes and other specific information for inpatient visits. Both clinical and financial users are interested in a multitude of reports based on the DRG number. This combination of clinical and financial resources helps to determine a facility's case mix, which is often used to describe the severity of cases being treated within an institution.

APC Number Data Field

The APC number is the outpatient counterpart of a DRG. Although a relatively new type of payment classification, the APC is as important during this century as the DRG at its inception in the early 1980s. Outpatient reimbursement will be increasingly tied to APCs. Thus, users throughout a facility will seek to create reports describing outpatient service activities based on the APC number.

CPT Code Data Field

Like ICD-9-CM codes, CPT codes are used throughout a facility to create reports that depict the services provided and the resources expended to provide them. Coders generally assign surgical CPT codes, although some nonsurgical codes are assigned through the item charge process.

Other Data Fields

Other, less-standard data fields are defined by users throughout a facility as fields that must be abstracted for a variety of purposes. For example, nursing administration representatives might ask to have a field collected to indicate whether restraints were used on a patient. This information then could be used to find cases to study for agencies such as the Joint Commission on Accreditation of Healthcare Organizations (JCAHO) that are interested in determining whether the application and maintenance of restraints are appropriate.

Role of the Coder in Abstracting

In many facilities, coders are responsible for abstracting required data elements. Some controversy exists in the health information field as to whether this is an efficient use of coder time. Some argue that staff other than coders can be used to find and extract data elements. Others argue that because coders have to read the record in its entirety to assign appropriate codes, it is more efficient for them to abstract the data elements as they encounter them in the record review process.

Admission Coding versus Discharge Coding

In certain facilities, codes are applied prior to, or at the time of, admission to the facility. This is particularly true in long-term care and other types of facilities that obtain preapproval for the patient to stay in the facility for a prescribed length of time. The approved length of stay (LOS) is often determined based on the admission diagnosis code.

In some facilities, a coding professional determines the admission diagnoses codes; in others, admitting or utilization management personnel or case managers perform that task. In any case, a distinction is made to describe whether codes are admission codes or final codes. This distinction is important in the process of generating reports. Individuals who are building reports must be apprised of the difference between those code fields so that resulting reports are accurate and valid and clearly represent their intended uses.

Chargemaster Description Codes

Yet another distinction is necessary to ensure that all relevant codes are collected and available in the reporting process. A coder traditionally assigns ICD-9-CM procedure and diagnostic codes after the patient has been discharged. However, some CPT codes, particularly those not associated with a surgical procedure, are not assigned by a coder but, rather, are applied to an account through the routine hospital charging mechanism.

When a CPT code is associated with a procedure 100 percent of the time, it is much more efficient to have it applied through the charge description master (CDM) file process rather than have it reviewed by a coder and applied during the coding process. A code applied through the CDM file is sometimes referred to as a **hard code.** Using a hard code eliminates the possibility of missing a code assignment through human error. In essence, every time the ancillary department providing the service enters a specific charge, the system applies the corresponding CPT code. The combination of codes—those applied by coders and those entered in the CDM entry process—results in the patient bill. (See chapter 6 for a detailed discussion of the charge description master.)

In this scenario, it is important that the report creator understand this process. The user may wish to create a report of all CPT codes of a particular type for a specific time frame. In most systems, the user queries a CPT code field to find this information. However, a hard code may not be identified in this manner because it is not usually stored in the same field as a CPT code assigned by a coder. Sometimes a combination of reports or reporting systems must be used to obtain the desired result. As long as the individual creating the report understands the limitations of the system being used and the flow of coding within the facility, a comprehensive report can usually be designed.

System Interrelationships

As described previously, multiple data sources are joined to create a single, complex record used in the process of assigning codes. The validity of data received from disparate systems must be assessed routinely to ensure that all required data reach the final destination in their appropriate form.

If some type of routine verification process is not used to compare data sent from feeder systems with those stored in the primary HIS, the risk of inaccurate reporting is great. When reports are analyzed, the source of the data is generally unknown, which again lends credence to the importance of data integration.

Traditionally, HISs have been strong in their ability to store and process financial information, but weak in their ability to link it to clinical information. Facilities have dealt with this situation by purchasing stand-alone or networked database systems that collect and store clinical data. Integration of the HIS and the database systems results in the ability to create reports based on any collected element. Users are generally trained in extracting required data to create a usable report. Many systems make use of **Structured Query Language (SQL)** or other report-writing programs to pull and integrate data from various sources into a single, comprehensive report.

Uses of Coded Data

Coded data are a valuable resource used extensively throughout the healthcare organization. Users from virtually all areas of healthcare operations have an interest in coded data. Additionally, there are numerous external demands for coded and associated data elements.

Clinical versus Financial Uses

Some users' needs of coded data are clinical in nature; other users' needs are financial or administrative in nature. Regardless what the need is, individual codes or codes grouped into a DRG, APC, or other grouping category are the basic element used to provide the information needed.

This wide variety of grouping methods adds another level of complexity to the collection and analysis of information. Users comparing reports must understand the grouping system used in each report and base their conclusions on a comparison of like information. From the housekeeping department that analyzes codes on the spread of infectious disease to the hospital administration that plans for expansion of services, diagnostic and procedure codes are the underlying mechanism enabling appropriate case selection and analysis.

Frequency of Use

Daily users of coded data, such as the patient financial services (patient accounts) department, integrate the coded data with other patient-specific financial data such as insurance information to create a single, comprehensive bill of services provided. Other departments, such as the risk management department, need to assess coded data on a less-frequent basis. Nevertheless, in some way or another, all areas within a facility need information arising from coded data.

Use for Given Time Periods

Aggregated coded data succinctly identify the number of cases of each condition within the facility within a given time period. This factor alone is invaluable in scheduling staff resources. For example, a high frequency of cases of congestive heart failure is a cue to nursing administration on how to staff the cardiology unit. Knowledge of the frequency trend of a specific type of case over a significant time period can clarify when to expand certain nursing units or, conversely, when to reduce staff in certain areas. Because coded data are coupled with patient-specific LOS data, even more inferences can be made on how to staff within individual care units.

Use in Decision Making

Both long- and short-term decision making are based on coded data. Reports designed to present coded data are used to support the decision-making process. However, codes alone do not allow for appropriate analysis and management of information. Rather, it is the ability to select codes in conjunction with other significant clinical and financial data that results in reports that support user needs.

Users of Coded Data

Various user areas and departments within a typical acute care facility rely heavily on coded data to perform their functions. Indeed, the success of those departments is closely linked to appropriate analysis of reports depicting ICD-9-CM and CPT codes, as well as DRGs, APCs, and other code groupings.

Cost and Reimbursement Department

The cost and reimbursement department, also sometimes referred to as the cost accounting department, has the daunting task of correlating cost to charges and charges to reimbursement. It is responsible for budgeting, cost reporting, and, in many cases, cost accounting. Under the auspices of the finance division, the cost and reimbursement department is typically separate from the general accounting area, which is responsible for internal accounting practices such as payroll and the preparation of income statements and balance statements.

The integration of clinical and financial information is nowhere more important than in the cost and reimbursement department. Individuals with a strong background in finance are generally found in a hospital's cost and reimbursement department. In some facilities, individuals with an HIM background also are an invaluable component of this department. The department is often responsible for the charge description file that is closely related to the coding function within a facility. For this reason, HIM professionals are often involved with chargemaster development and maintenance.

Definitions of Cost, Charges, and Reimbursement

To understand how the cost and reimbursement department uses coded data, it is important to first define the terms *cost, charges,* and *reimbursement.* A detailed analysis of these elements is extremely important to the healthcare organization's financial well-being.

Cost

Cost is the dollar amount of a service provided by a facility. The term is closely associated with the accounting method called cost accounting. This accounting method attributes a dollar figure to every input required to provide a service. For example, a patient who receives chemotherapy treatment for a brain tumor will have direct costs, such as medication, and indirect costs, such as the electricity required to heat or cool the patient's room during the hospital stay. These direct and indirect costs are combined to arrive at the total cost per treatment. The total of all the treatments and procedures received by a single patient then can be grouped to arrive at a total cost per case. The CDM file links cost file information and code description.

Charges

Charges are the amount the facility actually bills for the services it provides. The actual charge for a service may be $3,500, but only $2,000 may be paid as a result of contractual allowances agreed on with managed care companies and other insurers. A **contractual allowance** is the difference between what is charged and what is paid. It is commonly known that self-pay patients are usually the only patient type that pays full price for services. Individuals do not have the same market power to negotiate reductions in bills that managed care companies representing millions of patients have. However, healthcare consumer groups are now advocating for more standardized payment arrangements for self-pay patients. When coupled with stronger federal requirements for charity care programs, current self-pay practices are changing.

Reimbursement

Reimbursement is the amount collected by the facility for the services it bills. Even though $1 million may be billed for a given period, some of this money will never be collected. Rather, it will be written off as charity care or as income that cannot be collected because of a variety of other circumstances.

Another concept to be considered is that of volume to reimbursement. Healthcare finance specialists attempt to build the volume of cases that increase reimbursement, while at the same time try to reduce the volume of reimbursement-losing services. Marketing programs designed to increase consumer awareness of high-income service generators are based on volume-to-reimbursement analyses.

Although high-activity levels are generally sought after, some services are known as "losers." That is, some services are not only unprofitable, but also actually cost the hospital to provide them. Nevertheless, community needs sometime dictate that those services be provided.

DRG Payment System

Prior to implementation of the DRG payment system, comparison of individual cases within a facility based on cost and resources used was difficult. The DRG system created the ability to integrate clinical and financial data. As a result, facilities now can compare costs across the healthcare spectrum.

Although the DRG system has been discredited for causing the financial demise of many a healthcare facility, DRGs actually provide an opportunity for healthcare facilities to more accurately predict their reimbursement for services provided. Even more important, the DRG payment system allows facilities to analyze their own efficiency. Patients now can be classified based on resource consumption. Although it might be obvious that a labor and delivery case is less resource-intensive than a cardiac catheterization case, it is not so easy to make comparisons among more similar types of services. For example, facilities now can analyze resource consumption among three or more different types of cardiac catheterizations, as shown in figure 10.1.

The ability to assess data by ICD-9-CM and CPT/HCPCS code numbers and by DRG, APC, and other groups enables facilities to participate in benchmarking. This allows across-the-board comparison among disparate facilities and even among providers and physicians within the same organization.

Case-Mix Reports

Case mix can be referenced to quickly assess the types and severity of cases treated within a facility. **Case mix** is a description of a patient population based on any number of specific characteristics, including age, gender, type of insurance, diagnosis, risk factors, treatment received, and resources used. Ideally, case-mix reports would include both cost- and revenue-based information. However, this is not always the case. Sophisticated cost-accounting systems have been developed and are providing increasingly popular methodologies for ensuring that case-mix reports include both cost and revenue details.

The case-mix index (CMI) is used to report the resources used in the patient care process. The CMI is often calculated based on DRGs and represents the average DRG weight of patients discharged from the hospital. The CMI is calculated by first multiplying the number of cases for each DRG by the relative weight of the DRG. Next, the sum of that calculation is divided by the total number of cases (LaTour and Eichenwald, 414). For example, if in a specific month, a facility reported 55 cases of DRG 143 (Chest Pain) with a relative weight of 0.5659, 10 cases of DRG 243 (Medical Back Problems) with a relative weight of 0.7658, and

Figure 10.1. Cardiac catheterization comparison report

Source: Anyplace Health Systems
Comparison of All Cardiac Surgeons—Inpatients
Quarter 1, Fiscal Year 06

DRG 104   CARDIAC VALVE PROCEDURES AND OTHER MAJOR CARDIOTHORACIC PROCEDURES WITH CARDIAC CATH

DR. ID #	# of Pts.	ALOS	Case-Mix Index	Estimated Net Revenue	Total Costs	Net Income (Loss)	Net Income % Gross Revenue
12554	3	14.0	7.1843	174,945	168,541	6,404	2.0
25874	5	19.8	7.1843	274,468	235,120	39,348	8.7
32682	3	2.7	7.1843	89,265	84,337	4,928	4.7
TOTAL	11	13.6	7.1843	538,678	487,998	50,680	

DRG 105   CARDIAC VALVE PROCEDURES AND OTHER MAJOR CARDIOTHORACIC PROCEDURES WITHOUT CARDIAC CATH

DR. ID #	# of Pts.	ALOS	Case-Mix Index	Estimated Net Revenue	Total Costs	Net Income (Loss)	Net Income % Gross Revenue
25874	10	10.6	5.6567	359,286	371,001	(11,715)	(1.7)
36589	1	8.0	5.6567	23,277	31,030	(7,753)	(14.0)
66482	2	12.0	5.6567	50,923	78,915	(27,992)	(19.0)
TOTAL	13	10.6	5.6567	433,486	480,946	(47,460)	

DRG 107   CORONARY BYPASS WITH CARDIAC CATH

DR. ID #	# of Pts.	ALOS	Case-Mix Index	Estimated Net Revenue	Total Costs	Net Income (Loss)	Net Income % Gross Revenue
25874	1	5.0	5.3762	22,467	19,124	3,343	7.9
36589	5	9.2	5.3762	122,525	124,070	(1,545)	(0.6)
66482	2	9.5	5.3762	64,599	52,492	12,107	11.5
TOTAL	8	8.8	5.3762	209,591	195,686	13,905	

3 cases of DRG 475 (Respiratory System Diagnosis w/Ventilator Support) at a relative weight of 3.6091, the CMI calculation would be:

Step 1: Multiply number of cases of each DRG by relative weight of each DRG

$$\# \text{ cases} \times \text{relative weight}$$
$$55 \times 0.5659 = 31.1245$$
$$10 \times 0.7658 = 7.658$$
$$3 \times 3.6091 = 10.8273$$

Step 2: Sum the relative weights from step 1

$$31.1245 + 7.658 + 10.8273 = 49.6098$$

Step 3: Sum of step 3 divided by total number of cases

$$49.6098/68 \text{ (total of cases)} = 0.7296 \text{ (rounded up from fifth decimal)}$$

The CMI can be used to indicate the average reimbursement for the facility (LaTour and Eichenwald). A cursory evaluation of a CMI report provides the reader with a general sense of how many resources are expended in the care process as well as the anticipated revenue based on the service provision.

Case mix is the broad category name for a variety of reports. The CMI is just one part of this category of reports. Some of the data elements included in a standard charge-to-reimbursement case-mix report are patient account number, patient name, assigned DRG, actual LOS, charges, predicted reimbursement, and variance (the difference between charges and reimbursement).

Case-mix reports can be run and sorted in a variety of ways. Most of them include the assigned DRG, principal diagnoses, principal procedure, charge per case, reimbursement per case, and physician information. For example, one type of case mix report might show the total number of DRGs sorted by DRG or major diagnostic category (MDC).

The significance of case mix within a healthcare facility is shown by the following example:

For a facility with a CMI of 1.47, an increase to an index of 1.62 would result in an average increase in reimbursement of about $600 per DRG-paid case. This increase would depend on the wage index and other factors influencing case-mix calculations. Personnel responsible for analyzing case-mix reports can predict the potential increase in reimbursement by finding the average number of DRG-paid cases within a given time period and multiplying it by $600 per case. Depending on the level of activity, this could result in a multimillion-dollar increase in revenue each year.

Physician Data

In addition to needing DRG information to compare payments received with bills submitted, the cost and reimbursement department also requires associated physician data. The following scenario clearly depicts the importance of assessment by physician:

Dr. Mitchellson (physician I.D. number 4769) is a nephrologist specializing in progressive kidney disease. At 65 years of age, he is the hospital's number one revenue-producing physician. An analysis of the physician data report also reveals that no other physicians are waiting in the wings to treat the kind of patients that Dr. Mitchellson does. The cost and reimbursement staff analyzing this type of data should recommend to administration the need to recruit a physician with a skill set similar to Dr. Mitchellson's to ensure the continuation of that revenue source when Dr. Mitchellson retires.

Decision Making and Case-Mix Reports

Major decisions are based on information found in a facility's case-mix reports. With limited funds, most institutions make decisions on whether to purchase major capital equipment or to curtail spending only after a thoughtful review of their case-mix reports. Generally, the cost and reimbursement staff summarizes information in the case-mix reports and forwards it to the administration and the board of directors. The administration and the board of directors then consider that information in determining how the facility will spend its limited resources.

In addition to the variety of daily and monthly case-mix reports produced for and used by the cost and reimbursement department, innumerable on-demand reports can be created either by the users or at their request to meet a specific—and often transient—need. For example, a facility that wishes to participate in a government-sponsored demonstration project must perform a full assessment of all the relevant information related to the DRGs falling within the project's scope. Although projects of this nature, such as Centers of Excellence programs, lend prestige to the selected organization by identifying it as a high-quality care provider at government-approved pricing, the project's financial cost may not be acceptable.

By evaluating on-demand case-mix reports, the facility can determine whether existing inefficiencies can be reduced to compensate for reduced payment from Medicare program recipients. If the analysis reveals that the facility is already operating as efficiently as it can, the facility can decide to reject or accept demonstration project status based on comparing expected financial losses with the expected benefits of participating in the program.

Knowing the magnitude of the decisions that are based on analysis of DRG and other code-based reports makes the issues related to the quality of coded data readily apparent. In addition to selecting and sequencing appropriate codes, associated quality issues must be addressed. Codes are entered into a system either manually or by automated methods. Manually entered codes are at risk of being miskeyed and subsequently misgrouped. Quality assessment (QA) programs should be in place to routinely compare keyed codes to the source document from which they were entered. Moreover, the routine use of more sophisticated QA mechanisms to validate code assignment and sequencing must be in place to ensure the appropriate collection and reporting of coded data.

Patient Financial Services Departments

The most obvious uses of code-based reports are those that detail the relationship of coded data to the billing process. Entire functional groups within the patient financial services (PFS) department are devoted to ensuring that bills are produced in a timely fashion. However, because the production of a bill largely depends on the presence of a coded final diagnosis, routine reports are required to track the status of accounts that have not been billed.

Accounts Not Selected for Billing

The accounts not selected for billing report is a daily report used to track the many reasons that accounts may not be ready for billing, as shown in figure 10.2. This report is also called the **discharged not final billed (DNFB)** report. (See figure 11.3 for an alternate format of a DNFB report.) Some billing takes place electronically; other bills are created and submitted in paper

Figure 10.2. Accounts not selected for billing (or discharged not final billed [DNFB] report)

Issue Date: 5/1/06
Issue Time: 0600

Source: Anyplace Health Systems
Accounts Not Selected for Billing—Inpatients
Patient Financial Services Version

Patient Name	Acct. #	Med Rec #	Status	Unbilled Charges	Days Since Disch.	Pt. Type	Insurance Verification			Final Dx	DRG	Open Orders	Fin. Class
							Ins. 1	Ins. 2	Ins. 3				
Axxxxxx, Rxxx	1452585	124785	Discharged	18,139.45	13	E-Inpt	Yes	Yes	Yes	No	000	No	J
Bxxxx, Vxxxx	4568972	258564	Discharged	1,173.75	26	Inpt	No	No	No	Yes	466	No	T
Cxxxx, Axxxx	7456594	256632	Discharged	10,286.70	5	E-Inpt	Yes	Yes	Yes	Yes	277	Yes	Q
Fxxxx, Txxxxx	7458961	148965	Discharged	3,425.45	15	Inpt	No	Yes	Yes	No	000	Yes	F
Plxxxxx, Gxxxxx	8585964	745321	Discharged	15,452.25	8	Inpt	Yes	Yes	Yes	Yes	321	Yes	J
Sxxxxxxx, Cxxxx	8569741	154428	Inpt-In-house	52,846.25	0	E-Inpt	No	No	No	No	000	Yes	T
Zxxx, Mxxxxxxx	7458946	147589	Discharged	25,584.55	20	E-Inpt	Yes	Yes	Yes	No	000	No	B

Totals

		Unbilled Charges	Reason for Rejection				
I/P Discharged	6	74,062.15	Insurance Not Verified	4	No Final Dx	4	4
I/P In-House	1	52,846.25	Open Orders	4	Invalid DRG	0	0

Issue Date: 5/1/06
Issue Time: 0600

Anyplace Health Systems
Accounts Not Selected for Billing—Outpatients
Patient Financial Services Version

Patient Name	Acct. #	Med Rec #	Status	Unbilled Charges	Days Since Disch.	Pt. Type	Insurance Verification			Final Dx	DRG	Open Orders	Fin. Class
							Ins. 1	Ins. 2	Ins. 3				
Cxxxx, Jxxx	5869751	586462	O/P—Recur.	1,377.50	34	Recur.	No	Yes	Yes	Yes	131	No	T
Dxxx, Axxx	7469832	154783	O/P—Surg	10,850.40	16	Surgical	Yes	Yes	Yes	Yes	479	Yes	L
Gxxx, Dxxxxx	7459831	852697	O/P	12,587.75	4	Out	Yes	Yes	Yes	No	000	No	Q

Totals

		Unbilled Charges	Reason for Rejection				
Recurrent Outpatients	1	1,377.50	Insurance Not Verified	1	No Final Dx	1	2
Outpatient Surgical	1	10,850.40	Open Orders	1	Invalid DRG	1	0
Outpatient General	1	12,587.75					

format. In either case, accounts that have not met all facility-specified criteria for billing are held and reported on this daily tracking list.

Some accounts are held because the patient has not signed the consents and authorizations required by the insurer. Others are held because a specific insurer may require a CPT code that has not been assigned. Still others are not billed because the primary and secondary insurance benefits have not been confirmed.

One of the major delays in billing accounts is the lack of final diagnosis and procedure codes. The reasons for that type of delay are varied. In some cases, a physician has not documented the diagnosis. In other cases, test results required to support the written diagnosis may not yet be on the record.

Purposes of the Accounts Not Selected for Billing Report

The purposes of the Accounts Not Selected for Billing Report are to:

- Monitor the total dollars not yet billed

- Monitor the age of accounts not yet billed

- Attribute the delay to one or more circumstances

- Provide a mechanism for users to prioritize their resources for getting accounts billed

Both the HIM and PFS departments receive daily copies of this report. However, the report may be modified to show various types of information based on each department's needs.

For example, the HIM department may be interested in accounts not billed based on the responsible physician number. In that way, the department can strategize how to elicit cooperation from a physician who is not providing sufficient documentation for coding. In another example, the HIM department may wish to sort the list by health record location so that a needed record can be found quickly and supplied for completion. The PFS department, on the other hand, may be more interested in knowing which accounts are being held because the appropriate payment authorization forms are not yet available. Both departments, however, keep close track of the highest-dollar cases and the oldest cases because billing those accounts is their highest priority.

Matching Payments to Billed Amounts

In addition to simply billing the account, ICD-9-CM coding–based reports are required to match payments to billed amounts. An account is often billed at a specific amount, but the payment received and accepted by the facility is less than the billed amount. This situation arises because agreements have been made with managed care companies and other insurers to pay certain DRGs at a lower rate.

For example, a facility may have a contract with a managed care company to carve out DRG 104 for payment at a rate of 60 percent to charges. A **carve-out** occurs when a payer cuts the applicable service from the contract and pays it at a different rate. Instead of receiving the full, expected payment, the facility receives only 60 percent of the amount it charged. The carve-out process is commonplace and is used as a mechanism to control costs for the managed care company. The facility agrees to the carve-outs to increase the volume of patients it treats. Thus, even though the facility receives less money per case, it receives more money in total.

Reports designed to show payments by case and payer include fields for charges compared with payments. An analysis of those reports over time can reveal whether carve-outs are effective in meeting the facility's financial goals.

The fact that so many insurers exist, each with its own rules for billing, makes for numerous complications in the prebill process. Some insurers require CPT codes for certain nonsurgical procedures and others do not. To complicate matters further, insurers do not always communicate their billing requirements before receiving the bill, which results in a duplication of work and in delays in receipt of payment for services provided. Tracking such occurrences and entering them in a database can generate reports that identify trends in information requested by payers after the fact. Once reported, process or system interventions can be put in place on the front end of the process to ensure that the required elements are coded before a bill is generated.

Nonstandard Reasons for Bill Holds

Reports also can facilitate communication between departments. Not every issue that causes a bill to be held is included on the daily Accounts Not Selected for Billing Report. Those issues that occur less frequently are generally more difficult to manage. Their infrequency means that no procedure is in place for reaching an efficient resolution to a problem. Some facilities have created automated programs to deal with those types of issues.

Examples of situations that could require extensive communication on a less-than-routine basis might include:

- The need to assign specific accounts to an APC group instead of a DRG

- The need to code a preventative treatment using an ICD-9-CM procedure code. For example, a code might be needed to report a Vitamin B injection as this is not a routine procedure.

- The need for a nonstandard E/M code to be applied to a specific account based on individual agreements with insurers

In such instances, the PFS and HIM staffs enter system-generated standard notes, or customized notes, into a specific account file with directions for what must occur to process the bill. The note stays with the account until it is billed, thus providing an efficient account management process. Each department then can generate reports grouping all accounts-pending billing based on a specific note type. This permits processing en masse, which is more efficient than resolving situations on a case-by-case basis.

Rebilling Process

The HIS usually generates the bill, and the data from the HIS are often passed on to other systems for future reporting of integrated clinical and financial information. At times, certain accounts are manipulated or revised after the bill has been produced. The process of rebilling is an important concept that relies heavily on reports of coding revisions. The timing of data transfer from one system to another is essential for accuracy in reporting.

Report Validation

Medicare program requirements include provisions for self-auditing of billed accounts. In some cases, Medicare outlines the specific CPT codes to be audited. At times, the CPT code might be applied through the CDM charge process. In many facilities, the CDM codes are not stored in the abstract file of the HIS but, rather, are printed directly on the UB-92/UB-04 claim form. In such cases, pulling together a full listing of accounts to be audited becomes difficult.

Moreover, reporting in these situations becomes difficult, and the need to validate the report contents becomes critically important. Whenever data are drawn from multiple, disparate sources, the results must be reviewed to ensure that the report creator selected the appropriate data elements to appear on the report. Moreover, even if the correct elements were selected, the results must be further validated to ensure that technical issues did not result in report discrepancies.

Rigorous testing of system interfaces and data exchange protocols is essential to ensure that valid data are being reported. First-time reports must be reviewed thoroughly to confirm data validity. After a critical assessment of the report has been performed, the report can be considered reliable. However, subsequent random reviews of reports for the purpose of ensuring data validity must be performed, particularly after any system change that might affect the report's results.

Quality Management Departments

The quality management (QM) department interprets a variety of code-based reports. Issues of current significance being reviewed by JCAHO include rates of cesarean sections and of vaginal deliveries after cesarean sections within a facility. Both of these statistics are inferred from ICD-9-CM procedure codes. Reports designed to clarify the frequency of those procedures help the QM department prepare summarized data for JCAHO review purposes.

Another area of concern is patient LOS by diagnosis. QM data analysts review LOS reports to determine whether physicians are deviating from the mean LOS. After a deviation is noted, the department implements performance improvement initiatives to bring outliers within an acceptable standard deviation for the specific LOS indicator. This type of information also is used in the physician reappointment process as a reflection of how physicians compare with their peers or with a national standard.

Code Validation

In many facilities, the QM department staff acts as a secondary level to ensure coding accuracy within the facility. Although it may be an inefficient use of resources to have the QM department staff validate every code assigned by the HIM department staff, random validation can be considered a judicious use of staff time.

By identifying trends in code assignment errors, the QM department can focus on areas of concern. Code validation becomes particularly important when physician discipline is based on deviation from acceptable care standards, as identified by diagnosis and procedure codes combined with other clinical details.

Work Lists

Facilities with electronic patient record systems can use codes to create work lists for secondary users in departments such as QM. Rather than retrieving paper records to review the assigned codes, the records to be reviewed can be retrieved based on the assigned codes. This is a subtle difference, but one that makes for an efficient use of staff resources.

Source Documents

Reports alone do not always provide enough detail to support QM practices. Sometimes the QM staff must review the actual source documents to fully evaluate the indicator being assessed. For example, a facility wishing to determine its risk-adjusted mortality rate would have to review each mortality case to ascertain comorbid conditions because these types of conditions are not generally detailed in standard mortality reports.

Ancillary Departments

Various ancillary departments use coded data for different reasons. Generally, ancillary users of coded data are interested in CPT codes to assess the volume of procedures provided in their area. For example, the clinical laboratory management staff might be interested in assessing the frequency with which glycohemoglobin tests are performed. Patients with diabetes should have at least one glycohemoglobin test each quarter. By determining the volume of this type of test and by performing a correlated assessment of ordering practices of physicians for this type of test, a laboratory can prepare a marketing plan to ensure that diabetic patients and their physicians are aware of the standard recommended protocol for the assessment and treatment of diabetes.

CPT code assessment also lends itself particularly well to comparisons across the healthcare spectrum. Laboratory test profiles can vary from facility to facility, but because a CPT code is applied to each test, a national standard of comparison becomes available. This enables users to compare provisions of like services, regardless of the ordered laboratory test profile. Using an external database such as that of the College of American Pathologists allows laboratories to compare their staffing efficiency against other laboratories, as well as across shifts within their own facility.

With continued movement toward case management, further extrapolation of code-based data can be expected. For example, laboratories might want to evaluate coded data from all hospital-affiliated sources. This might include home healthcare and facility-managed physician offices. In that way, clinical laboratories could ensure that appropriate disease management and clinical pathway methodologies are being followed. (Radiology, diagnostic, and other ancillary departments use reports that detail CPT codes for reasons similar to those for clinical laboratories.)

Managed Care Departments

Summarized reports of ICD-9-CM codes are valuable in determining the scope of managed care contracts. Analyzing codes as an isolated data element is rarely useful. However, when assessed with other data elements using demographic assessment software, trends can be identified and programs developed to meet a specific population's needs. For example, certain areas of the country are at a higher risk than others for cardiovascular diseases. Cancer rates are higher in highly industrialized areas where air pollution is more common than in less-industrialized areas. Analysis of ICD-9-CM codes can help to identify these types of trends.

Strategically, facilities should provide the product lines most needed by the community they serve. For example, a facility located in a community with an aging population should provide an appropriate level of geriatric services. In that type of situation, the managed care program manager would assess coded data to identify conditions associated with the aging process. Then the manager would recommend development of product lines such as adult exercise and rehabilitative services. Employers who represent the community's patient population contract with facilities that are strategically committed to providing needed services.

A variety of code-based reports, such as the Net Income by Product Line (figure 10.3), Physician Profile, and Managed Care Summary, are used to assess business efficiencies and contract success. Managed care departments generally receive coding data through system collection processes. They further manipulate those data by using spreadsheet programs to develop scenarios that compare best practices in managed care with the practices within their specific facility.

Medical Staff Departments

The medical staff department requires access to information for a variety of reasons. Reports required by physicians often include demographic information about patients that falls into the realm of protected health information as outlined in the HIPAA privacy rule. The HIPAA regulations support physician access to their own patient data for purposes related to treatment, payment, or healthcare operations. Other uses of data (for example, publication of physician-based research) do require specific authorization from the patient or, in some cases, from the institutional review board (IRB) within the organization. The HIM practitioner's role in providing the requested reports requires a clear understanding of why the data are needed and how they ultimately will be used.

Certification Reports

Physicians seeking to become board certified in their area of medical expertise must provide evidence of the number of cases and the outcome of each case of the specified type in which they participated. Cases identified on reports of this type are found by using case-finding programs. Such programs search abstracted or indexed fields to find cases that match the entered selection criteria.

Many physicians request reports that identify all their cases for a specific time period; others request only specific cases based on a particular ICD-9-CM diagnosis or procedure code, CPT code, or DRG. Those reports then are compared to the codes submitted by the physicians' office billing staff to ensure that appropriate coding practices are taking place in their office.

Physician Reappointment Summaries

The medical staff department is particularly interested in the ICD-9-CM codes associated with each physician. Because diagnostic codes can identify untoward events that occur during hospitalization, the quality of a physician's services can be identified through reports called physician reappointment summaries. These summaries outline the number of cases by diagnosis and procedure type, LOS, and infection and mortality statistics.

At initial credential confirmation (generally referred to as credentialing), initial appointment, and reappointment to a facility's medical staff, code-based reports are required. These reappointment reports identify all cases and procedures in which a specific physician was involved as an attending physician, a consultant, a surgeon, or a surgical assistant.

Reappointment reports are available by specific code number or by narrative description of a code. When such reports are combined with information regarding the physician's previous utilization of hospital facilities, quality improvement actions, and insurance claims, the full picture of a physician's history becomes clearer. The medical staff department accumulates these reports and works with the elected or appointed medical staff leadership to ensure that a thorough analysis of each physician's activities takes place before he or she is reappointed to the staff.

Figure 10.3. Net income by product line of four selected product lines

Anyplace Health Systems
Net Income by Product Line—Inpatients and Outpatients
Quarter 1, Fiscal Year 2006

Product Code (MDC)	Description	# of Patients	ALOS	Case-Mix Index	Total Charges	Deductions	Est. Net Revenue	Variable Costs	Contribution Margin	Cont. Margin %	Fixed Costs	Net Income	Net Income %
001	Cardiac Cath	302	1.1	1.2043	2,070,907	880,809	1,190,098	653,758	536,341	25.9	348,569	187,771	9.1
005	Cardiology	938	3.4	1.1516	8,309,282	3,778,766	4,530,515	3,426,684	1,103,831	13.3	1,545,018	−441,186	−5.3
055	Neonatology	158	8.4	1.9519	2,320,429	568,621	1,751,808	835,249	916,559	39.5	276,314	640,245	27.6
160	OP and ER	26,286	.0	.0000	16,679,820	6,087,147	10,592,673	3,834,331	6,758,342	40.5	2,791,237	3,967,105	23.8

Preceptor Programs

Preceptor programs also make use of code-based reports. In many organizations, when new physicians join the staff, they are appointed a preceptor. A preceptor is an experienced physician responsible for ensuring that the new physician has appropriate on-the-job experience to perform certain types of medical procedures. As part of the preceptor program, the experienced physician must work alongside the new staff member in surgery. When surgical procedures are abstracted, the new physician is credited with performing the procedure, but the experienced physician's number also is abstracted. When a preceptor relationship terminates, reports are generated by a specific ICD-9-CM procedure code to summarize the new physician's activity level.

Reports for Method of Approach

When a surgical innovation is first used in an organization, a procedure code may not always be available. For example, when laparoscopic tools first became widely used, the surgery could be coded, but there was no way to specify that it was a laparoscopic method of entry or approach. This detail was important because many studies were necessary to both ensure that postsurgical complications did not increase because of the new method of approach and give credit to physicians experienced in performing these "new" procedure types. To report on these details, some facilities chose to create a special modifier code. This special code was used with the procedure code number to identify the method of approach.

Corporate Compliance Departments

The corporate compliance department ensures that fraudulent coding and billing practices are not being performed within an organization.

Auditing Programs

The corporate compliance department uses record-auditing programs to review both source documents and summarized code-based reports. The record-auditing programs also identify trends in the frequency of high-profit tests and procedures that are coded and billed.

Coding audits can be performed by hospital-based staff or by agencies with which organizations contract for review. In either case, an objective review of the assigned codes is necessary to minimize the risk of civil and criminal penalties for inappropriate code assignment.

The MedPar Database

Each bill submitted to Medicare is tracked in the **MedPar database system.** All of the fiscal intermediaries in the country submit their information, including charges, DRG, and payment information, to this same database. The Office of Inspector General (OIG) analyzes this database to identify suspicious billing and charge practices. Medicare fraud and abuse investigations continue to increase as the efficiency of analyzing Medicare's MedPar file increases.

Hospitals typically do not have the resources to assess the information found in the MedPar file. However, for-profit reporting agencies have found them to be an area in which they can provide a useful service to healthcare facilities. These agencies have developed tools to create reports based on the MedPar file information. They then sell the reports to healthcare facilities that use them to compare their billing and charge practices with those of neighboring facilities.

Nursing and Infection Control Departments

Nursing services and infection control department staff members review code-based reports to identify specific patient records that must be evaluated for a variety of reasons. Quality improvement programs are developed and implemented based on cases that are identified through the process of electronically searching the record-abstracting software program.

Automated Case-Finding Programs

An automated case-finding program is an efficient way to locate specific records that meet selection criteria. The case-finding program should perform a search of the database based on the following elements:

- A specific time period

- A single patient visit type or a group of patient visit types

- A single or combined group of physician identification numbers

- ICD-9-CM diagnosis and procedure codes separated by principal and secondary code assignment levels and CPT codes

Additionally, user-defined fields should be eligible for use in case selection. For example, nursing staff might be interested in finding specific cases in which restraints were used. Infection control staff might want to identify cases with an elevated postoperative temperature. The output of those abstract searches can be either a screen display or a printed report.

Paper-Based Records

If a paper-based record system is being used, the health record's location also should appear on the report or the screen so that the HIM staff can more efficiently locate records to be pulled for study. Such reports are typically user generated and created on an ad hoc basis. Predesigned routine reports, on the other hand, can be prepared and run daily, monthly, or quarterly to track frequently requested health record review criteria.

The Reporting Process

In the early days of HIM, users requiring information on health records had nowhere to go but the HIM department. With the advances made in automated systems, this is no longer the case. Individual user departments now use departmental information systems to report on data elements stored within their own systems. However, it still is generally the function of the HIM department to assist users in creating reports based on an analysis of all types of information.

Security and Confidentiality Issues

Security access to report development programs should be limited. Such limited access ensures that only authorized users can create or receive reports based on protected health information. Therefore, departmental users generally have access to data only from their own departments' system. If users need integrated information detailing not only their department's input, but also other parts of the record, they must request such reports through the HIM department. In its role as guardian of patient information, the HIM department tracks requests for information and ensures that a legitimate need for access to it is present.

Frequency of Reports

Some ICD-9-CM code-based reports such as the Accounts Not Selected for Billing List are generated daily and often appear in the form of large, paper-based reports. Other reports such as case-mix and physician-profile reports are run on demand, or as needed, by the user or the HIM department representative. Still other reports are created through the use of ad hoc reporting programs that allow users to customize reports based on any collected data element.

Report information can be requested through many automated systems that produce the output and store it in a "queue." The output queue then can be downloaded onto stand-alone or networked personal computer (PC) programs. The PC user can format the data in the desired fashion.

Verification of Report Data

Verification of report data is essential. Random checks of the selected data must be performed. Ensurance of data validity requires that selected data be compared with the source documents and that all system integration elements be functional.

External Reporting

In addition to the many users and uses of system-based reports within healthcare facilities, numerous external entities receive data for a variety of reasons, including program approval, research, treatment, payment, quality improvement, benchmarking and other purposes.

For example, the Centers for Medicare and Medicaid Services (CMS) offer a variety of demonstration project opportunities to organizations that have sound data to support their participation in such projects. One such program is the Health Aging Initiative. This federal research project is intended to evaluate how a variety of factors influence the aging population. The three separate efforts in this initiative include:

- Assessment of the use of standing orders in influenza immunization programs

- Development of a smoking cessation program for seniors

- Implementation of a senior risk-reduction program to determine how personal choice in matters such as diet, exercise, and other health-related activities can positively influence senior health status

To participate in such initiatives, providers are required to report massive amounts of data related to each of the content areas described above. Although the data may be available within the patient record systems of many healthcare organizations, the challenge for most is to efficiently extract the required information in the report format outlined by CMS. Generally, provider organizations find these demonstration programs appealing because grants or other federal monies are available to assist in program development. In some cases, greater financial rewards accrue for providers who are identified by CMS as a Center of Excellence for a specific specialty area. Therefore, participation in these programs is often worth the added effort and expense to the organization, even though the data collection and extraction process can be grueling. This is one area in which the value of coded data becomes apparent. Searching the database for uncoded data is a cumbersome and unreliable process. However, with coded data, a report of cases can be easily identified and further analyzed for ultimate reporting to CMS or other interested entities.

CMS has also implemented a wide variety of quality initiatives that rely heavily on data reported by healthcare providers. In addition to the hospital quality initiative program, CMS evaluates data submitted by home health, end stage renal disease, physician, nursing home, dialysis, and ambulatory care facilities. Each of these provider settings is required to submit data for evaluation and comparison purposes. Although the quality evaluation is not entirely based on diagnostic and procedure codes, it is the combination of this coded information and other important data elements that allow CMS to assess the quality of services provided to Medicare recipients.

Another example of an external entity with an interest in specific content reports is The Leapfrog Group. This consortium is charged with the formidable task of improving patient safety. With numerous federal and private initiatives now underway to promote patient safety, The Leapfrog Group seeks to voluntarily collect data about medical errors and quality improvement processes that can reduce the number of preventable medical errors. Much of the data analyzed by this group stems from reports of coded diagnoses and procedures.

JCAHO, the National Association on Healthcare Quality, and the Healthcare Facilities Accreditation Program are just a few of the many other external agencies who demand timely and sophisticated data reports from healthcare providers.

No discussion of reporting from coded data can be considered complete without mentioning its importance to public health authorities. Public health reporting was the initial and primary function of medical classification and coding systems. For example, communicable disease reporting is generally required at the state level. When disease reports indicate an abnormal increase in a specific communicable disease, action is taken to understand the reason for the increase and to develop corresponding prevention and/or awareness programs. With the prevalence of the DRG payment system, the original purpose of coded data has become rather secondary in nature. Currently, however, through the use of coded data, federal and state health initiatives are developed and implemented for the good of the public. State-level cancer registries are a prime example of how coded data is used to monitor cancer incidence by geographic location. Other, specific statewide registries request coded data from hospitals and other providers to monitor and evaluate a wide variety of diseases and conditions. Ultimately, these data reported by hospitals and other provider settings serve as a key building block of public health policy. For this reason, the accuracy and validity of the reporting function, and the underlying coding process is of critical importance.

Conclusion

The massive amounts of data stored in automated systems create a plethora of information. However, unless reports are thoughtfully designed and distributed, the information may not be comprehensible. For that reason, users must develop the skills necessary to succinctly define the information they really need. The creators of reports must become equally skilled in developing reports to meet users' needs.

Formatting reports for readability and ease of use is an important step in presenting code-based data in an organized and useful manner. A report's length should guide its creator in determining the spacing, font size, and other advanced formatting options. The flexibility afforded by automated report-writing programs allows users to sort, group, and summarize information, as needed. Some reports require great detail; others provide summaries. Sometimes reports are printed in code-number or DRG-number order. At other times, they are sorted by code within a specific medical staff specialty and then grouped by physician number. Some data lend themselves well to summarizing features such as totaling, subtotaling, or counting.

As the information age continues to advance, new and more efficient reporting mechanisms will become available. However, the essential process of ensuring appropriate access to and use of code-based health information will become even more challenging. With each new system, another integration element will be required. With each new integration element, the need for data validation will become even more important. Finally, HIM practitioners will be evaluated on their ability to create a flexible and secure system that generates reports to meet the needs of every user.

Part III

Financial Implications

Chapter 11

The Revenue Cycle

Mia M. Isbell, CPC, CCS-P, ACS-EM

Over the years, most healthcare facilities' patient accounts departments were the "back-end," cleanup departments for everything to do with the submission of clean claims and the collection of revenue. For example, after a claim had been rejected because of incorrect information, the patient accounts staff corrected errors in insurance and demographic information collected during the registration process. The staff responsible for patient preregistration for elective services did not understand the concepts of referral numbers, prior authorizations, or insurance verification and coverage determination. No one informed the patient of his or her financial responsibilities before elective surgery, which meant that the recuperating patient received a bill he or she had never anticipated. Coding errors and inaccuracies were identified after the third-party payer had received the claim. Coding by health information management was often based on the availability of the information or the staff to do the work, with little understanding of the impact accounts receivable (A/R) or discharged not final billed (DNFB) amounts. Clinical departments had little idea of the impact of "late charges" or poor documentation on the collection of revenue; they thought their charges were actually reimbursed. The situation was characterized by delays in reimbursement, lost reimbursement, new programs that did not generate payment, and finger-pointing in all directions.

This chapter defines the organizational framework within which coders function. It introduces the revenue cycle management model and defines the key terms with which coders need to be familiar. Finally, the chapter examines the key players and their roles in the revenue cycle.

Revenue Cycle Management Model

The concept of the revenue cycle originated out of the healthcare facilities' need to structure services to meet the changing and challenging demands for reimbursement from third-party payers, compliance, patient and physician satisfaction, and demands for greater efficiencies to enhance revenue. The restructuring consisted of a realignment of departments as well as a new concept for how those departments interrelate. The emphasis is on best practices, the use of the most appropriate resources for the most appropriate functions, and performance metrics, all enveloped in the performance improvement model of "do it right the first time."

Figure 11.1 depicts the new revenue cycle management model. Many facilities have organized work groups of the managers of each of the departments in the revenue cycle. Departments normally involved include patient registration, utilization review, case management, HIM (coding), charge entry, A/R up to the chief financial officer (CFO). Discussions first focused on helping

Figure 11.1. Revenue cycle management model

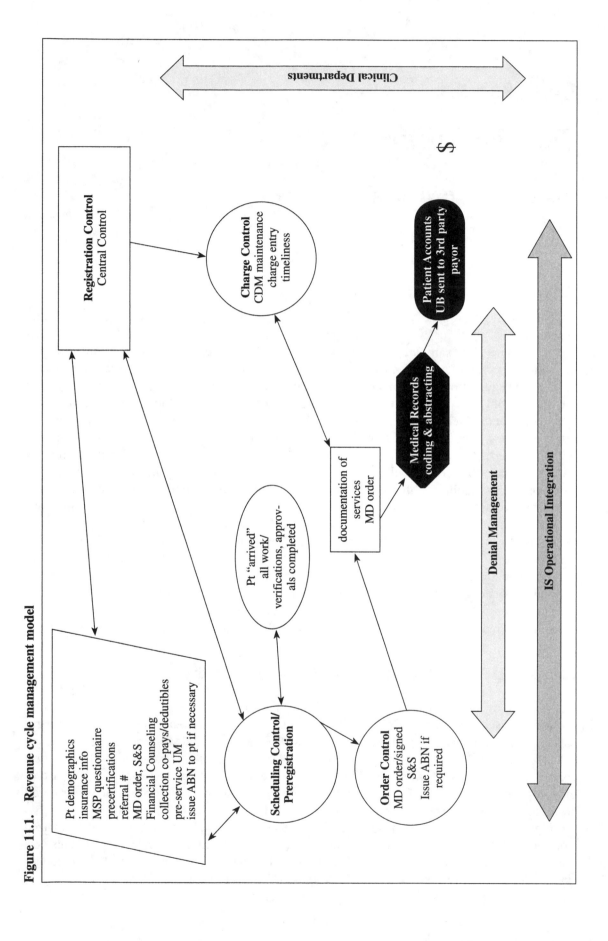

everyone understand the key concepts used by patient accounts. When everyone was able to "speak the same language," the building of a new culture began, followed by discussions of opportunities for improvements.

Key Concepts and Best Practices

The following sections provide definitions of basic concepts that are key to the revenue cycle. In many cases, the definitions are followed by the measures that are considered best practice for each.

Accounts Receivable

Accounts receivable (A/R) refers to the charges for patient services for which the healthcare facility is awaiting payment. In other words, the third-party payers and/or patients have received the claim, but the healthcare facility has not yet been paid. Patient accounts staff members speak of A/R but rarely use the words "accounts receivable," and it is important that HIM directors and coding managers speak the same language. The total A/R charges include: in-house patient charges, discharged unbilled patients, billed charges, and patient-responsible bills. Credit balances are reductions in the value of A/R because the facilities owe the patient or the insurers the credit balance. A/R is money owed to the facility.

AR is categorized by payer type (Medicare versus commercial insurers and other possible categories) and by actual payer source (for example, Blue Cross, Aetna, patient responsibility) to allow the production of reports based on these categories.

Days in A/R

The term **Days in A/R** refers to the total A/R (minus credit balances) divided by the average daily revenue for the accounting period (usually 1 month, 6 months or 1 year). The equation that expresses this is:

$$Days\ in\ A/R = \frac{Ending\ accounts\ receivable\ balance\ for\ the\ period}{Average\ revenue\ per\ day}$$

Example:
Ending A/R = \$200,000
Total A/R for the month of April = \$150,000
Days in April = 30

$$\frac{\$200,000}{\$5,000} = 40\ Days$$

This statistic measures approximately how many days it takes to collect any dollar placed into A/R. Best practice for days in A/R is less than 50 days but varies regionally and based on the types of services provided by the facility.

Credit Balances

Credit balances are the balances on an account that are to be refunded to an insurer or the patient. This occurs, for example, when a patient has paid a portion of the claim and that portion is later paid through another source, secondary insurance, or a state reimbursement program (for example, Free Care).

Dollars in A/R

The term **Dollars in A/R** refers to the total dollar amount of A/R, with or without credit balances. The Gross Dollars in A/R does not include the credit balances. Net Dollars in A/R uses the total amount of A/R minus the credit balances.

Aging of Accounts

The term aging of accounts refers to the aging of the A/R after the claim has been dropped for billing. The aging "buckets," as they are often called, are usually in 30-day increments and broaden as the age of the account gets older: 0–30, 31–60, 61–90, 91–180, 181–360, 360+. The best practice is no more than 15 to 20 percent of final billed A/R greater than 90 days. (Figure 11.2 shows an example of an account aging report.)

Cash versus Revenue

Revenue and charges are synonymous. All charges that are created on a patient's account become the A/R for the account. The term **cash versus revenue** refers to the ratio of charges (revenue) for goods and services to the actual reimbursement (cash) based on a percentage of those charges. It is important for staff in all departments to understand that charges, or revenue, are rarely collected at 100 percent of their value.

Contractual Allowances

When charges are not collected at 100 percent of their value, it is because a contract has been signed with a payer to provide the payer with a reduction in the charges. The difference between the actual charge and the contracted amount is termed **Contractual Write-off** or **Contractual Allowance.** A write-off or allowance removes a specific amount of the balance due from the A/R account and makes it uncollectible. For Medicare, the contractual allowance is the difference between the charges and the approved amount for the service, such as the DRG rate, APC rate or resource-based relative value scale (RBRVS) amount. Patients are not responsible for any of the contractual allowance.

Cash

Cash is the actual money collected of the A/R. Point of service (POS) cash is the cash collected at the point of service, such as copays and payments on account.

Patient Responsibility or Self-Pay

When all third-party payments have been received and contractual allowances have been written off, the remaining balance is categorized as patient responsibility. Best practice is patient responsibility balances that are less than 15 percent of the total balance.

Bad Debt

The term **bad debt** refers to accounts that show money owed by the patient and that healthcare facility policy has defined as uncollectible. When serious attempts have been made to collect but when no money has been paid, these charges are written off to bad debt approximately 120 days from the issue of the first patient statement.

Figure 11.2. Account aging report

PT #	AT	ADM/SER	DIS	STATUS	0–30	31–60	61–90	91–180	181–360	361+
ZZ746153153	E/D	04/15/03	04/15/03	BD		148.84				
ZZ746160492	E/D	07-06-03	07-06-03	BD	25					
ZZ746162518	REC-THRY	07/29/03	07/31/03	FB				10		
ZZ746162874	REC-THRY	08-05-03	08/31/03	FB				30		
ZZ746163484	E/D	08-07-03	08-07-03	BD	165					
ZZ746162580	E/D	07/30/03	07/30/03	BD	114					
ZZ746125122	OP	06/19/02		FB						16
ZZ746160520	E/D	07-06-03	07-06-03	BD		50				
ZZ746169245	OP	10-09-03		FB			175			
ZZ746165628	REC-THRY	09-03-03	09/30/03	FB				266		
ZZ746163713	OP	08-12-03		BD	52					
ZZ746166048	E/D	09-04-03	09-04-03	FB				280		
ZZ746161964	OP	07/23/03		FB				93.5		
ZZ746162506	OP	07/30/03		FB				93.5		
ZZ746164953	OP	08/25/03		FB				52		
ZZ746169231	E/D	10-09-03	10-09-03	FB			25			
ZZ746157104	E/D	05/29/03	05/30/03	BD		50				
ZZ746124652	OBV	06/14/02	06/15/02	FB						83.93
ZZ746126673	OP	07-09-02		FB						147.19
ZZ746122161	OP	05/20/02		BD		207				
Total $					**1440.19**	**16450.8**	**1613.22 3**	**3365**	**13156**	**3754.2**
Total Accts					**157**	**221**	**10**	**395**	**129**	**32**

Late Charges

Late charges are any charges that have not been posted to the account number within the healthcare facility's established bill hold time period. Best practice is 4 days from the date of service/discharge. Late charges particularly affect reimbursement in outpatient areas when Medicare is the payer and the payment is based on APCs. Late charges can affect modifier assignment and/or the calculation of the APC and are, therefore, not accepted by Medicare. To be paid for these charges, an adjusted claim must be sent to Medicare.

Timely Filing Limit

Many insurance contracts have a provision called Timely Filing Limit, or the time period within which a valid claim may be sent to the insurer to be considered for payment. This limit is usually 90 days but can vary from 60 days to more than 1 year based on the insurance contract. Claims that are not submitted within this time period are denied and must be written off to contractual allowance, because the terms of the contract were not met. The patient cannot be billed for charges not submitted within the timely filing limit.

Bill Hold

Bill hold is an established time between the date of service and the date the claim is sent to the payer. This time is to allow all charges to be entered and all coding to be completed. The best practice for bill hold is 4 days from the date of service/discharge.

Discharged Not Final Billed

DNFB refers to accounts where the patient has been discharged but the charges have not been processed and have not been billed. The DNFB report is usually "owned" by the HIM department. Because the HIM department codes the records, any uncoded records, for whatever reason, become the responsibility of the HIM department. Unfortunately, the reason why an account cannot be coded has little to do with HIM operations. More often, uncoded accounts are due to untimely documentation, misposted charges, registration for the wrong service area, services provided under an incorrect revenue code, lost paperwork, and myriad issues that fall to the HIM director to resolve. (Figure 11.3 shows a sample DNFB report. See figure 10.2 on p. 339 for an alternate format.)

Local Coverage Determination

Local coverage determination (LCD) refers to coverage rules, at a fiscal intermediary (FI) or carrier level, that provide information on what diagnoses justify the medical necessity of a test. If diagnoses or signs/symptoms do not justify medical necessity, Medicare will not pay for the test. Payment becomes the patient's responsibility, but only when the patient is informed before the test that he or she will have to pay for it. This information must be provided to the patient in writing, using an advance beneficiary notice (ABN). (See figure 11.4.) If the ABN is not completed, there is no payment for the testing.

National Coverage Determinations

National coverage determinations (NCDs) are the equivalent of LCDs at the national level. They exist for laboratory testing, although Medicare is moving toward making many existing LCDs into NCDs. Both LCDs and NCDs may be found on the Centers for Medicare and Medicaid Services (CMS) Web site and/or the Web sites of the Medicare carriers or FIs. Links to some of these Web sites are listed in table 11.1.

Medicare Parts A and B

Medicare Part A is the federal program that provides coverage for Medicare beneficiaries for services provided at a healthcare facility inpatient level of care. Medicare (under CMS) contracts with a FI to pay claims. The UB-92/UB-04 is the claim form currently in use. For facilities that comply with Health Insurance Portability and Accountability Act (HIPAA) regulations, the claims are submitted as electronic claims using the 837I transaction standards.

Medicare Part B is the federal program under which physician's claims and healthcare facility outpatient diagnostic testing services are paid. FIs and carriers are required to respond to all claims within fourteen days of their receipt. Each claim is subjected to a number of edits. These edits are used to determine if the claims in a batch meet the basic requirements of the HIPAA standard for electronically submitted claims. If these claims pass the initial, first-level

Figure 11.3. DNFB report

BILL GRP	ACCOUNT ##	UNIT#	LOCATION	BILL TYPE TYP	ATT'ER	PREM INS	ADM DAT	DIS DAT	BILL#	CUT DAT	BILL CHGS	UR CHGS FROZEN?	DAYS PRIM CLAIM CL STATUS	PRO HOLDS	HOLD VALUE
E/D	ZZ000181xx51	ZZ00xx635xx	ZZ-ED	E/D	SCH,ER	MCD-PZZ	03-01-04	03-01-04	1	03-0xx-2004	3,525	3,525	8	CHG CAT & PROC	Charge Cat should ha
E/D	ZZ000182670	ZZ0084430	ZZ-ED	E/D	MUL,MAR	TUFTS SH	03-08-04	03-08-04	1	03/16/04	3 5xxw.11	35xxw.11	1	CHG CAT& CPT	Charge Cat needs Cpt
IP	ZZ0001w2542	ZZ0006w4w	ZZ-2MS	IP	RAM,AL	MCR-A	03-07-04	03-11-04	1	03/15/04	11xx77.xx3	11xx77.xx3	2	DRG ST	FAIL
IP	ZZ0001w1727	ZZ00ww715	ZZ-2MS	IP	NAV,KA	MCR-AB	02/w04	03-03-04	1	03-07-04	12,214	12,214	10	DRG ST	FAIL
OP	ZZ0001w2653	ZZ00wx406	ZZ-LABD	OP	ANT,RI	TUFTS-HMO	03-0w-2004		1	03/16/04	325	325	1	DX1	FAIL
OP	ZZ0001w2657	ZZ00w7013	ZZ-LABD	OP	NAV,KA	FALLON-SEL	03-0w-2004		1	03/16/04	1w0	1w0	1	DX1	FAIL
OP	ZZ0001w2675	ZZ00xxw5xx2	ZZ-LABD	OP	KAN,LU	COMA-UH/GM	03-0w-2004		1	03/16/04	7w	7w	1	DX1	FAIL
OP	ZZ0001w2210	ZZ0054466	ZZ-ORC	OP	PHI,JE	BC-MA HMO	03-0w-2004		1	03/16/04	5xx	5xx	1	DX1	FAIL
OP-MCR	ZZ0001w15xx7	ZZ00217w7	ZZ-PREOP	OP	HOR,WL	MCR-A	03-0w-2004		1	03/16/04	115	115	1	DX1	FAIL
OP	ZZ0001w2303	ZZ0072117	ZZ-PREOP	OP	HOR,WL	FALLON SR	03-0w-2004		1	03/16/04	115	115	1	DX1	FAIL
OP	ZZ0001w230w	ZZ007wwxx1	ZZ-PREOP	OP	HOR,WL	BC-MA HMO	03-0w-2004		1	03/16/04	115	115	1	DX1	FAIL
OP-MCR	ZZ0001w2310	ZZ00xx5645	ZZ-PREOP	OP	HOR,WL	MCR-AB	03-0w-2004		1	03/16/04	115	115	1	DX1	
OP	ZZ0001w231w	ZZ00xx7030	ZZ-RAD	OP	NAV,KA	MCD-PZZ	03-0w-2004		1	03/16/04	2w35	2w35	1	DX1	FAIL
OP-MCR	ZZ0001w263w	ZZ000002w	ZZ-RAD	OP	FIN,ST	MCR-AB	03-0w-2004		1	03/16/04	3,002	3,002	1	DX1	FAIL
OP-MCR	ZZ0001w2432	ZZ0074051	ZZ-LABD	OP	MON,AT	MCR-AB	03-05-04		1	03/13/04	545	545	4	DX1	FAIL
OP-MCR	ZZ0001w21xx0	ZZ001w477	ZZ-PREOP	OP	HOR,WL	MCR-AB	03-05-04		1	03/13/04	115	115	4	DX1	FAIL
OP	ZZ0001w21xx3	ZZ00x6026	ZZ-PREOP	OP	STE,SV	BC-MA HMO	03-05-04		1	03/13/04	115	115	4	DX1	FAIL

Figure 11.4. **ABN form**

Patient's Name: _____   Medicare # (HICN): _____

ADVANCE BENEFICIARY NOTICE (ABN)

NOTE: You need to make a choice about receiving these health care items or services.

We expect that Medicare will not pay for the item(s) or service(s) that are described below. Medicare does not pay for all of your health care costs. Medicare only pays for covered items and services when Medicare rules are met. The fact that Medicare may not pay for a particular item or service does not mean that you should not receive it. There may be a good reason your doctor recommended it. Right now, in your case, **Medicare probably will not pay for –**

Items or Services:

Because:

The purpose of this form is to help you make an informed choice about whether or not you want to receive these items or services, knowing that you might have to pay for them yourself. Before you make a decision about your options, you should **read this entire notice carefully.**

x Ask us to explain, if you don't understand why Medicare probably won't pay.
x Ask us how much these items or services will cost you (**Estimated Cost: $**_____),
   in case you have to pay for them yourself or through other insurance.

PLEASE CHOOSE **ONE** OPTION. CHECK **ONE** BOX. **SIGN & DATE** YOUR CHOICE.

Option 1. YES. **I want to receive these items or services.**
I understand that Medicare will not decide whether to pay unless I receive these items or services. Please submit my claim to Medicare. I understand that you may bill me for items or services and that I may have to pay the bill while Medicare is making its decision. If Medicare does pay, you will refund to me any payments I made to you that are due to me. If Medicare denies payment, I agree to be personally and fully responsible for payment. That is, I will pay personally, either out of pocket or through any other insurance that I have. I understand I can appeal Medicare's decision.

Option 2. NO. **I have decided not to receive these items or services.**
I will not receive these items or services. I understand that you will not be able to submit a claim to Medicare and that I will not be able to appeal your opinion that Medicare won't pay.

_____   _____
Date   **Signature of patient or person acting on patient's behalf**

NOTE: Your health information will be kept confidential. Any information that we collect about you on this form will be kept confidential in our offices. If a claim is submitted to Medicare, your health information on this form may be shared with Medicare. Your health information which Medicare sees will be kept confidential by Medicare.

OMB Approval No. 0938-0566   Form No. CMS-R-131-G   (June 2002)

Table 11.1.   Online resources for coders

Organization	Web Site Address
American Health Information Management Association	http://www.ahima.org
American Medical Association	http://www.ama-assn.org/ama/pub/category/4555.html
Associated Hospital Services Medicare FI	http://www.ahsmedicare.com/
BC/BS of MA	http://www.bcbsma.com/common/en_US/medical_policies/medcat.htm
California QIO	http://www.lumetra.com/
CMS	http://www.cms.hhs.gov/
CMS MedLearn	http://www.cms.hhs.gov/MLNGenInfo/
CMS NCDs	http://www.cms.hhs.gov/ncd/default.asp?
CMS Office of the Inspector General	http://www.oig.hhs.gov/
CMS State Operations Manual: Site of the Conditions of Participation	http://www.cms.hhs.gov/manuals/IOM/list.asp
Iowa QIO	http://www.ifmc.org/
IPRO	http://providers.ipro.org/index/coding-corner
Massachusetts QIO	http://www.masspro.org/
Mutual of Omaha Medicare: FI link to Medicare Reason Codes and LMRPs	http://www.mutualmedicare.com/
National Blue Cross/Blue Shield site	http://www.bluecares.com/
National Heritage Insurance Co, Part B Carrier for New England and California	http://www.medicarenhic.com/cpt_agree.shtml
Northeast Health Care Quality Foundation	http://www.nhcaf.org
Quality Net	http://www.qualitynet.org
Texas Medical Foundation/TX QIO	http://www.tmf.org/

edits or preedits, they are then edited against implementation guide requirements in HIPAA claim standards. Once the first levels of edits are passed, each claim is edited for compliance with Medicare coverage and payment policy requirements. Other edits include the National Correct Coding Initiative to promote correct coding methodologies and to control improper coding leading to inappropriate payment under Part B claims. The result is that either the FI or carrier pays the claim, or the claim is returned to the provider with an edit. In the latter scenario, additional follow-up may be necessary to receive payment. HIM directors and coders should be reasonably familiar with the edits generated by coding issues. These are available on the FI Web sites or the CMS Web site.

Office of the Inspector General

The **Office of the Inspector General** (OIG) is the department under Health and Human Services (HHS) responsible for monitoring compliance with the Medicare and Medicaid programs. The OIG issues an annual work plan that contains the areas of focus. It is essential that all members of the revenue cycle know the plan and understand its impacts. For example, the OIG monitored the billing submitted by teaching physicians against the documentation in the hospital medical records and concluded that the physicians were billing inappropriately. These audits—Physicians at Teaching Hospitals, or PATH—resulted in significant fines and penalties for some teaching hospitals. Another area of focus is the higher-paying DRGs in audits to determine upcoding, the practice of assigning a reimbursement code expressly for the purpose of obtaining a higher payment.

Front End

The term "front end" refers to preregistration, prebooking, scheduling, and registration activities that perform collection of patient demographic and insurance information, verification of patient insurance, and determination of medical necessity. Best practice is 98 percent accuracy.

Revenue Cycle Management Model: The Players, Their Roles, the Impact

The concept of the revenue cycle or revenue cycle management (RCM) requires that departments abandon a mindset frequently seen in healthcare organizations called "silo thinking," in which the narrow concerns of the department come before the good of the larger organization. Each department/player has an impact on the generation of revenue in the organization and meeting the performance metrics as described above.

Patient Access Services

Often referred to as admitting, the patient access services department encompasses all of the front-end processes, including obtaining information before the patient even arrives at the facility for services. The preregistration/booking/scheduling processes address the following:

- Capture of the correct patient demographics

- Verification of insurance coverage for the patient

- Determination of the appropriate level of care (for example, does the patient need services at an inpatient or ambulatory level of care despite the physician's requests?)

Insurance verification is essential to determine whether the patient actually has the insurance he or she claims to have, whether the insurance covers the services the patient will have, and whether the patient must pay a deductible or copayment. Nonverification of some or all of this information can result in claims either being sent to an insurance company that will not pay, being returned to patients accounts staff to try to determine the actual insurance, or reverting to the patient for payment. In the first case, resubmission of the claim to the correct insurer may be delayed beyond the timely filing limit, which results in the claim not being paid. If the patient is responsible for payment due to lack of insurance and no financial arrangements have occurred, the claim is written off as bad debt and the healthcare facility receives almost no reimbursement for the services provided.

The registration process for patients whose services are not prescheduled has the same requirements as for prebooked patients, with the additional challenge of time constraints. The demographics must be accurate, the insurance information must be verified, and patients who have no insurance or are underinsured must receive financial counseling before they leave the building. As in the case of the prescheduled patients, a failure in any of these areas can result in payment delays and/or no payment.

The registration process for patients sent to the healthcare facility for ambulatory diagnostic testing (for example, laboratory tests or cardiology services) is even more complex. Most insurers have medical necessity requirements based on the model of Medicare NCDs and LCDs. Registration staff must be certain that the patient arrives for services with an order signed by his or her physician certifying that the services are medically necessary. The concept that a test ordered by a physician may be deemed unnecessary by a payer is difficult for physicians and patients to accept. Many facilities have front-end software that serves as a compliance checker and allows registration staff to enter the narrative of the sign/symptom to determine whether it meets the requirements for medical necessity. If the test is performed when the order does not meet medical necessity, the claim for payment is denied. Although possible, appeals are time-consuming and costly and do not always result in payment. Best practice is for HIM coders to assign the codes used for billing.

Medicare does have a provision that a patient may be billed for a test that is not medically necessary if he or she receives an ABN before the test is performed. Therefore, not only must the registration staff determine whether the sign/symptom is sufficient, they may contact the patient's physician to obtain a new order or, if a new order is not provided, to issue an ABN. Success in the patient registration process involves a thoroughly educated staff with the tools to determine medical necessity, the processes in place to clarify orders, and the ability to obtain signatures on ABNs.

Utilization Management

Front-end utilization management (UM) is essential to the prevention of **denials** for inappropriate levels of care. UM staff work with the physician to ensure that the requested services meet medical necessity requirements and are provided in the most appropriate setting. Managed care companies follow the Medicare guidelines in these areas, although far more aggressively. When the insurer denies the claim, it may be possible to appeal it. However, as mentioned above, denial management (application of the appeals process) after the fact is time-consuming and costly and does not always result in payment of the claim. UM staff also are key in obtaining documentation during an inpatient stay. Immediate access to the physicians while a patient is in-house enables the UM staff to obtain clarification. For this process to benefit the coding staff, there must be communication between coders and UM staff to define what is needed to support coding decisions. Joint monthly meetings would facilitate communication between the two areas, as would mutual understanding of the documentation guidelines for the problem DRGs. Appendix 11.1 provides an example of standards issued by a state quality improvement organization (QIO).

Third-Party Payers

The companies that pay claims are referred to as third-party payers. Medicare and Blue Cross/Blue Shield (BCBS) are examples of third-party payers. In the past, many payers reimbursed healthcare organizations based on a percent of the charges. After implementation of the Inpatient Prospective Payment System in 1983 and the growth of managed care, a set rate of pay based on DRGs became the norm. Now, CMS has issued the hospital inpatient prospective payment system (IPPS) final rule for fiscal year (FY) 2007. This rule is a first step to improve the accuracy of Medicare's payment for inpatient stays by better reflecting costs rather than charges and by adjusting payment to better account for the difference in severity of illness and risk of mortality of the patient's condition. The final IPPS rule is available in the August 18, 2006, *Federal Register* at www.access.gpo.gov/su_docs/fedreg/a060818c. html (CMS 2006). In FY07, 20 new DRGs (12 medical, 8 surgical) have been implemented by subdividing existing DRGs through diagnosis codes, subdividing DRGs based on specific surgical procedures and selecting cases with specific diagnosis and/or procedure codes to account for resource use and severity. Eight DRGs were deleted and 32 modified DRGs are created to better capture the differences in patient severity. This is a start at moving forward with a severity-based DRG system.

The proposed consolidated severity (CS) adjusted DRGs as proposed were not approved for FY07. These CS DRGs were developed by CMS and based on the APR-DRGs. CMS stated that further adjustments are needed to CS DRGs, and that no other alternatives were evaluated and that a proprietary DRG system was involved. An independent contractor will assist in evaluating alternative severity adjustment systems, and CMS intends to implement such system FY08.

Several versions of DRGs are currently in use, and HIM coding staff, patient accounts staff, and reimbursement staff must be aware of each version. In some cases, again following the Medicare payment pattern, third-party payers and the reimbursement staff in healthcare organizations contract for "carve-outs." Carve-outs are services that are not paid under the usual rate but, rather, at a special rate. Reimbursement staff calculate conditions/services for carve-outs based on the coding and the charges. For example, expensive drugs used in chemotherapy or high-cost implantable devices are often carve-outs. Thus, the coding must be of the highest degree of specificity and accuracy.

In the physician setting, many third-party payers, including Medicare, have code-sequencing requirements for payment that are also inconsistent with coding guidelines from the AHA *Coding Clinic* or the AMA *CPT Assistant*. Most facilities will need to check with each contracted payer to find out how they want certain services or procedures coded, increasing the complexity of coding compliance. In these cases, the HIM coding policy and procedure manual must contain documentation from the payer about these requirements. An example of this is the Medicare requirement that ICD-9-CM category 585 be the principal diagnosis for dialysis, rather than the appropriate V code. See Bowman (2004) for more information on the correct way to handle payers who do not follow coding guidelines.

Third-party payers also prefer to delay payment as long as possible. Prompt payment laws can help prevent frivolous delays. The State Commissioner of Insurance monitors actions of insurance companies and can assist facilities and physicians in obtaining payments if delay tactics are suspected.

Charge Description Master

As covered in chapter 6, the charge description master (CDM) is a translation table that puts the appropriate codes on the UB-92/UB-04 claim form or the 837I file. Proper maintenance of the CDM is vital to the RCM. Many facilities make oversight of the CDM update process part of the duties of the revenue cycle team. (Chapter 6 discusses the CDM in detail.)

Clinical Departments/Physicians

As noted previously, clinical departments in healthcare organizations traditionally focused on the care they provided to patients and were not involved in the financial aspects of service provision. Typically, they understood their role in generating revenue as "we treat patients and the bill is paid." Physicians operated with much the same understanding in both their hospital activities and their office practices.

The RCM concept brings clinical providers into an integrated team in the healthcare organization's financial well-being. It attempts to ensure clinical provider awareness of documentation requirements, scheduling requirements, and third-party payer rules in a manner that is supportive and promotes teamwork. Frequently, in an effort to ease the burden of the documentation requirements and to promote more timely billing, healthcare organizations have developed encounter forms, or so-called superbills. (See figure 11.5.)

The intent is to provide a simple checkoff form of the diagnoses used most frequently by physicians. The corresponding ICD-9-CM and CPT/HCPCS codes are transmitted directly to the billing system, without the intervention of trained coders. Although this method is efficient, best practice is to have CPT codes in the 10,000–69,999 range assigned by HIM coders. When physicians/providers complete an encounter form or superbill that is not verified by a coder, revenue may be lost because of missing coding and/or lack of specificity.

Health Information Management

Although most chief financial officers and patient accounts directors consider coding to be the HIM department's most significant function, the department's other functions are equally essential if coders are to have accounts coded in a timely manner, that is, with 98 percent accuracy. The activities of the entire HIM staff must be performed in a complementary, unified process. If one piece is "broken," coding cannot meet the requirements for DNFB, bill holds, **clean claims,** and quality.

Unless a healthcare organization is totally automated, the health records from which the coders code must be assembled. It is unusual for the HIM department to receive all the documents for an occasion of service, whether inpatient or ambulatory, all together and on the same day. The staff members who manage this paper flow are the backbone of the coding effort. Many payers require copies of medical records before they pay. In this case, the release-of-information staff must have established turnaround times to provide copies and must know all the applicable laws, statutes, and HIPAA regulations. The staff members who manage incomplete records and report transcriptions are key players in the revenue cycle management within the HIM department. Records must be analyzed for physician completion requirements immediately, and physicians must be held accountable for the timely completion of their patients' health records.

Although high in the salary range, coders also are high (just behind the HIM director) in the accountability for timely, accurate coding. Determination of the quality of coding requires audits, and many healthcare organizations engage outside companies to perform them. Quality audits can be positive experiences for the coding staff but also can be frustrating because of variations in interpretation of the documentation. The most beneficial coding audits are those that include a concluding discussion of the findings with all the coders and the auditors. When presented as an educational session, the frustrations of having coding decisions challenged are mitigated.

As discussed in chapter 1, the physician query form provides for additional clarification of physician documentation in the health record. The healthcare facility must have written policies and procedures in place for use of this tool, based on guidelines established by CMS and the American Health Information Management Association (AHIMA).

As noted previously, the coding professional must know the details of managed care contracts and each payer's coding and sequencing requirements. This ensures that clean claims are submitted the first time.

Coding software/computer applications are an integral part of the coder's tools for successful coding. Such programs enable application of many of the coding edits before the claim is sent to the patient accounts system. Web-based reference tools and links to the Web sites of third-party payers also support quality coding. Although many coding staff use an encoder and software that calculates a DRG, the APC, and the payment, coders must never completely rely on these tools. The most effective coding is done using coding books with the computer tools as supports.

Figure 11.5. Extract from an encounter form/superbill

✓	Code	Administration	Fee	✓	Code	Therapeutic Rx	Fee
		INTRAVENOUS INFUSIONS			J0133	Acyclovir, 5mg (Zovirax)	
	90760	Intravenous infusion, hydration; initial, up to 1 hour			J0289	Amphotericin B, liposomal 10 mg (AmBisome)	
	90761+	Intravenous infusion, hydration; ea add'l hour, up to 8 hrs			J3490155	Ascorbic Acid 500 mg	
	90765	Intravenous infusion, therapeutic; initial, up to 1 hour			J3490111	Bumetamide 1 mg (Bumex)	
	90766+	Intravenous infusion, therapeutic; ea add'l hour, up to 8 hrs			J0610	Calcium gluc, 1 g	
	90767	Intravenous infusion, therapeutic; add'l sequential inf up to 1hr			J0637	Caspofungin 5mg (Cancidas)	
	90768	Intravenous infusion, therapeutic; concurrent infusion			J0696	Ceftriaxone, 250 mg (Rocephin)	
		THERAPEUTIC INJECTIONS			J0740	Cidofovir 375mg (Vistide)	
	90772	Therapeutic injection; subcutaneous or intramuscular			J1070	Depotestosterone up to 100mg	
	90774	Therapeutic injection; IV push, single or initial			J1100001	Dexamethasone, 1 mg (Decadron)	
	90775+	Therapeutic injection; ea add'l sequential IV push of **new** substance			J1200	Diphenhydramine, 50 mg (Benadryl)	
		CHEMOTHERAPY/IMMUNOTHERAPY ADMINISTRATION			J0881	Darbepoetin alpha, 1 mcg, non-ESRD (Aranesp)	
	96401	Chemotherapy administration; subQ or IM, non-hormonal antineoplastic			J1335	Ertapenem 500 mg (Invanz)	
	96409	Chemotherapy administration; IV push, single or initial			J1650	Enoxaparin, 10 mg (Lovenox)	
	96411+	Chemotherapy administration IV; each additional drug			J3490007	Famotidine, 20 mg inj (Pepcid)	
	96413	Chemotherapy administration; up to 1hr single or initial			J3010	Fentanyl Citrate 100 mcg	
	96415+	Chemotherapy administration; up to 1hr single or initial			J1440	Filgrastim (G-CSF), 300 mcg (Neupogen)	
		PUMPS			J1441001	Filgrastim (G-CSF), 480 mcg (Neupogen)	
	NC	Pump for Medicare Patient			J1450	Fluconazole 200 mg (Diflucan)	
	96416	Pump Initiation			J1940	Furosemide, 20 mg (Lasix)	
	96425	Chemo infusion pump >8hrs			J1570002	Ganciclovir, 500 mg (Cytovene)	
	96521	Refill/Maint Portable Pump			J1626	Granisetron, 100 mcg (Kytril IV)	
	E0781	Pump Rental			J1644	Heparin, 1000 units	
	Z735	Pump Supplies			J1642	Heparin, 10 units	

Another key tool is Internet access. Coding staff need to know the online resources that are available and how to use them. Some of these Web sites are listed in table 11.1.

Patient Accounts

The staff in the patient accounts department need a wealth of knowledge about each payer's billing rules, requirements, and contract details. Further, they need to know how to analyze the estimate of benefits (EOB) received, and know and understand the Medicare Reason Codes. Patient accounts staff post the receivables to each account and determine delays in reimbursement based on the information in the EOBs. They also analyze the claims rejections and communicate them back to the appropriate departments.

In addition to the actual bills, the computer applications used by the patient accounts department generate the DNFB, A/R, late charge, and denial reports. The patient accounts staff can utilize a number of "canned text codes" when generating these tracking reports. (See figures 11.6 and 11.7.) These reports provide feedback to the revenue cycle management team from the patient accounts staff as they work on improving their processes.

Figure 11.6. Canned text examples

Code		Description	Code	Description
1	M20	CHARGES PREVIOUSLY CONSIDERED	W-OFFSET	AUTO OFFSET (DIFFERENT BILLS)
2	M201	NONPROVIDER PHYSICIAN	WADMIN	ADMINISTRATIVE ALLOWANCE
3	M202	NOT WORK-RELATED INJURY	WAUDIT	AUDITOR W/O
4	M204	PATIENT INELIGIBLE	WCL-CLNT	CLIENT ADJUSTMENT
5	M208	INSURANCE PAID PATIENT	WHADMIN	HOSPITAL ADJUSTMENT
6	M209	PATIENT MUST SUBMIT INFO TO INS.	WHINJ	HOSPITAL ADJUSTMENT
7	M210	OVER THE FILING LIMIT	WHPFS	PATIENT FINANCIAL SERVICES W/O
8	M211	RETURN CHECK	WLIVDONR	LIVING DONOR ALLOWANCE
9	M212	INS REQ INFO FROM PROVIDER	WMCR-LC	M'CARE LATE CHARGES UNBILLED
10	M26	DEPENDENT NOT COVERED	WMCR/MCD-X	M'CARE/M'CAID CROSSOVER ADJ
11	M28	SERVICE NOT COVERED	WMCRA	MEDICARE PROVIDER LIABLE
12	M3	PATIENT COPAYMENT	WMCRAB-LC	MCRAB LATE CHARGES UNBILLED
13	M30	BENEFITS LIMITED	WMCRABMCDX	MCRAB/M'CAID CROSSOVER ADJ
14	M301	PIP EXHAUSTED	WMCRABP	MEDICARE PROVIDER LIABLE
15	M34	INVALID POLICY NUMBER	WMCRR-LC	MCR RR LATE CHARGES UNBILLED
16	M48	COVERAGE TERMINATED		
17	M5	PRIOR TO EFFECTIVE DATE		
18	M57	NO MEDICARE PART B BENEFITS		
19	M58	SERVICE AFTER TERMINATION		
20	M59	PATIENT HAS OTHER INSURANCE		

Figure 11.7. Use of canned text in report

PROCEDURE	COUNT	AMOUNT	PT LC	TXN.DATE	ACCT #	ADM/SER	ACCT TYPE	PT	PRIMARY INS
WMCRA	1	21	CC-ED	02-05-04	ZC0001XTXT229	01-07-04	E/D	O	MCR-A
WMCRA	1	40	CC-ED	02/17/04	ZC0001XT8430	01/21/04	E/D	O	MCR-A
WMCRA	1	20	CC-LABD	02-06-04	ZC0001XTXT08XT	01/13/04	OP	O	MCR-A
WMCRA	1	20	CC-LABD	02-12-04	ZC0001XT8153	01/19/04	OP	O	MCR-A
WMCRA	1	52	CC-LABD	02/24/04	ZC0001XT9128	01/29/04	OP	O	MCR-A
WMCRA	1	162	CC-OTH	02/25/04	ZC000109440	10-11-03	REC-THRY	O	MCR-A
WMCRA	1	801	CC-PTH	02-11-04	ZC000108421	10-02-03	REC-THRY	O	MCR-A
WMCRA	1	1,452	CC-PTH	02-11-04	ZC000108441	10-03-03	REC-THRY	O	MCR-A
WMCRABP	1	20	CC-ED	02-04-04	ZC0001XTXT491	01-11-04	E/D	O	MCR-AB
WMCRABP	1	21	CC-ED	02-05-04	ZC0001XTXT585	01-12-04	E/D	O	MCR-AB
WMCRABP	1	20	CC-ED	02-06-04	ZC0001XTXT041	01/13/04	E/D	O	MCR-AB
WMCRABP	1	20	CC-ED	02-11-04	ZC0001XT8002	01/17/04	E/D	O	MCR-AB
WMCRABP	1	112	CC-ED	02-11-04	ZC0001XT8009	01/17/04	E/D	O	MCR-AB
WMCRABP	1	20	CC-ED	02-11-04	ZC0001XTXT843	01/15/04	E/D	O	MCR-AB
WMCRABP	1	20	CC-ED	02/17/04	ZC0001XT831XT	01/20/04	E/D	O	MCR-AB
WMCRABP	1	20	CC-LABD	02-06-04	ZC0001XTXT031	01/13/04	OP	O	MCR-AB
WMCRABP	1	92	CC-LABD	02-06-04	ZC0001XTXT084	01/13/04	OP	O	MCR-AB
WMCRABP	1	52	CC-LABD	02/17/04	ZC0001XT8033	01/23/04	OP	O	MCR-AB
WMCRABP	1	128	CC-LABD	02/17/04	ZC0001XT85XT5	01/23/04	OP	O	MCR-AB
WMCRABP	1	20	CC-LABD	02/17/04	ZC0001XT8544	01/22/04	OP	O	MCR-AB
WMCRABP	1	20	CC-LABD	02/23/04	ZC0001XT8802	01/27/04	OP	O	MCR-AB
WMCRABP	1	20	CC-LABD	02/24/04	ZC0001XT911XT	01/29/04	OP	O	MCR-AB
WMCRABP	1	128	CC-LABD	02/24/04	ZC0001XT9014	01/28/04	OP	O	MCR-AB
WMCRABP	1	52	CC-LABD	02/24/04	ZC0001XT9202	01/30/04	OP	O	MCR-AB
W-OFFSET	-1	-649	CC-ED	02/15/04	ZC0001XT0292	12/29/03	E/D	O	MCD-PCC
W-OFFSET	1	1,422	CC-LABD	02-08-04	ZC000139XT52	11/15/02	OP	O	G-HMO-NET
WSMBAL	1	8	CC-ED	02/14/04	ZC0001584XT8	06-12-03	E/D	O	BC-MA HMO
WMCRABMCDX	1	625	CC-2MS	02/23/04	ZC0001XT0353	12/29/03	IP	I	MCR-AB
WMCRABMCDX	1	840	CC-2MS	02/23/04	ZC0001XT04XT3	12/30/03	IP	I	MCR-AB
WMCRABMCDX	1	840	CC-2SCU	02-11-04	ZC0001XT0143	12/26/03	IP	I	MCR-AB
WMCRABMCDX	1	770	CC-3PSY	02-06-04	ZC000105920	09-03-03	IP-PSY	I	MCR-AB

Impact of Electronic Health Records on Revenue Cycle Management

With the implementation of electronic health records, it is important to analyze how this will affect reimbursement. Real-time collection and interfacing of data will improve and speed information flow but care must be taken to replace all manual charge collection processes with accurate electronic processes.

What does this mean to the HIM department? CMS is evaluating the shift from the DRG system in use for hospital inpatient since 1983 to a severity-adjusted system. In order to identify all conditions for reporting, documentation in the medical record will become even more crucial. Use of this new grouping software will provide new opportunities for coders to assist physicians in documentation improvement. Severity-adjusted DRG systems require documentation and coding of different types of complications and co-morbid conditions without the guidance of a preset list of these CCs. In some of these systems V codes, history of certain conditions, even a family history, have an impact on reimbursement. Improved data capture will be facilitated by the use of electronic health records using clinical terminologies and updated classifications.

Conclusion

The most significant concept in the revenue cycle is that of integrated teamwork. In most organizations, this is a fundamental change in their culture. It can be achieved only when all the players understand their roles and the impact of their actions on the entire process, and all receive positive reinforcement for a "job well done."

The HIM department and its coders play a vital role in the education, training, and support of both the clinical and nonclinical departments. They frequently bridge the clinical area and the purely financial area. Straddling the two worlds, they bring clarity and understanding of documentation challenges with an in-depth knowledge of interrelationships and regulations.

References and Resources

Bowman, S. *Health Information Management Compliance: A Model Program for Healthcare Organizations,* 3rd ed. Chicago: AHIMA.

Centers for Medicare and Medicaid Services. 2006 (Aug. 18). Changes to the Hospital Inpatient Prospective Payment Systems and Fiscal Year 2007 Rates. *Federal Register* 71(160):47870–48351.

TMF Health Quality Institute. 2006. DRG 243: Medical back problems ICD-9-CM coding guidelines. Available online from http://www.tmf.org.

Appendix 11.1

DRG 243 – Medical Back Problems ICD-9-CM Coding Guidelines

The below listed medical back problem guidelines are not inclusive. The coder should refer to the applicable *Coding Clinic* guidelines for additional information. The Centers for Medicare and Medicaid Services considers *Coding Clinic*, published by the American Hospital Association, to be the official source for coding guidelines. Hospitals should follow the *Coding Clinic* guidelines to ensure accuracy in ICD-9-CM coding and DRG assignment.

Definition of Principal Diagnosis

The principal diagnosis is that condition established after study to be chiefly responsible for occasioning the admission of the patient to the hospital for care.

Two or more diagnoses may equally meet the definition for principal diagnosis. This is in terms of the circumstances of admission, diagnostic workup and/or therapy provided. Be aware that there is a difference between admitting a patient to treat two conditions and two conditions being present at the time of admission. The principal diagnosis is always the reason for admission.

Documentation to Support Medical Back Problem Diagnoses

When reviewing these charts, determine whether or not the medical record documentation substantiates the principal diagnosis as the reason for admission and treatment.

The presence or absence of myelopathy (a functional disturbance and/or pathological change in the spinal cord that is often due to compression) effects the selection of some of these codes. Do not assume the presence of myelopathy. It is important to follow the excludes notes.

If the underlying cause effects the code selection, the documentation needs to include this information.

Coding Guidelines

Aspiration core needle biopsy T11-T12

Aspiration core needle biopsy of the T11-T12 disk space is coded 80.39, biopsy of joint structure (includes the aspiration biopsy) and 88.38, other computerized tomography, for the CT guidance. (See *Coding Clinic,* third quarter 2005, page 14.)

Category 805/Category 806/Category 952

Category 805 is used for a fracture of the vertebral column without spinal cord injury, category 806 is used for a fracture of the vertebral column with spinal cord injury, and category 952 is used for a spinal cord injury without evidence of spinal bone injury. (See ICD-9-CM, volume 1.)

Excludes notes under categories 723, other disorders of cervical region, and 724, other and unspecified disorders of back

Symptoms and signs associated with (due to) spondylosis and allied disorders, 721.0-721.91, or intervertebral disc disorders, 722.0-722.93 are included in the 721-722 code series. If the physician states the symptoms and signs are not attributed to the conditions noted in the excludes note, then use two codes; one from category 723 or 724 and one for the condition. Spinal stenosis due to degenerative disc disease is classified to the 722 category. Spinal stenosis, congenital or NOS, is classified within the 723-724 categories. (See *Coding Clinic,* third quarter 1994, page 14 and *Coding Clinic,* second quarter 1989, page 14.)

Revised: March 2006

Source: TMF Health Quality Institute 2006. This material was prepared by TMF Health Quality Institute, the Medicare Quality Improvement Organization for Texas, under a contract with the Centers for Medicare and Medicaid Services (CMS), an agency of the U.S. Department of Health and Human Services. The contents presented do not necessarily reflect CMS policy.

Far lateral disc herniation

This is coded using the appropriate code from the 722.0-722.2 series for displacement of intervertebral disc. (See *Coding Clinic,* first quarter 1988, page 10.)

Fracture/dislocation

A fracture-dislocation of the same site is coded using the fracture code. It is incorrect to use an additional code for the dislocation. Likewise, reduction of the fracture-dislocation is coded using only the code for the reduction of the fracture. (See *Coding Clinic,* third quarter 1990, page 13.)

Healing fracture/admitted for other acute condition

A patient treated three weeks ago for a hip fracture is admitted to a hospital for treatment of congestive heart failure (CHF). During hospitalization the hip fracture received minimal treatment. The secondary diagnosis of the fracture is coded to V54.9, unspecified orthopedic aftercare. (See *Coding Clinic,* third quarter 1995, pages 3 and 4.)

Intervertebral disc space infection

This is coded to discitis, 722.90, intervertebral disc disorder, other and unspecified disc disorder, unspecified region. (See *Coding Clinic,* November-December 1984, page 19.)

Multiple fractures

Multiple fractures of specified sites are coded individually. Combination categories for multiple fractures are only used when there is insufficient documentation, limited space on a reporting form, or there is insufficient specificity at the fourth-digit or fifth-digit level. Multiple fractures are sequenced in order of severity. (See *Coding Clinic,* September-October 1986, pages 5-9.)

Occipital neuralgia

Occipital neuralgia involves nerve entrapment or impingement and is characterized by pain in the back of the head and suboccipital region. Treatment depends on the symptoms or if the cause is known the treatment is directed toward the cause. Code 723.8, other syndromes affecting cervical region, for occipital neuralgia. If a nerve block is performed, code 04.81, injection of anesthetic into peripheral nerve for analgesia. (See *Coding Clinic,* first quarter 2000, pages 7 and 8.)

Ocular torticollis

Visual problems causing tilting of the head is referred to as ocular torticollis. Coding depends on the ocular condition causing the torticollis; i.e., nystagmus, code 379.50, strabismus, code 378.9, fourth nerve palsy, code 378.53. The ocular condition is the principal diagnosis with a secondary diagnosis of torticollis, coded 723.5, torticollis, unspecified. (See *Coding Clinic,* second quarter 2001, page 21.)

Pathologic fracture

A pathologic fracture is a break in a diseased bone due to weakening of the bone structure by pathologic processes, such as osteoporosis or neoplasm, without any identifiable trauma or following only minor trauma. A physician must determine when a patient has severe bone disease if the level of injury is in accordance with the degree of trauma suffered by the patient, so as to determine if the fracture should be coded as a traumatic or pathologic fracture. (See *Coding Clinic,* fourth quarter 1993, pages 25 and 26.)

Revised: March 2006

Spinal cord injury from a pathological compression deformity of T8 with identified vertebral body metastatic carcinoma. This is coded 733.13, pathological fracture of vertebrae (principal diagnosis), 336.3, *myelopathy in other diseases classified elsewhere,* and 198.5, secondary malignant neoplasm of other specified sites, bone and bone marrow. (See *Coding Clinic,* third quarter 1999, page 5.)

Postlaminectomy syndrome

Postlaminectomy syndrome is a buildup of scar tissue after a laminectomy has been performed. This can be coded (722.8x) when the physician documents a patient's pain is due to scar tissue formed following disk surgery. If an MRI is done that shows a new herniated disc then the code for the herniated disc should be used. (See *Coding Clinic,* second quarter 1997, page 15 and *Coding Clinic,* January-February 1987, page 7.)

Radiofrequency neuroablation for pain reduction

Radiofrequency neuroablation or neurolysis performed to reduce the amount of pain in a patient with a history of L1 compression fracture is coded 04.2, Destruction of cranial and peripheral nerves. The treated nerve normally repairs itself in three to six months. (See *Coding Clinic,* third quarter 2002, page 11.)

Sandifer syndrome

Sandifer syndrome is synonymous with gastroesophageal reflux and torticollis. Code 530.81, esophageal reflux and 723.5, torticollis. (See *Coding Clinic,* first quarter 1995, page 7.)

Spinal arachnoiditis due to postoperative scarring

Spinal arachnoiditis due to postoperative scarring following back surgery is manifested by chronic back pain or leg pain. The code assignment is found under postlaminectomy syndrome, 722.8x, or kyphosis, postlaminectomy, 737.12. (See *Coding Clinic,* January-February 1987, page 7.)

Spontaneous fracture

A spontaneous fracture is one occurring as the result of disease of a bone or from some undiscoverable cause and not due to trauma. These fractures are always pathologic and coded to classification 733.1, pathologic fracture.

A physician diagnosis of spontaneous fracture is always coded to classification 733.1, pathologic fracture, regardless of whether or not the documentation includes the underlying condition.

(See *Coding Clinic,* September-October 1985, page 13.)

Stress fracture

Stress fractures are caused by overuse or repetitive jarring of the bone. The most common sites for stress fractures are the metatarsal bones in the feet, the lumbar spine, the neck of the femur and the tibia and fibula.

Stress fractures are coded to codes 733.93-5. These codes were new as of October 1, 2001. Previously stress fractures were classified with pathological fractures in classification 733.1, pathologic fracture. (See *Coding Clinic,* fourth quarter 2001, pages 48 and 49.)

Subluxation of spine/chiropractor

The 839.xx series, other, multiple, and ill-defined dislocations, are not used for conditions treated by a chiropractor. When a subluxation of the spine is treated

Revised: March 2006

by a chiropractor, the 739.x series, nonallopathic lesions, NEC, should be used.
(See *Coding Clinic*, fourth quarter 1995, page 51.)

Revised: March 2006

Chapter 12

Case-Mix Management

Lou Ann Schraffenberger, MBA, RHIA, CCS, CCS-P

The case mix of a patient population is a description of that population based on any number of the following characteristics:

- Age

- Gender

- Type of insurance

- Diagnosis

- Risk factors

- Treatment received

- Resources used

Case mix has been defined in the following ways:

- "The method by which patients are grouped together based on a set of characteristics, e.g., resource consumption, diagnosis or procedure" (Abdelhak 2001)

- "The categories of patients (types and volumes) treated by a hospital representing the complexity of a hospital's caseload" (Amatayakul 1985)

- "An interrelated but distinct set of patient attributes which include severity of illness, prognosis, treatment difficulty, need for intervention and resource intensity" (3M 2000)

This chapter introduces various case-mix methodologies. It then elaborates on the uses of the CMI and how comparative data are used in case-mix analyses.

Case-Mix Methodologies

Coding professionals use various methodologies to perform case-mix analysis. The specific methodology used to develop a case mix depends on the nature and intended purpose of the grouping of the patients and any further analyses that might be performed. Case-mix analyses may be performed for the following reasons:

- To determine reimbursement

- To describe a population to be served

- To identify differences in practice patterns or coding complexity

In some instances, a classification of patients may be based simply on one variable, such as type of insurance. That kind of case-mix analysis may reveal a great deal of information about a patient population. In a more complex approach, an analysis may be performed using several variables. That type of case-mix analysis develops distinct patient groups (Carpenter et al. 1999; National Health Information 1997).

The key factor that distinguishes each case-mix methodology is based on the type of data used, including the following data sets:

- Claims data

- Demographic characteristics

- Disease- and procedure-based classifications

- Severity-of-illness systems

Using Claims Data

In some methodologies, only claims data are provided for the case-mix analysis. This information is limited to all charge-related data for both inpatient and outpatient visits to the provider. Claims data also include all diagnostic and procedural codes.

In more complex methodologies, additional clinical information supplements claims data. This additional information might include findings from the patient's health history, physical examination, and laboratory, radiology, and pathology results. Because the additional data elements provide a more complete view of each patient, the ultimate analysis of each group of patients may be more accurate.

Using Demographic Characteristics

A number of case-mix methodologies include demographic characteristics such as age, gender, race, type of insurance, level of education, level of income, employment status, and place of residence—urban, suburban, or rural area (Zaslavsky et al. 2000; National Health Information 1997; Hofer et al. 1999). Those characteristics are included routinely in case-mix analyses because they are readily available, lend themselves to analysis, and are objective in nature. Moreover, a wealth of information may be gained from a minimal set of those data elements.

Age and Gender Data

A case-mix analysis of a patient population limited simply to age and gender data may prove quite revealing. For example, it might show a concentration of elderly patients. From this information, the healthcare facility could plan for a greater incidence of chronic diseases, such as emphysema and hypertension.

In another example, the case-mix analysis might show that children younger than 15 years of age are a significant part of the population. Accordingly, the healthcare facility might conclude that this group will require more well-child visits and routine immunizations. Such services follow a rather prescribed schedule. From this analysis, the facility could plan the use of resources, such as examination rooms and personnel, for well-child visits.

As a third example, the case-mix analysis also might reveal a large group of women of childbearing age. From that information, the facility might conclude that more gynecological, obstetrical, and family planning services will be needed. Because obstetrical services also follow a regular schedule, the facility could appropriate its resources to the best advantage (Muldoon, Neff, and Gay 1997).

Racial and Socioeconomic Data

A case-mix analysis limited to racial and socioeconomic data may prove illuminating, as well. For example, it might reveal that cultural or linguistic factors are creating barriers that result in some patients not receiving the healthcare they need (Zaslavsky et al. 2000).

Studies have noted that the use of certain healthcare services varies across racial groups, educational levels, and areas of residence. This is true of services such as mammograms and immunizations (Zaslavsky et al. 2000).

Type of Insurance Coverage Data

A number of studies have correlated types of insurance coverages to resource use. Because managed care organizations routinely offer preventive services, their members generate more well-child and routine vaccination visits. A healthcare facility could anticipate decreased use of emergency department (ED) services from a patient population covered by managed care organizations. This population uses preventive services for health problems before they reach the point that warrants a visit to the ED.

Decreased use of ED services for nonemergent care also has been noted among populations covered by specific types of insurers. These insurers include financial disincentives to minimize nonemergency visits to the ED. Thus, members of those insurance plans may be more inclined to arrange care through a visit to their primary care provider (Peabody and Luck 1998).

Case-mix analyses have revealed that populations covered by specific insurers demonstrate different kinds of health issues. For example, Medicaid populations differ from patient groups that are not covered by Medicaid. Medicaid is administered at the state level to a state's indigent population. This section of the population is routinely associated with a number of health risk factors, including increased prevalence of chronic conditions such as diabetes and asthma (Muldoon, Neff, and Gay 1997). Moreover, some studies have shown that the length of stay for the Medicaid population is longer after inpatient admission to an acute care hospital (Arndt et al. 1998).

In contrast, a private insurance plan may have fewer members with neuromuscular conditions, such as muscular dystrophy and paralytic syndromes, because patients suffering from these illnesses are typically covered by Supplemental Security Insurance (SSI) for the disabled (Muldoon, Neff, and Gay 1997).

Using Disease- and Procedure-Based Classification Systems

Many of the more familiar case-mix classification systems, such as diagnosis-related groups (DRGs) and ambulatory payment classifications (APCs), group patients according to diagnoses and/or procedures reported in claims data. (See chapter 5, Uses of Coded Data in Risk Adjustment and Payment System) for an explanation of DRGs and APCs.) Diagnosis- and procedure-based classification **case-mix systems** are often criticized. Critics believe these methodologies do not distinguish between different levels of a specific illness (Carpenter et al. 1999). For instance, although two patients may carry a diagnosis of diabetes mellitus, a patient who presents with well-controlled diabetes will have very different issues than one with fluctuating glucose levels.

Because the DRG system was designed to classify patients into groups based on clinical and hospital resource-consumption patterns, the level of an illness may not be directly related to the use of services. Clearly, a patient with end-stage breast cancer has a much more severe form of the disease than a patient presenting with stage I breast cancer. However, the patient with stage I cancer may actually require more resources for workup of the disease. The patient with end-stage breast cancer may only need supportive services (3M 2000). Because the DRG system includes complications and comorbidities in calculating the DRG, this methodology tends to minimize the effect of the severity of the illness.

Using Severity-of-Illness Methodologies

Some case-mix methodologies address the weakness inherent in the DRG system. Those methods group and analyze patient data according to the following variations (Estaugh 1998; 3M 2000):

- Extent of the disease

- Risk of death

- Need for intervention

- Urgency of care

- Intensity of resources

- Difficulty of treatment

One CMI approach, developed by Jefferson Medical College and SysteMetrics, Inc., uses disease staging as the basis for classifying patients with similar conditions. The CMI determines patterns of resource use (Plomann 1984). The CMI is covered in more detail later in this chapter.

Adjusted Clinical Groups

After implementation of the DRG system, physicians repeatedly criticized the DRG methodology for not adequately addressing severity-of-illness differences among provider caseloads. In response to that criticism, Johns Hopkins University Hospital developed the **adjusted clinical groups** (ACGs). This software application classifies individuals into groups that are likely to have similar resource requirements. Then it maps diagnostic codes into 1 of 106 diagnostic groups based on age, gender, and number and type of diagnostic-group morbidity clusters.

NACHRI Classification

The National Association of Children's Hospitals and Related Institutions (NACHRI) has developed a classification of congenital and chronic health conditions. This **NACHRI classification** uses disease progression factors for case-mix analysis that are based on the anticipated course of the disease, as well as on the treatment goal, disease progression, and severity of the disease (Muldoon, Neff, and Gay 1997).

The Medical Outcomes Study Short-Form Health Survey

The **Medical Outcomes Study Short-Form Health Survey** also uses such factors as the severity of the disease and health status measures. In this survey, patients are asked to report on their disease and symptom intensity to characterize the total burden of the disease (Hofer et al. 1999).

The Atlas System

The **Atlas System,** formerly referred to as the medical illness severity grouping system (MedisGroups), is perhaps the most commonly used severity-of-illness system employed by hospitals in the United States and Canada. In fact, as a result of the Health Care Cost Containment Act, all acute care providers in the Commonwealth of Pennsylvania must provide an Atlas score for all discharges. The score is based on claims data supplemented by key clinical findings abstracted from the health record and includes data from the following sources:

- Health history

- Physical examination

- Laboratory, radiology, and pathology results

The Atlas System specifically excludes the patient's diagnosis in the scoring process (Abdelhak 2001).

Using Other Clinical Characteristics

In addition to diagnosis and procedure information or severity-of-illness factors, some methodologies include other clinical characteristics in the case-mix analysis.

The Resource Utilization Group Version III

The resource utilization group, version III (RUG-III) is such a case-mix classification system. It is used for reimbursement of skilled nursing services for Medicare patients (Mueller 2000). Because of the unique nature of patients in a nursing home setting, this case-mix methodology includes clinical factors such as:

- Cognition

- Sensory deficits

- Psychological well-being

- Nutrition patterns

- Medications taken

This case-mix methodology also considers clinical conditions such as complications or comorbidities that may affect the level and extent of care provided to the patient.

The Functional-Related Group System

The functional-related group (FRG) system is a case-mix methodology used in rehabilitation settings. Clinical factors considered for case-mix analysis in the rehabilitation setting include the patient's ability to perform activities of daily living and the patient's level of spinal cord injury (Tesio, Bellafa, and Franchignoni 2000).

The Home Health Resource Grouping System

The home health resource grouping (HHRG) system includes the following clinical attributes in the case-mix analysis:

- Extent of pain
- Respiratory status
- Integrity of the integumentary system (as indicated by the presence of stasis ulcers, for example)

Moreover, in determining the HHRG assigned to a patient, the following social factors are considered as key factors (HCFA 1999, 2001):

- The caregiver who has primary responsibility for the patient
- The current residence of the patient
- The principal residence of the primary caregiver

Case-Mix Index

After the patient population has been classified into groups based on one of the case-mix methodologies previously described, the professional coder can analyze the groupings and compare the results to those of other facilities. From this comparison, the coding professional arrives at the facility or physician's CMI.

The CMI is the average of the relative weights (RWs) of all cases treated at a given facility or by a given physician. It is calculated by adding the relative weights of all cases and then dividing that total by the number of cases in the population. A CMI score, or RW, reflects the resource intensity or clinical severity of a specific group in relation to the other groups in the classification system. The theoretical "average" CMI is 1.00. (See chapter 5, Uses of Coded Data in Risk Adjustment and Payment System.)

Morbidity Index in the ACG System

In the ACG system, a key factor in the physician profile is the specific physician's morbidity index. This figure indicates the severity of the physician's case mix compared with his or her peers (National Health Information 1998). The overall peer-group morbidity index, or the overall average weight, is valued as 1.00. Each physician then is compared with this average to determine his or her morbidity index relative to that of the overall peer group. If the physician's morbidity index is greater than 1.00, he or she has a more severely ill group of patients than his or her peers. Conversely, a morbidity index of less than 1.00 indicates that a physician has a healthier pool of patients than the average physician.

The RW also indicates variance from the norm. If a physician has a morbidity index of 1.10, his or her pool of patients has a morbidity rate 10 percent higher than the peer group.

Case-Mix Index in the DRG System

In a hospital setting, the CMI is usually based on the relative weights assigned to DRGs. (An explanation of assigning relative weights to DRGs appears later in this chapter.) To calculate the CMI for a group of DRGs, multiply the relative weight of each DRG by the number of discharges in that DRG. Add all of the RW results to determine the total RW. Divide the total RW by the total number of discharges included to determine the CMI. Table 12.1 presents an example of this calculation.

Case-Mix Index as a Measure of Resource Use and Severity of Illness

The coding professional can calculate an overall score that reflects the resource intensity of the service provided, or the population's severity of illness. For example, DRG 127, heart failure and shock, has a relative weight of 1.0345. DRG 552, other permanent cardiac pacemaker without major cardiovascular diagnosis, has a RW of 2.0996. In this example, the resource intensity and subsequent Medicare reimbursement for DRG 552 is approximately twice that of DRG 127.

A typical Medicare DRG CMI for a university hospital that provides heart surgery, organ transplants, and neurosurgery might be approximately 2.00. On the other hand, a community hospital that does not offer such complex services and provides more routine care, such as general surgery and medicine, might have a CMI of 1.15. The difference between those indices reflects that the average case at the university hospital is more resource intensive than the average case at the community hospital.

Table 12.1. Typical community hospital's Medicare DRG case mix

DRG	DRG Title	RW*	Discharges	ALOS**
127	Heart failure and shock	1.0345	818	5.2
089	Simple pneumonia and pleurisy age >17 with CC	1.0320	512	5.7
088	Chronic obstructive pulmonary disease	0.8778	399	4.9
544	Major joint replacement or reattachment of lower extremity	1.9643	359	4.5
014	Intracranial hemorrhage or cerebral infarction	1.2456	356	5.8
518	Percutaneous cardiovascular procedure without acute myocardial infarction without coronary artery stent implant	1.6544	309	2.1
430	Psychoses	0.6483	273	7.9
462	Rehabilitation	0.8700	251	10.8
174	GI hemorrhage with CC	1.0060	237	4.7
296	Nutritional and miscellaneous metabolic disorders age >17 with CC	0.8187	235	4.8
182	Esophagitis, gastritis and miscellaneous digestive disorders age >17 with CC	0.8413	235	4.4
Case-Mix Index		**1.1066**	**3,984**	

*RW: Relative weight
**ALOS: Average length of stay

CMI as a Basis for Reimbursement

Some case-mix systems use the CMI as a basis for reimbursement. In that way, the CMI also is a measure of the average revenue received per case. Many hospitals closely monitor the movement of their CMI for inpatient populations for which payment is based on DRGs and for outpatient populations for which payment is based on APCs.

Influences on a Facility's Case-Mix Index

A host of factors influences a facility's CMI (Holland 1998). Coding managers must be aware of the following influences on their facility's CMI:

- Changes made by the Centers for Medicare and Medicaid Services (CMS) to DRG relative weights
- Changes in services offered by the facility
- Accuracy of documentation and coding when assessing changes in the CMI

Changes Made by CMS to DRG Relative Weights

Annually, CMS reviews and then increases or decreases, as appropriate, the RWs for DRGs. Those changes are based on predictions of variations of resource consumption caused by technological advances in medicine.

For example, during the 1980s, surgical methods for a number of procedures shifted from an incisional to a laparoscopic approach. A laparoscopic approach is significantly less invasive and usually requires a shorter recovery period, or length of stay. Therefore, an admission for such a procedure is considered less resource intensive. Accordingly, CMS reevaluated the RW for the DRG associated with the procedure to reflect the change in resource consumption.

Sometimes a substantial proportion of a facility's inpatient admissions is associated with a DRG that was revised. In that case, the overall CMI for the facility also would be altered.

Changes Caused by Shifts in Services

In addition to modifications in the CMI that may be imposed by CMS, changes in services rendered by a facility also may impact its CMI. For instance, surgical DRGs tend to have higher relative weights than medical DRGs. If a facility shifts from a medical to a predominantly surgical caseload, its CMI will be higher.

Table 12.1 presents a list of the 11 most frequently used DRGs for Medicare patients in a hypothetical hospital. The CMI for that hospital is depicted as 1.1066. If a large orthopedic practice responsible for caring for a majority of patients assigned to DRG 544 were recruited by a competing facility, the CMI would be lower.

Table 12.2 displays the effect of reducing the patient volume for DRG 544 by 229 patients, from 359 (as shown in table 12.1) patients to 130. Such a change in the DRG distribution for the facility results in a drop in the hospital's CMI from 1.1066 to 1.0543.

Table 12.3 displays the effect on the hospital's CMI if those 229 orthopedic patients (from table 12.1) became internal medicine patients and were divided among the medical DRGs 127, 089, and 088. The CMI for the scenario with the increase in internal medicine patients is 1.0501. The increase in the number of internal medicine patients in medical DRGs is still insufficient to compensate for the loss of the surgical patients. In other words, even though the

Table 12.2. Medicare case mix with decline in orthopedic patient populations

DRG	DRG Title	RW*	Discharges	ALOS **
127	Heart failure and shock	1.0345	818	5.2
089	Simple pneumonia and pleurisy age >17 with CC	1.0320	512	5.7
088	Chronic obstructive pulmonary disease	0.8778	399	4.9
544	Major joint replacement or reattachment of lower extremity	1.9643	130	4.5
014	Intracranial hemorrhage or cerebral infarction	1.2456	356	5.8
518	Percutaneous cardiovascular procedure without acute myocardial infarction without coronary artery stent implant	1.6544	309	2.1
430	Psychoses	0.6483	273	7.9
462	Rehabilitation	0.8700	251	10.8
174	GI hemorrhage with CC	1.0060	237	4.7
296	Nutritional and miscellaneous metabolic disorders age >17 with CC	0.8187	235	4.8
182	Esophagitis, gastritis and miscellaneous digestive disorders age >17 with CC	0.8413	235	4.4
Case-Mix Index		**1.0543**	**3,755**	

*RW: Relative weight
**ALOS: Average length of stay

Table 12.3. Medicare case mix with increase in internal medicine patients

DRG	DRG Title	RW*	Discharges	ALOS **
127	Heart failure and shock	1.0345	895	5.2
089	Simple pneumonia and pleurisy age >17 with CC	1.0320	588	5.7
088	Chronic obstructive pulmonary disease	0.8778	475	4.9
544	Major joint replacement or reattachment of lower extremity	1.9643	130	4.5
014	Intracranial hemorrhage or cerebral infarction	1.2456	356	5.8
518	Percutaneous cardiovascular procedure without acute myocardial infarction without coronary artery stent implant	1.6544	309	2.1
430	Psychoses	0.6483	273	7.9
462	Rehabilitation	0.8700	251	10.8
174	GI hemorrhage with CC	1.0060	237	4.7
296	Nutritional and miscellaneous metabolic disorders age >17 with CC	0.8187	235	4.8
182	Esophagitis, gastritis and miscellaneous digestive disorders age >17 with CC	0.8413	235	4.4
Case-Mix Index		**1.0501**	**3,984**	

*RW: Relative weight
**ALOS: Average length of stay

patient volume is unaffected, the shift in the caseload to a more medical orientation resulted in a reduction in the CMI—from 1.1066 in table 12.1 to 1.0501 in table 12.3.

As mentioned previously, surgical DRGs typically have higher RWs than medical DRGs and thus can increase a hospital's CMI. Orthopedic, vascular, and general surgical cases typically have DRG RWs greater than 1.25. However, higher RWs are not apparent for urologic and gynecologic procedures (Holland 1998).

Effect of Coding Accuracy on CMI

Accurate documentation and subsequent coding also can affect a hospital's DRG CMI. Incomplete documentation or **undercoding**—missing diagnoses or procedures that should be coded—could result in a CMI lower than that warranted by the actual service intensity of the facility. It is especially crucial to code all surgical procedures accurately to assure the correct assignment of a higher weighted surgical DRG. For example, a patient with a chronic respiratory condition is intubated, placed on mechanical ventilation but then requires a temporary tracheostomy for continued ventilation. The most likely DRG assigned is DRG 542, Tracheostomy with mechanical ventilation 96 or more hours with a relative weight of 12.8719. If the coder would not have assigned the ICD-9-CM procedure code of 31.1, the DRG for this same patient would have changed to DRG 475, respiratory system diagnosis with ventilator support with a RW of 3.6091. This one procedure code accounts for more than nine points in RW.

Risk Adjustment

Often the purpose of a case-mix analysis is to identify differences among patient populations. To compare diverse populations, coding professionals must adjust the data to make a fair comparison. Such an adjustment may be referred to as a risk adjustment, a case-mix adjustment, or a severity-of-illness adjustment (Hagland 2000).

Risk adjustment is defined as "any method of comparing how sick one group of patients is, compared with another group of patients. The compared group might be defined as all patients of individual doctors, physician groups, or hospital systems, or they might be membership of different health plans" (Hagland 2000).

Risk adjustment is applied to prevent providers with more severely ill populations of patients from being unfairly penalized (Berlowitz et al. 1998). For example, physician A sees a predominantly aged population that presents with a host of chronic conditions and comorbidities. Physician B's practice is primarily composed of patients between the ages of 20 and 60 years who present for routine visits or for acute illnesses of limited duration. Accordingly, a comparison between physician A's and physician B's patient population would be unfair: Physician A's patient population consumes more resources because of the severity of their illnesses (Hagland 2000).

Age and Gender Adjustments

Typically, a managed care program provides a fixed rate per month to a primary care provider for each **capitated patient** in the practice. A capitated patient is one who, upon enrollment in a managed care program, selects his or her primary care provider. Based on this selection, the managed care program directs the fixed monthly payment to the identified primary care provider. This patient is considered a capitated patient for that primary care provider.

The managed care program may adjust the fixed rate slightly based on a patient's age and gender. This risk adjustment method has been criticized because age and gender attributes account for only 5 percent of the variability in anticipated resource use for a patient (National Health Information 1997).

Clinical Risk Adjustments

Sophisticated approaches using clinical data for risk adjustment also have been developed. For example, a method based on patient treatment episodes relies on the following clinical data:

- Physician charges
- Number of outpatient visits
- Number of inpatient days
- Prescription drug charges
- Laboratory and radiology charges

From those data, **adjustments** are made to the capitated payments of the primary care physician. The adjustments are based on the patient's severity-of-illness level (National Health Information 1997).

Situation-Specific Risk Adjustments

Risk adjustment also may be applied to specific clinical conditions and specialty providers.

Risk Adjustment for Specific Clinical Conditions

A study reviewed the medical outcomes for patients with the following specific clinical conditions:

- Blood pressure $\geq$ 160/90 mm Hg for hypertension
- Glucose level of $\geq$ 240 mg/dL for diabetes mellitus (DM)
- Hospitalization for chronic obstructive pulmonary disease (COPD)

The study revealed that exacerbation of those conditions in the prior year indicated patients with a poorly controlled disease. Such patients had more complex conditions and would be expected to have poorer clinical outcomes than patients with well-controlled diseases (Berlowitz et al. 1998).

Some criticism has been directed at disease-specific risk adjustment methods applied at the provider level. For those methods to be administered appropriately, the provider must have a sufficiently large group of patients with a particular disease. This ensures that a risk adjustment is statistically sound. Because primary care providers see a diverse population, the issue of insufficient patient volume for disease-specific risk adjustment may be more prevalent in that setting (Hofer et al. 1999).

Risk Adjustment for Specialty Providers

Situation-specific risk adjustment also may be applied to specialty providers. For example, a hospital's rate of cesarean sections is an outcome that is often analyzed from both quality and cost perspectives (Whitsel et al. 2000). **Outcomes measures** assess what happens or does not happen to a patient as a result of healthcare processes provided.

The following situations are high-risk factors for cesarean sections:

- Multiple gestation

- Malpresentation of the fetus

- Preterm labor

- No trial of labor permitted for medical reasons

In one study, the crude rate of cesarean sections for a hospital-based practice versus a community-based practice was estimated at 24.4 and 21.5 percent, respectively. However, after adjusting for the high-risk factors, the adjusted cesarean rates were 20.1 and 21.5 percent, respectively. Those percentages showed no statistically significant difference between the two practices in cesarean section rates (Lieberman et al. 1998).

Use of Comparative Data in Case-Mix Analysis

Comparative data are provided by a host of sources, including the following:

- CMS

- State-mandated databases, such as the Health Care Cost Containment Council of the Commonwealth of Pennsylvania

- Professional associations, such as the Medical Groups Management Association (MGMA)

The data sets from those sources allow individual healthcare providers or organizations to identify other organizations with similar case mixes with which they may conduct comparisons. Alternatively, those comparative data may reveal the characteristics upon which one facility varies from seemingly similar ones. In turn, those differences may promote a more focused case-mix analysis. Such an analysis can assess variances among facilities in outcomes or in patterns of resource use.

For example, figure 12.1 lists comparative data provided by CMS for home healthcare agencies. A specific facility may generate a report in which the facility's case-mix profile is compared with a national reference sample. The report provides detailed information on patient characteristics, such as the following:

- Living situation

- Activities of daily living scores

- Presence of pressure ulcers

- Presence of acute and chronic conditions

- Length of time receiving home healthcare services

The report also identifies statistically significant differences between the specific facility and the reference sample.

Figure 12.1.   Comparative data provided for CMS for home healthcare organizations

Agency Name: Faircare Home Health Services Agency ID: HHA01 Location: Anytown, USA Medicare Number: 007001 Medicaid Number: 999888001	Requested Current Period: 09/2000–08/2006 Actual Current Period: 09/2005–08/2006 Number of Cases in Current Period: 601 Number of Cases in Reference Sample: 29983 Date Report Printed: 11/30/2006

All Patients' Case-Mix Profile at Start/Resumption of Care

	Current Mean	Reference Mean	Sig.		Current Mean	Reference Mean	Sig.
Demographics				**ADL Disabilities at SOC/ROC**			
Age (average in years)	70.75	72.78	**	Grooming (0–3, scale average)	1.02	0.86	**
Gender: Female (%)	69.4%	62.9%	**	Dress upper body (0–2,			
Race: Black (%)	1.7%	10.7%	**	scale average)	0.56	0.59	
Race: White (%)	97.5%	85.5%	**	Dress lower body (0–3,			
Race: Other (%)	0.8%	3.8%	**	scale average)	1.22	1.10	*
				Bathing (0–5, scale average)	2.15	2.03	
Payment Source				Toileting (0–4, scale average)	0.63	0.57	
Any Medicare (%)	80.4%	82.6%		Transferring (0–5, scale average)	0.64	0.70	**
Any Medicaid (%)	12.9%	14.3%		Ambulation (0–5, scale average)	1.05	1.07	
Any HMO (%)	3.0%	5.8%	*	Eating (0–5, scale average)	0.33	0.32	
Medicare HMO (%)	1.3%	2.2%					
Any third party (%)	19.9%	21.9%		**ADL Status Prior to SOC/ROC**			
				Grooming (0–3, scale average)	0.66	0.52	**
Current Residence				Dress upper body (0–2,			
Own home (%)	74.7%	78.7%		scale average)	0.35	0.35	
Family member home (%)	20.5%	14.1%	**	Dress lower body (0–3,			
				scale average)	0.70	0.63	
Current Living Situation				Bathing (0–5, scale average)	1.33	1.20	
Lives alone (%)	28.6%	29.4%		Toileting (0–4, scale average)	0.39	0.38	
With family member (%)	66.7%	64.2%		Transferring (0–5, scale average)	0.38	0.44	**
With friend (%)	1.3%	1.6%		Ambulation (0–5, scale average)	0.70	0.71	
With paid help (%)	2.3%	3.3%		Eating (0–5, scale average)	0.22	0.21	
Assisting Persons				**IADL Disabilities at SOC/ROC**			
Person residing in home (%)	57.0%	55.9%		Light meal prep (0–2, scale average)	1.02	0.90	**
Person residing outside				Transportation (0–2, scale average)	1.05	0.99	**
home (%)	44.3%	53.0%	**	Laundry (0–2, scale average)	1.62	1.51	**
Paid help (%)	9.3%	14.1%	**	Housekeeping (0–4, scale average)	2.89	2.68	**
				Shopping (0–3, scale average)	2.10	2.06	
Primary Caregiver				Phone use (0–5, scale average)	0.63	0.72	
Spouse/significant other (%)	31.0%	33.6%		Mgmt. oral meds (0–2,			
Daughter/son (%)	33.0%	26.4%	**	scale average)	0.69	0.70	
Other paid help (%)	3.7%	6.1%	*				
No one person (%)	21.7%	20.2%		**IADL Status Prior to SOC/ROC**			
				Light meal prep (0–2, scale average)	0.65	0.56	*
Primary Caregiver				Transportation (0–2, scale average)	0.78	0.69	**
Assistance				Laundry (0–2, scale average)	1.10	0.96	**
Freq. of assistance (0–6,				Housekeeping (0–4, scale average)	1.93	1.73	*
scale average)	4.11	4.10		Shopping (0–3, scale average)	1.45	1.32	
				Phone use (0–5, scale average)	0.49	0.59	
Inpatient DC within				Mgmt. oral meds (0–2, scale average)	0.53	0.54	
14 Days of SOC/ROC							
From hospital (%)	69.1%	68.4%		**Respiratory Status**			
From rehab facility (%)	7.2%	6.4%		Dyspnea (0–4, scale average)	1.33	1.19	
From nursing home (%)	1.8%	3.3%					
				Therapies Received at Home			
Med. Reg. Chg. w/in				IV/infusion therapy (%)	4.3%	3.7%	
14 Days of SOC/ROC				Parenteral nutrition (%)	0.5%	0.3%	
Medical regimen change (%)	67.7%	81.2%	**	Enteral nutrition (%)	2.2%	1.8%	
Prognoses				**Sensory Status**			
Moderate recovery				Vision impairment (0–2,			
prognosis (%)	85.3%	85.9%		scale average)	0.32	0.30	
Good rehab prognosis (%)	62.6%	68.2%	*	Hearing impair (0–4, scale average)	0.38	0.45	**
				Speech/language (0–5,			
				scale average)	0.45	0.47	

(Continued on next page)

Figure 12.1. (Continued)

	Current Mean	Reference Mean	Sig.		Current Mean	Reference Mean	Sig.
Pain				**Home Care Diagnoses**			
Pain interf. w/activity (0–3, scale average)	0.95	0.98		Infectious/parasitic diseases (%)	13.0%	4.5%	**
Intractable pain (%)	14.0%	137%		Neoplasms (%)	11.8%	12.3%	
				Endocrine/nutrit./metabolic (%)	29.0%	27.1%	
Neuro/Emotional/Behavioral Status				Blood diseases (%)	8.2%	6.7%	
Moderate cognitive disability (%)	10.8%	11.9%		Mental diseases (%)	20.1%	9.9%	**
Severe confusion disability (%)	5.7%	6.9%		Nervous system diseases (%)	13.8%	9.4%	**
Severe anxiety level (%)	16.7%	11.7%	**	Circulatory system diseases (%)	61.6%	55.3%	*
Behav probs > twice a week (%)	14.0%	5.7%	**	Respiratory system diseases (%)	24.3%	19.5%	*
				Digestive system diseases (%)	13.8%	12.0%	
Integumentary Status				Genitourinary system diseases (%)	10.7%	10.4%	
Presence of wound/leson (%)	31.6%	31.2%		Pregnancy problems (%)	0.5%	0.2%	
Stasis ulcer(s) present (%)	3.7%	2.9%		Skin/subcutaneous diseases (%)	6.2%	7.4%	
Surgical wound(s) present (%)	21.1%	22.3%		Musculoskeletal system diseases (%)	26.1%	23.5%	
Pressure ulcer(s) present (%)	8.2%	5.4%		Congenital anomalies (%)	1.8%	0.8%	
Stage 2–4 ulcer(s) present (%)	6.5%	4.5%		Ill-defined conditions (%)	24.1%	19.6%	*
Stage 3–4 ulcer(s) present (%)	4.0%	1.4%		Fractures (%)	12.0%	9.1%	
				Intracranial injury (%)	0.2%	0.3%	
Elimination Status				Other injury (%)	9.5%	5.9%	**
UTI within past 14 days (%)	22.5%	9.7%	**	Iatrogenic conditions (%)	2.2%	3.1%	
Urinary incont./catheter present (%)	12.6%	16.7%	**				
Incontinent day and night (%)	10.0%	9.3%		**Length of Stay**			
Urinary catheter (%)	6.0%	5.9%		LOS until discharge (average in days)	49.52	40.35	**
Bowel incont. (0–5, scale average)	0.29	0.23		LOS from 1 to 31 days (%)	46.6%	54.0%	**
				LOS from 32 to 62 days (%)	28.0%	30.0%	
Acute Conditions				LOS from 63 to 124 days (%)	17.8%	11.8%	**
Orthopedic (%)	18.5%	21.5%		LOS more than 124 days (%)	7.7%	4.3%	**
Neurologic (%)	13.1%	9.3%	*				
Open wounds/lesions (%)	33.0%	31.8%					
Terminal condition (%)	5.7%	5.6%					
Cardiac/peripheral vascular (%)	27.0%	30.9%					
Pulmonary (%)	17.3%	16.9%					
Diabetes mellitus (%)	7.7%	8.4%					
Gastrointestinal disorder (%)	12.5%	11.5%					
Contagious/communicable (%)	9.8%	3.0%	**				
Urinary incont./catheter (%)	6.0%	8.1%					
Mental/emotional (%)	9.3%	3.1%	**				
Oxygen therapy (%)	11.2%	11.2%					
IV/infusion therapy (%)	4.3%	3.7%					
Enteral/parenteral nutrition (%)	2.7%	2.0%					
Ventilator (%)	0.0%	0.1%					
Chronic Conditions							
Dependence in living skills (%)	42.1%	35.9%	*				
Dependence in person care (%)	37.9%	22.9%	**				
Impaired ambulation/mobility (%)	14.0%	13.4%					
Eating disability (%)	4.2%	3.2%					
Urinary incontinence/catheter (%)	13.1%	13.7%					
Dependence in med. admin. (%)	44.1%	39.9%					
Chronic pain (%)	7.7%	5.7%					
Cognitive/mental/behavioral (%)	28.6%	23.5%	*				
Chronic pt. with caregiver (%)	40.4%	34.0%	**				

*The probability is 1% or less that the difference is due to chance, and 99% or more that the difference is real.
**The probability is 0.1% or less that the difference is due to chance, and 99.9% or more that the difference is real.

Conclusion

There are many approaches to and uses for case-mix data. Case-mix analyses have been used for outcomes analysis, strategic planning, budget forecasting, and staffing analysis. Moreover, results of case-mix analyses can be applied to assign patients more appropriately to disease-management programs, to provide more equitable compensation to providers, and to track quality indicators. The key factor in case-mix analysis is to select a case-mix methodology that is most appropriate to the analysis under consideration.

References and Resources

Abdelhak, M., ed. 2001. *Health Information: Management of a Strategic Resource*. Philadelphia: W.B. Saunders.

Amatayakul, Margret. 1985. *Finance Concepts for the Health Care Manager*. Chicago: American Health Information Management Association.

Arndt, M., et al. 1998. A comparison of hospital utilization by Medicaid and privately insured patients. *Medical Care Research and Review* 55(1):32–53.

Averill, R.F., et al. 2002 (January). A closer look at all-patient refined DRGs. *Journal of American Health Information Management Association* 73(1):46–50.

Berlowitz, D.R., et al. 1998. Profiling outcomes of ambulatory care: case mix affects perceived performance. *Medical Care* 36(6):928–33.

Boucher, A., et al. 2006 (July/August). Evolution of DRGs. *Journal of American Health Information Management Association* 77(7):68A–C.

Bowman, S. 2006 (July/August). New DRG system for IPPS: CMS proposes severity-adjusted DRG system based on APR DRGs. *Journal of American Health Information Management Association* 77 (7):18, 20

Carpenter, C.E., et al. 1999. Severity of illness and profitability: a patient-level analysis. *Health Services Management Research* 12(4):217–26.

Castro, A., and E. Layman. *Principles of Healthcare Reimbursement*. Chicago, IL. AHIMA, 2006.

Centers for Medicare and Medicaid Services. 2006 (May 18). Acute inpatient PPS. Available online from www.cms.hhs.gov/AcuteInpatientPPS.

Estaugh, S.R. 1998. *Health Care Finance: Cost, Productivity, & Strategic Design*. Gaithersburg, Md.: Aspen Publishers.

Hagland, M. 2000. Risk adjustment: Medicare's latest move to tinker with your income. *Medical Economics* 77(16):126–28.

Health Care Financing Administration. 1999 (November 29). *Medicare Fact Sheet: The Home Health Prospective Payment System*. Accessed on-line from http://www.hhs.hcfa.gov/medicare/hhfact.htm.

Health Care Financing Administration. 2001 (January 19). *Sample Case Mix and Adverse Event Report*. Satellite broadcast.

Hofer, T.P., et al. 1999. The unreliability of individual physician "report cards" for assessing the costs and quality of care of a chronic disease. *Journal of the American Medical Association* 281(22):2098–2105.

Holland, R.P. 1998. Case-mix index. *For the Record* (July 27):40–41, 43.

Lieberman, E., et al. 1998. Assessing the role of case mix in cesarean delivery rates. *Obstetrics and Gynecology* 92 (1):1–7.

Mueller, C. 2000. The RUG-III case-mix classification system for long-term care nursing facilities: is it adequate for nursing staffing? *Journal of Nursing Administration* 30(11):535–43.

Muldoon, J.H., J.M. Neff, and J.C. Gay. 1997. Profiling the health service needs of populations using diagnosis-based classification systems. *Journal of Ambulatory Care Management* 20(3):1–18.

National Health Information. 1997 (May). Use this statistical tool to analyze practice patterns and develop capitation rates. *Capitation Management Report,* pp. 77–81.

National Health Information. 1998 (February). Adjust utilization for case mix and make physician responsible for remaining variation. *Data Strategies & Benchmarks,* pp. 25–28.

Peabody, J.W., and J. Luck. 1998. How far down the managed care road? A comparison of primary care outpatient services in a veterans affairs medical center and a capitated multispecialty group practice. *Archives of Internal Medicine* 158(21):2291–2299.

Plomann, M.P. 1984. Understanding case-mix classification systems. *Topics in Health Record Management* 4(3):77–87.

Tesio, L., A. Bellafa, and F.P. Franchignoni. 2000. Case-mix in rehabilitation: a useful way to achieve a specific goal. *Clinical Rehabilitation* 14(4):112–14.

3M Health Information Systems. 2005. *Diagnosis Related Groups Version 18.0: Definitions Manual* (prepared under Center for Medicare and Medicaid Services [formerly HCFA] Contract 500-99-0003).

3M Health Information Systems. 3M APR-DRG classification system. Available online at www.3m.com/us/healthcare/his/products/coding/refined_drg.jhtml

Whitsel, A.I., et al. 2000. Adjustment for case mix in comparisons of cesarean delivery rates: university versus community hospitals in Vermont. *American Journal of Obstetrics and Gynecology* 183(5):170–75.

Zaslavsky, A.M., et al. 2000. Impact of sociodemographic case mix on the HEDIS measures of health plan quality. *Medical Care* 38(10):981–92.

Part IV

Future Considerations

Chapter 13

The Changing Landscape of the Professional Coding Community

Rita A. Scichilone, MHSA, RHIA, CCS, CCS-P, CHC

As conditions in the healthcare industry have become more challenging, many positions within the health information management (HIM) profession have evolved, making management of the coding process a dynamic undertaking. In a variety of ways, coding professionals continue to serve important roles in a rapidly evolving workplace with more technology and automation of data management possible than ever before.

Forces inside and outside the profession have profoundly affected the work at hand. In fact, some find it challenging to navigate the evolving changes (Scichilone 2004). To be effective, those who manage clinical data in healthcare organizations must recognize and make use of new tools and technologies. Along with rapid changes in coding system requirements there is a major revolution in healthcare delivery systems and claims processing that affect the administrative use of code sets.

This chapter focuses on how new tools and technologies are changing the roles of coding professionals and expanding employment opportunities for HIM professionals within the healthcare industry.

In Search of the "Good Record"

"The only fee for which the doctor pays for the use of a thoroughly equipped and serviced workshop, the hospital, is the good medical record," wrote Betty Wood McNabb (1958, 8). Coding professionals have always had to contend with records that are not "good" for optimal data capture, and this is still true. Healthcare organizations still strive to paint an accurate clinical picture from code assignments for external agencies and internal use. Coding professionals work with good records of bad patient care, bad records of good care, bad records of bad care, and, most often, excellent records of excellent care. The form and formats of the records are different than they were in 1958, and keeping up with changes still ahead will keep coding managers busy for quite awhile.

Clinical coding in the United States continues to be a process of piecing together data elements to create a consistent and uniform data set that accurately represents health services. At one time, the uniform data set was the CMS-1500 or the UB-92 (CMS-1450) form used for health insurance processing. The Health Insurance Portability and Accountability Act (HIPAA) of 1996 created standards for the electronic transmission of health data that transcend former requirements and further refine data elements and data requirements. In many ways, the contemporary mandates and the adoption of voluntary standards create a better process for a more consistent application of coding and reporting guidance.

McNabb warned prospective coding professionals that the "career you have chosen is a career; it is complex, responsible, and professional in caliber—you are not a clerk. Decide to learn as much as you can about medical record science, and you will find every medical record librarian, everywhere, ready to help you" (1958, 20). HIM and clinical coding professionals are still distinguished by their dedication and willingness to innovate and supply the industry with high-quality data. As a group, they have developed unique skills to meet the specific requirements of their jobs.

Transition of Coding Education and Employment Potential

In the past, many coders were trained on the job. Even though coding education moved from the workplace to the academic setting more than 30 years ago, the on-the-job training process continues even now because of a continuous influx of new technology and tools and a shortage of qualified coding professionals. According to the Bureau of Labor Statistics, of the top 10 occupations expected to show the strongest growth in jobs by 2014, eight of them are in the healthcare field (BLS 2006). From 2004 to 2014, medical records and health information technicians are expected to exhibit a 27 percent increase. According to the BLS web site, "technicians with a strong background in medical coding will be in particularly high demand. Changing government regulations and the growth of managed care have increased the amount of paperwork involved in filing insurance claims. Additionally, healthcare facilities are having difficulty attracting qualified workers, primarily because of the lack of both formal training programs and sufficient resources to provide on-the-job training for coders. Job opportunities may be especially good for coders employed through temporary help agencies or by professional services firms" (BLS 2006).

In 2002, the American Health Information Management Association (AHIMA) commissioned an independent national workforce research study from the Center for Health Workforce Studies (CHWS), State University of New York at Albany. The AHIMA member survey aimed to gather information about the membership of AHIMA and about the HIM workforce.

More than 10,000 surveys were sent to a random sample of AHIMA members, with responses received from 5,333 members, representing a 55 percent response rate. Almost 30 percent of the respondents identified themselves as being coders or clinical data specialists.

Among the coders who responded, more than 60 percent worked in hospital inpatient settings, 18 percent in hospital outpatient facilities, and 7 percent in clinicians' offices. According to this research, 58 percent of American coders had an associate degree, 22 percent held a bachelor's degree, 18 percent had no further education beyond high school, and 1 percent attained postgraduate qualifications. Nearly 60 percent of AHIMA-credentialed coders held an RHIT, another 14 percent held an RHIT with mastery-level coding credentials (such as CCS or CCS-P), 16 percent held an RHIA, and 9 percent held a CCS/CCS-P only. The average annual salary of clinical coders was approximately $37,000, with coders with an RHIT and mastery-level coding credentials attaining the highest average annual salary of more than $40,000.

In 2006, AHIMA surveyed employers of coding professionals and of the 1,105 responses to the question, "Are you currently recruiting for clinical coding positions?" more than 29% said "yes." Employers indicated that they are looking for experienced, highly skilled individuals to fill the vacancies. This survey of salary levels shows that income rises with experience and remains consistent with the 2002 workforce data. Almost half (49%) of the respondents indicate coders with 2 to 3 years of experience have a salary between $37,000 and $40,000 per year (Scichilone 2006).

Health Information Technology Programs

The traditional 2-year program awarding an associate's degree in health information technology (HIT) has produced many clinical coders. In the past, most graduates of HIT programs accepted coding positions in hospitals. Currently, HIT graduates have diverse career opportunities, and fewer of them are interested in jobs that are strictly limited to hospital coding. Complicating the situation, many HIT programs are struggling to fill their traditional day-program enrollment. To be more attractive to working individuals, many HIT programs have transitioned to evening and weekend programs. Yet, the demand for coders still exceeds the supply of HIT graduates. In the 2002 AHIMA survey, approximately 96 percent of American coders reported that there were some or many jobs available in their regions, so those within the profession are challenged to keep qualified personnel in these positions. The 2006 AHIMA survey with 1,106 responses revealed that more than 58% had open coding positions to fill within the past year. The shortage of experienced coders is a wake-up call for the profession to do a better job at recruitment. The leading response from the 2006 question about the reason for the vacancies indicated that "no experienced coding professionals have applied" so employers are still very interested in job experience before hire (Scichilone 2006).

Many HIT programs have added 1-year certificate programs in clinical coding and/or reimbursement. A 1-year program usually consists of 24 to 30 semester hours and focuses on the knowledge and skills required for entry-level coding in both hospital and physician-office settings. Although programs of this type are new, they have increased the supply of clinical coders ready to enter the marketplace. However, employers may not perceive these individuals to be potential coding employees because most employers want coders to be "certified." AHIMA offers three categories of coding credentials: certified coding associate (CCA), certified coding specialist (CCS), and certified coding specialist-physician based (CCS-P). For the specialist credentials it is recommended that candidates have several years of experience before attempting either examination. The CCA credential offers the graduates of coding certificate programs or individuals with some, but not significant, experience an avenue for obtaining a respected credential at the entry level. Some employers understand that the new certificate graduate will require time to prepare for specialist examinations and have placed new coders with the CCA credential in "junior coder" or "coding assistant" positions. This practice enables the employer to take advantage of the new coder's knowledge and skills and at the same time gives the new coder time to gain the coding experience necessary to pass the mastery-level examination for CCS and CCS-P.

Internet-Based and On-Site Training

Because the academic setting has not met the needs of all employers, many have been forced to look for alternatives. Many organizations now provide Internet-based training to help employees develop skills in coding systems. In this way, persons with clinical backgrounds in radiology, laboratory, nursing, and other areas are learning how to assign codes. This may seem to be a return to the early days of on-the-job training for coders. However, many organizations have recognized the advantage of a structured training program and have worked with local colleges and remote companies to bring that training on-site to their facility or to the computer desktops of the employees in remote locations. Because of the growing market for coding and billing support across all healthcare settings, a variety of "boot camp" programs and other types of short-cut programs have arisen that are attractive to many individuals looking for a quick way to get into the profession. Managers of the coding function have the responsibility to evaluate graduates of these programs carefully to make sure they are prepared for the discipline and complexity of the job and possess the knowledge base required to perform coding at an acceptable rate of accuracy.

Boom Times for Coders

The expansion of prospective payment systems (PPSs) from acute and psychiatric care hospitals into skilled nursing facility care, long-term care hospitals, rehabilitation services, home health agencies, hospital outpatient services, and physician professional services has created a universal theme of "what you code is what you get"—in reimbursement, that is. All government-sponsored healthcare reimbursement is now linked to the reported clinical codes that describe the services and conditions of the encounter or stay.

In the hospital setting, coders traditionally have been employed in the HIM department where traditional medical records were filed. As more information is stored in computers and electronic health records are available, many hospitals are decentralizing clinical coding in an effort to locate coders closer to patients so that health information can be translated into diagnosis and procedure codes for immediate use. Coders now work in emergency departments, primary care clinics, admitting and scheduling departments, patient accounting or business offices, and off-site patient care centers. From these settings, coders can have coded data ready for billing as well as for use by their healthcare facility for future patient encounters. Rather than working from paper records, the coding process in an electronic health record system requires coders to view documentation on a computer screen and it is commonplace for coders to work remotely from patient care sites, or even from home using secure transfer methods via the Internet.

Healthcare facilities other than hospitals are hiring clinical coders for their internal data needs. Home health agencies and physician group practices have been the most active in recruiting and hiring clinical coders. These facilities have come to understand the importance of coded data to their financial bottom line.

Other organizations that use clinical data also are recognizing the value of clinical coders and are starting to recruit them. Such organizations include coding software developers and marketers, health insurance companies, and pharmaceutical companies. With the new demand for coders outside the traditional hospital setting, the boom time for coders continues.

New Roles, New Opportunities in an E-HIM World

As the healthcare industry moves away from paper records to electronic systems, HIM professionals are the best candidates for the emerging data management and reimbursement coordinator roles. They possess the knowledge of disease processes and reimbursement principles and have been trained in documentation requirements in a variety of media. The role of the coding professional is no longer that of literal translator of diagnostic statements into codes. The coding professional's new and widening role is that of clinical coding advisor for correct code selection based on clinical evidence in the health record. This new role is expanding with the implementation of natural language processing (NLP) systems that automatically assign clinical codes to text documents Even though these NLP systems are now emerging and taking over some of the manual processes that previously required a coder's skill, HIM professionals are needed in oversight and editing roles. Professional insight is required to ensure that the software is interpreting the source of the data appropriately and that the resulting code assignments are accurate and complete. Clinical terminology use is expanding beyond administrative code sets used for claims reporting and this creates another emerging role for managing use of controlled medical vocabulary and terminologies in an electronic environment and the maps that link one terminology to another for specific use cases.

Technology has changed coding practice and secondary clinical data use significantly. At one time, a few reference sources kept coders current with coding principles and reimbursement requirement. Now coders must use a variety of resources just to keep abreast of constant changes in reporting guidelines, reimbursement methods, advanced therapies, and new health conditions. There will be a time when coders will no longer use any type of "coding manual." Instead, they will download code sets from an Internet site. Because coding systems of the future are expected to be much larger in size and complexity than can be contained in book form, computer skills and Internet data retrieval skills are essential, and knowledge and management of the "maps" between systems may be an addition to job descriptions.

Analysis and use of coded data have revolutionized the industry by providing consistent and reliable clinical data that are accessible in electronic formats. Coding professionals have learned how to be real "detectives," finding data within health records that legitimately improve reimbursement by DRG, APC, ASC, or RBRVS. Coders analyze abnormal findings, medications, and surgical therapies so that complications, comorbidities, or valid operating room procedures overlooked by a physician in a final diagnostic statement can be used to optimize hospital reimbursement. They also apply guidelines to physician documentation for professional services so they can assign the appropriate level of service or validate levels assigned by physicians, thus helping physicians avoid audits and overpayment.

In the 21st century, diagnosis and procedure code numbers became the universal product code of the healthcare service marketplace. Coding professionals can expect coding systems to become increasingly sophisticated as they evolve to take advantage of new informatics tools. Use of a universal procedural coding system will likely replace the dual reporting now common for hospital outpatients. It is inevitable that the current systems, which were developed in a pre-electronic age, will not endure much longer in their current form. Initiatives such as the National Health Information Network, Regional Health Information Organizations, HL7 messaging standards, and Consolidated Health Informatics national standards will advance the use of a variety of controlled medical vocabulary tools, including SNOMED CT, to serve an industry poised for an electronic revolution. Rapid movement towards creating a language of health data exchange is creating a new framework for health care delivery systems to consider.

The use of ICD-10-CM is expected to be adopted in a few years to create a more universal language that can be used throughout the international community for mortality and morbidity reporting on a global scale. Classifications systems and terminologies used as data structures in electronic health records will continue to be harmonized through standards adoption as technology enables adoption. A new procedural coding system, ICD-10-PCS, is expected to be introduced for hospital inpatient reporting in the United States when ICD-10-CM is introduced. As political unrest unfolds and threats of bioterrorism emerge, a more sophisticated public health system will require greater uniformity and granularity in clinical data reporting than the current systems allow.

A Crystal Ball for Coding

Seven years ago an AHIMA Coding Futures Task Force was convened to study how several dominant forces in the area of medical vocabularies and enabling technologies could affect the domain of coding practice. **Enabling technologies** produce innovative devices that facilitate data gathering or information processing in ways not previously possible. For example, a handheld computer that works with a wireless network enables clinicians to collect health data at the point of care in a new manner that is more efficient than dictation, transcription, and filing pages in a paper health record. Composed of nationally recognized authorities in the development of medical vocabularies, standards development, and use of coded data, the task force looked beyond current frames of reference to illuminate what the future will likely hold. A complete report of its findings was published in the January 2000 issue of the *Journal of AHIMA* (Johns 2000). All current and future coding professionals and managers should read this important information to provide a foundation for what is happening today.

The task force evaluated the effect of the following three forces on coding:

- The evolution and growth of medical vocabularies

- The development and application of information and enabling technologies for coded data

- The emergence of the information economy

To assess the combined effects of these forces, the task force used a process called scenario planning to create stories about the future based on environmental variables. The results are a provocative collection of scenarios about the future of the coding industry. These scenarios forecast changes in the way HIM professionals will work with data, technology, standards, and patients. The task force also developed recommendations for the best actions for HIM professionals and AHIMA to take in the future so that the profession benefits no matter which scenario proves to be true.

The task force's crystal ball yielded four scenarios that developed around the key factors of technology, standards development, the cost-driven environment, and consumer demands.

Rapid Changes in Technology

The first scenario is dominated by rapid changes in technology that include a better technology infrastructure and the development of electronic health record systems. In this scenario, forward-thinking organizations anticipate technological breakthroughs and accordingly reengineer to capitalize on them. Conversely, professional organizations that do not anticipate, shape, and stake their positions feel the aftershocks of technological change. It is interesting to watch the emergence of computer-assisted coding software use and a 2005 survey confirms a trend toward wider acceptance of process changes that automate the coding process (Frieman 2006).

Standards Development

The second scenario is dominated by development and implementation of standards—a "virtual" approach to data management. Organizations that cling to inefficient practices and have not developed methods for data and knowledge management are left behind. Similarly, professions that have not transformed themselves and are overly invested in old conceptual frames of reference suffer. Data mapping is an essential component of standards building to facilitate health information exchange, so "HIM professionals not involved with data mapping now will be soon" (McBride 2006). Terminology standards in electronic health records including the adoption of the standard reference terminology SNOMED CT enable maps between clinical data expressions (source) and administrative code sets (targets), so there are increasing demands for support personnel and managers who understand how the systems interact and how to assure data quality when data maps are used.

Coding professionals are also called upon to evaluate clinical data management systems in many organizations and standards adoption is creating a strong case for data quality management and structure data submission standards. Data dictionaries are used as building blocks that support communication across business processes in an electronic world and coding professionals should understand there purpose and how they function. The *Journal of AHIMA* February 2006 issue includes a practice brief with Guidelines for Developing a Data Dictionary that is helpful for coding managers to better understand its role in contemporary health systems.

Cost-Driven Environment

In the third scenario, cost drives the healthcare industry. Financial, consumer, and professional interests clash over new, cost-efficient delivery models that have little or no room for negotiation with payers and regulators. Algorithmic technologies for interpreting coded data support best practices and compliance with fraud and abuse regulations. Failure to deploy such technology sounds alarms. For all parties, hindsight reveals that misplaced and misordered priorities resulted in costly mistakes. In 2005, AHIMA conducted research for the Office of the National Coordinator for Health Information Technology concerning the potential of computer-assisted coding systems to enhance antifraud activities that impact the cost of healthcare services payment. "The impact of fraud can be mitigated, however, with appropriate technology, fraud prevention and detection processes, and ongoing educational efforts" illustrating that this projection was on target. The 2005 research reports are available from the Office of the National Coordinator at http://www.hhs.gov/healthit/documents/AutomaticCodingReport.pdf and http://www.hhs.gov/healthit/documents/ReportOnTheUse.pdf (FORE and University of Pittsburgh 2005; FORE 2005).

Consumer Demand for Information and Quality

In the final scenario, a consumer demand for better information and a better quality of life dominates. Healthcare yields to the preferences and purchasing decisions of millions of people. In this scenario, what originally was a private fiduciary relationship between doctors and patients now looks and feels more like a relationship between suppliers and customers at multiple levels. Only organizations that listen, hear, and respond to their customers' collective voice survive. There is increased interest in personal electronic health records and the coding profession has a role to play, as healthcare system users take a more active role in managing their information and healthcare transactions. Increasingly, there are more healthcare services using coding systems than ever before, including code assignment for services such as medication therapy management services used by pharmacists.

Preparations for the Future

What do these scenarios tell about the future of coding practice? In a sense, they offer a mixed bag. On the one hand, the convergence of forces and major trends in technology, medical vocabularies, and the information economy offers many new opportunities for HIM professionals who specialize in coding. On the other hand, these opportunities will only be available to those who are prepared to develop and assess technology at deeper levels. Those who wish to take advantage of these opportunities must develop new skills, especially in the development of areas such as:

- **Algorithmic translation:** This process involves the use of algorithms to translate or map clinical nomenclatures among each other or to map natural language to a clinical nomenclature or vice versa (Johns 2000, 33).

- **Concept representation:** A concept is a unit of knowledge created by a unique combination of characteristics. The SNOMED-CT is a clinical terminology based on clinical concepts represented by unique numbers. Concept representation is a methodology that has been used in the construction of the Unified Medical Language System (UMLS) developed by the National Library of Medicine (Johns 2000, 33).

- **Vocabulary mapping processes:** These processes occur especially among clinical nomenclatures and reimbursement methods. A clinical vocabulary is a dictionary containing the terminology of a particular subject field. A vocabulary mapping process would connect or cross-walk one clinical vocabulary to another.

According to the task force, in the future, the critical shortage of individuals to assign diagnostic and procedural codes will all but disappear thanks to the development of enabling technologies, computer-assisted or automatic coding systems, and the maturity of natural language processing. Instead, an acute urgency will arise for leadership in the creation, maintenance, and oversight of the vocabulary mapping process. Many individuals will be needed to monitor the output of these processes and to ensure overall data quality. Individuals with the knowledge and skills to position themselves as authorities on the cutting edge of healthcare **nosology** (the classification of diseases) also will be needed.

Ultimately, the task force's findings show that the HIM profession must define itself in an open-ended way to take full advantage of opportunities in the electronic world. First and foremost, HIM professionals who specialize in coding must define themselves as information managers with a focus on data as opposed to records. According to the task force, HIM professionals must position themselves as visible agents of change in coded data activities and in furthering new methods of concept representation, extraction, and use of clinical data.

The academic preparation and training for coding professionals must prepare them to go beyond the assignment of diagnostic and procedural codes from a code book. With the implementation of advanced technologies and informatics tools common in electronic health records and transactions, the code assignment will occur through internal software processes subject to validation. HIM professions who manage coding must be trained and/or retrained in **coding formalization principles** broader than ICD and CPT codes as a number of special purpose terminologies are used in contemporary systems. Coding formalization refers to the transition from analysis of health records to a process that involves data analysis using more sophisticated tools such as algorithmic translation, concept representation, and vocabulary or reimbursement mapping. Skills and knowledge in the creation, development, and research validation of new coding systems are premium competencies currently sought by the marketplace. See figure 13.1 for a sample job description for a clinical data manager.

A New Trajectory of Practice

Having analyzed the possible scenarios, the 1999 task force offered insights about factors that were expected to have a direct and lasting impact on HIM professionals who specialize

Figure 13.1. Sample job description: Clinical data manager

Build your career and experience the advantages that come with working for the "World's Most Admired Company" (Fortune Magazine) offering significant opportunities for growth and career advancement! Ensure the delivery of accurate, flexible, and evidence-based clinical decision support tools used by physicians at the point of care and manage data administration for secondary clinical data reporting requirements.

Open Position Title: Clinical Data Manager

Business:	**Salary (range):** $40K–$118K
Subbusiness:	**Currency:** US Dollar
Reports To	**Location:** Anywhere
Career Band:	**Relocation:** No
EEO Type (Exempt/Non-Ex): Exempt	**# Openings:** 1 **Shift:** Day

Add/Replacement:

Primary Responsibilities include:

- Clinical content oversight—cataloging of all encounter forms, functions, clinical lists and other content that contain medical information that may require correction and updates to stay current and enhance patient safety
- Track medical knowledge sources to be sure that guidelines are kept current and suggest improvements in the current approach to this discipline.
- Update and monitor XXXXX Protocols and other clinical recommendations made by the base EHR and enhance to support quality patient care.
- Provide consulting to support a robust workflow for administrative coding.
- Work directly with customers to analyze workflows, identify requirements and design clinical content solutions for a variety of specialties

Additional responsibilities may include:

- Monitor and research the application of documentation templates to monitor data integrity
- Monitor third-party sources of clinical reference data (i.e. medications, ICD and CPT codes, formularies) and recommend new sources or improvements
- Promote the development of an easy to deploy demo and training system including realistic use cases and demo data that best displays the capabilities of the system

Qualifications/Requirements: (Basic Qualifications): These elements are required to perform the role. Any candidate who does not possess the basic criteria will be screened out of the candidate pool. Please ensure that your criteria are specific but be careful not to disqualify desirable candidates.

- Credentials, RHIA, RN, NP, PA, MD or other healthcare discipline with foundational knowledge of clinical data standards and CCS or CCS-P certification.
- Requires a minimum of 2 years of direct work experience in an ambulatory or inpatient clinical setting with data administration responsibilities
- Working knowledge of data content and data standards used in electronic health records

Desired: (Desired Characteristics)

- Experience in clinical coding guidelines, use case and performance measurement including documentation requirements and regulatory compliance
- Excellent interpersonal, communication, and presentation skills
- Demonstrated quality in written communication
- Basic skills in data quality analytics and tools
- Experience writing ad hoc SQL queries
- Proficient developer of clinical encounter forms and reports used in clinical data management
- Familiarity with computer-assisted coding software applications

in coding. The most fundamental insight is that merging external forces are producing a new trajectory for HIM practice. This "trajectory" is a way of describing a fundamental change from a records management focus to a data management focus. The trajectory depends on a number of corresponding critical initiatives that are unfolding as this decade passes its midpoint.

The task force projected that the new trajectory of practice would affect numerous parts of the coding picture in the following ways:

- Innovative methods of professional development training and retraining: The evolution of HIM practice is producing a critical need for new training (and retraining) of HIM professionals who carry out coding functions. At each level of practice, new tasks along the growth trajectory must be identified, and opportunities for special skills training must be developed for newly and rapidly evolving roles. Coders must be prepared to develop and assess technology at deeper levels than they currently can, especially in areas of data security, data structures, system implementation, data integrity, process flow, information modeling, and concept representation. **Information modeling** involves the use of clinical code sets with application software to create information meaningful to the end user. Concept representation is a methodology being used in the construction of medical language systems.

- Certification title changes: As the trajectory continues to move away from records management, current certification titles must change to reflect the movement toward data and information management. AHIMA's 1999 House of Delegates approved the new credential titles of registered health information administrator (RHIA) and registered health information technician (RHIT), which replace RRA and ART, respectively. With this step, the profession has already recognized the new trajectory of practice. Mastery level certifications such as CCS and CCS-P will begin to reflect new practice roles as job analyses indicate new skills and job requirements.

- A need for leadership in standards development: To be a valued and competitive player in the new roles, HIM professionals who specialize in clinical data management must expand their participation in standards and vocabulary groups. The merging of external forces will create new roles, but these roles will require a broader and deeper knowledge in areas of information modeling and concept representation. HIM professionals must be actively involved in this process and also must contribute to the development of nomenclatures.

- An opportunity for leadership in compliance activities and ethics: Coding professionals should take advantage of opportunities created by regulatory mandates and organizational compliance programs. Ethical practices and the integrity of patient and coded data are major areas of future practice that coding professionals should aggressively pursue.

- An opportunity for leadership in the creation, maintenance, and oversight of the vocabulary mapping process: Coders should be educationally prepared to go well beyond assigning diagnostic and procedural codes. In the future, leadership in the creation, maintenance, and oversight of the vocabulary mapping process will be critical. For example, HIM professionals who specialize in coding should be leading enterprise-wide efforts to design and implement systems that provide a set of nonoverlapping controlled vocabularies that together cover the concepts needed to document patient problems and the process of care.

New Learning Tactics: Capitalizing on Opportunities

Because data management has traditionally been an information systems function, HIM professionals who specialize in coding now must emphasize their unique contributions to this area. In that way, they can maintain and create new value for their role in the marketplace. How can HIM professionals do this? Capitalizing on current and future opportunities requires:

- Special skills training and retraining in newly and rapidly evolving roles

- A long-term strategy for credential management that reflects a general core of competency complemented with subspecializations

- Expanded leadership and volunteer activity in standards and classification systems development and in oversight of vocabulary mapping processes

- Transformational organizational change that makes AHIMA's organizational structure and its component parts sufficiently nimble to provide new services and products ahead of the curve

Coding specialists can prepare to capitalize on these opportunities by applying lifelong learning strategies and updating their knowledge and skills in technology application and healthcare vocabularies. Some specific informal learning tactics include:

- Keeping current on technology and vocabulary issues such as those covered in the *Journal of AHIMA*

- Expanding their knowledge of medical vocabularies beyond ICD and CPT by becoming knowledgeable about the content, construction, use, and development of healthcare vocabularies. More than 100 vocabularies are currently contained in the National Library of Medicine's Unified Medical Language System (UMLS) *Metathesaurus.*

- Widening their reading horizons through key sources of information, such as the *Journal of the American Health Informatics Association, Proceedings of the American Medical Informatics Association, Nursing Informatics, Perspectives in Health Information Management,* and *Methods of Information in Medicine*

- Attending conferences and symposia that focus on medical vocabulary issues and terminology tools

- Visiting the National Library of Medicine's Web site at http://www.nlm.nih.gov and investigating issues related to development and use of the Unified Medical Language System

- Updating their knowledge and skills by reading books devoted to topics related to nosology, technology, and healthcare vocabularies and terminologies

- Participating in national and international clinical data management, and/or vocabulary and terminology standards groups

No one is able to predict the future due to the rapid changes made possible by information technology. However, one thing is clear: For HIM professionals who specialize in coding, the future will be very different from the present. Those who succeed will be those who are prepared—and the time for preparation is now.

What the Future Holds

The use of handheld computers and "palm" devices has already shown coding managers a glimpse of the health record of the future. Some insurance companies now market personal health records for consumers in the form of smart cards. Smart cards provide healthcare professionals with the information needed to provide appropriate healthcare services and to receive the appropriate reimbursement according to the patient's/card carrier's health insurance plan. Can it be long before Medicare adopts this type of system to simplify coverage and better serve its beneficiaries?

The health record of the future increasingly will be an audio or video image rather than a text-based account of care. These dynamic media will provide more useful healthcare observations. However, the clinical data specialist will continue to be an essential member of the healthcare team—managing and displaying clinical data sets, evaluating clinical trends, and ensuring data quality. The clinical skills that currently serve coding professionals will continue to serve them in this new role. By determining to learn all they can, coding professionals will remain gainfully employed for years to come.

Technology now makes it possible to perform coding from remote locations—the "coding-from-home" phenomenon is in full swing. Imaging and Internet-based platforms are now commonplace for moving health information to knowledge workers for analysis, whether it is across the street or across the ocean. Just as transcription is increasingly outsourced to companies providing specialized service under contract, so also are coding and other forms of data management being performed more often in this manner rather than only within HIM departments.

The sheer complexity of the systems required to manage these new processes will keep clinical data system managers in demand well into the middle of the 21st century. Although the coding systems will change and the technology will support better ways of collecting, storing, and reporting clinical data, the future is very bright for roles that require managing clinical data and vocabulary use.

"Due to the complexities involving coding and reimbursement, physicians, allied health professionals, reimbursement specialists, and third-party payers become focused on that 'piece' of the healthcare environment in which they directly work," wrote Denise Stace-Naughton, RHIA, CPC (1999, xiii). There are many pieces in the puzzle called healthcare delivery. Management of the clinical coding process is an essential part of the puzzle. For that reason, teams of dedicated HIM professionals will still be needed to deliver consistent, accurate results that satisfy the requirements for clinical information in a form easily digested by information systems and data warehouses.

Conclusion

Effective Management of Coding Services was intended to explore what is currently known about clinical coding models, the coding function, and the professional practice aspect of clinical code assignment and reporting. The authors have included material about related issues such as process improvement, quality control, documentation, and compliance monitoring. They hope this textbook will be a useful tool for managing data systems and clinical code sets and the personnel who use them well into the future.

References and Resources

Bureau of Labor Statistics, U.S. Department of Labor. 2006 (Aug. 4). *Occupational Outlook Handbook, 2006-07 Edition.* Medical Records and Health Information Technicians section Available online from http://www.bls.gov/oco/ocos103.htm#outlook.

Foundation for Research and Education. 2005 (Sept. 30). Report on the Use of Health Information Technology to Enhance and Expand Health Care Anti-Fraud Activities. Prepared for the Office of the National Coordinator, U.S. Department of Health and Human Services, contract number: HHSP23320054100EC.

Foundation for Research and Education and the University of Pittsburgh. 2005 (July 11). *Automated Coding Software: Development and Use to Enhance AntiFraud Activities.* Prepared for the Office of the National Coordinator, U.S. Department of Health and Human Services, contract number: HHSP23320054100EC.

Frieman, B. 2006 (April). Coding technology today. *Journal of American Health Information Management Association* 77(4):66–68.

Johns, M. 2000 (January). A crystal ball for coding. *Journal of American Health Information Management Association* 71(1):26–33.

HIM professionals vital in transition to e-HIM. 2003 (September). *AHIMA Advantage* 7(6).

McBride, S., R. Gilder, R. Davis, and S. Fenton. 2006 (February). Data mapping. *Journal of American Health Information Management Association* 77(2):44–77

McNabb, B.W. 1958. *Medical Record Procedures in Small Hospitals.* Chicago: Physicians' Record Co.

MacKenzie, S. 2003 (July/August). Coders today: Where they work, what they earn—Work force study finds credentials influence setting, salary. *Journal of American Health Information Management Association* 74(7):20–27.

Scichilone, R.A. 2006 (September). Coders wanted, experience required. *Journal of American Health Information Management Association* 77(8):46, 48.

Scichilone, R. 2004 (June). Navigating your HIM career: Beware of churns and roundabouts. *Journal of American Health Information Management Association* 75(6):68–70.

Stace-Naughton, D. 1999. *Coding and Reimbursement: The Complete Picture within Health Care.* Chicago: American Hospital Association Press.

Glossary

Abstracting: 1. The process of extracting information from a document to create a brief summary of a patient's illness, treatment, and outcome   2. The process of extracting elements of data from a source document or database and entering them into an automated system

Accounts Not Selected for Billing Report: A daily financial report used to track the many reasons why accounts may not be ready for billing [*See* **Discharged not final billed (DNFB) report**]

Accounts receivable (A/R): Records of the payments owed to the organization by outside entities such as third-party payers and patients

Activity date or status: The element in the chargemaster that indicates the most recent activity of an item

Adjusted clinical groups (ACGs): A classification that groups individuals according to resource requirements and reflects the clinical severity differences among the specific groups; formerly called ambulatory care groups

Adjustment: The process of writing off an unpaid balance on a patient account to make the account balance

Aggregate data: Data extracted from individual health records and combined to form deidentified information about groups of patients that can be compared and analyzed

Algorithmic translation: A process that involves the use of algorithms to translate or map clinical nomenclatures among each other or to map natural language to a clinical nomenclature or vice versa

Ambulatory surgical center (ASC): Under Medicare, an outpatient surgical facility that has its own national identifier; is a separate entity with respect to its licensure, accreditation, governance, professional supervision, administrative functions, clinical services, record keeping, and financial and accounting systems; has as its sole purpose the provision of services in connection with surgical procedures that do not require inpatient hospitalization; and meets the conditions and requirements set forth in the Medicare Conditions of Participation

Assumption coding: The practice of assigning codes on the basis of clinical signs, symptoms, test findings, or treatments without supporting physician documentation

Atlas System: A severity-of-illness system commonly used in the United States and Canada

Bad debt: The receivables of an organization that are uncollectible

Benchmarking survey: A survey in which a healthcare facility compares elements of its operation with those of similar healthcare facilities

Bill drop: The point at which a bill is completed and electronically or manually sent to the payer

Bill hold period: The span of time during which a bill is suspended in the billing system awaiting late charges, diagnosis and/or procedure codes, insurance verification, or other required information

Brainstorming: A group problem-solving technique that involves the spontaneous contribution of ideas from all members of the group

Capitated patient: A patient enrolled in a managed care program that pays a fixed monthly payment to the patient's identified primary care provider

Carve-outs: Applicable services that are cut out of the contract and paid at a different rate

Case mix: A description of a patient population based on any number of specific characteristics, including age, gender, type of insurance, diagnosis, risk factors, treatment received, and resources used

Case-mix index (CMI):   The average relative weight of all cases treated at a given facility or by a given physician, which reflects the resource intensity or clinical severity of a specific group in relation to the other groups in the classification system; calculated by dividing the sum of the weights of diagnosis-related groups for patients discharged during a given period divided by the total number of patients discharged

Case-mix system: A system for grouping cases that are clinically similar and ordinarily consume similar resources; used to provide information about the types of patients treated by a facility

Cash versus revenue: The ratio of charges (revenue) for goods and services to the actual reimbursement (cash) based on a percentage of those charges

Charge code: The numerical identification of a service or supply that links the item to a particular department within the charge description master

Charge description master (CDM):   *See* **chargemaster**

Chargemaster: A financial management form that contains information about the organization's charges for the healthcare services it provides to patients

Chargemaster coordinator: The person responsible for the chargemaster document, mentoring other staff, and assisting each department with its annual line-item updates

Charges: The dollar amounts actually billed by healthcare facilities for specific services or supplies and owed by patients

Classification system: 1. A system for grouping similar diseases and procedures and organizing related information for easy retrieval   2. A system for assigning numeric or alphanumeric code numbers to represent specific diseases and/or procedures

Clean claim: A claim that has all the billing and coding information correct and can be paid by the payer the first time it is submitted

Clinic cases: Patient encounters that take place on an outpatient basis in a clinic within a teaching environment

Clinical abstract: A computerized file that summarizes patient demographics and other information, including reason for admission, diagnoses, procedures, physician information, and any additional information deemed pertinent by the facility

Clinical terminology: A set of standardized terms and their synonyms that can be mapped to broader classifications; *See* **nomenclature**

Code look-up: A computer file with all of the indexes and codes recorded on magnetic disk or CD-ROM

Coder: A person assigned solely to the function of coding

Coder/biller: A person in an ambulatory care or a physician office setting who is generally responsible for processing the superbill

Coding formalization principles: A set of principles referring to the transition of coding from analysis of records to a process that involves data analysis using more sophisticated tools (for example, algorithmic translation, concept representation, or vocabulary or reimbursement mapping)

Comorbidity: A medical condition that coexists with the primary cause for hospitalization and affects the patient's treatment and length of stay

Complication: A medical condition that arises during an inpatient hospitalization (for example, a postoperative wound infection)

Concept representation: A methodology used in the construction of the Unified Medical Language System (UMLS) developed by the National Library of Medicine

Concurrent coding: A type of coding that takes place while the patient is still in the hospital and receiving care

Contract coder: A coder who is hired on a temporary basis to work on-site

Contractual allowance: The difference between what is charged by the healthcare provider and what is paid by the managed care company or other payer

Contractual write-off: *See* **contractual allowance**

Cooperating parties for ICD-9-CM: A group of organizations (the American Health Information Management Association, the American Hospital Association, the Centers for Medicare and Medicaid Services, and the National Center for Health Statistics) that collaborates in the development and maintenance of the *International Classification of Diseases, Ninth Revision, Clinical Modification* (ICD-9-CM)

Cost: The dollar amount of a service provided by a facility

CPT Level I: Current Procedural Terminology codes that constitute first level of the HCPCS coding system

CPT Level II: Current Procedural Terminology codes that are applicable to selected physician and nonphysician services, durable medical goods, drugs, and supplies

Credit balance: A balance on an account that is to be refunded to an insurer or to the patient

***Current Procedural Terminology, Fourth Edition* (CPT):** A comprehensive, descriptive list of terms and numeric codes used for reporting diagnostic and therapeutic procedures and other medical services performed by physicians; published and updated annually by the American Medical Association

Data quality review: An examination of health records to determine the level of coding accuracy and to identify areas of coding problems

Days in accounts receivable: The ending accounts receivable balance divided by an average day's revenues

Denial: The circumstance when a bill has been accepted, but payment has been denied for any of several reasons (for example, sending the bill to the wrong insurance company, patient not having current coverage, inaccurate coding, lack of medical necessity, and so on)

Discharged not final billed (DNFB) report: A report that includes all patients who have been discharged from the facility but for whom, for one reason or another, the billing process is not complete

Dollars in accounts receivable: The amount of money owed a healthcare facility when claims are pending

DRG creep: An increase in a case-mix index that occurs through the coding of higher-paying principal diagnoses and of more complications and comorbidities, even though the actual severity level of the patient population did not change

Drivers and passengers: The exploding charges wherein the driver is the item that explodes into other items and appears on the bill

Enabling technologies: Any newly developed equipment that facilitates data gathering or information processing not possible previously

Exploding charges: Charges for items that must be reported separately but are used together, such as interventional radiology imaging and injection procedures

Feeder system: An automated data system that feeds results into a comprehensive database

Fiscal intermediary (FI): An organization that contracts with the Centers for Medicare and Medicaid Services to serve as the financial agent between providers and the federal government in the local administration of Medicare Part B claims

General ledger (G/L) key: The two- or three-digit number in the chargemaster that assigns each item to a particular section of the general ledger in a healthcare facility's accounting section

Granularity: The relative level of detail or the smallest amount of discrete information that can be directly retrieved (higher granularity yields greater detail)

Grouper: A computer software program that automatically assigns prospective payment groups on the basis of clinical codes

Grouping: A system for assigning patients to a classification scheme via a computer software program

Hard code: A code applied through a healthcare organization's chargemaster

Hard coding: The process of attaching a CPT/HCPCS code to a procedure located on the facility's chargemaster so that the code will automatically be included on the patient's bill

HCPCS: *See* **Healthcare Common Procedural Coding System**

Healthcare Common Procedural Coding System (HCPCS): A classification system that identifies healthcare procedures, equipment, and supplies for claim submission purposes; the three levels are as follows: I, *Current Procedural Terminology* codes, developed by the AMA; II, codes for equipment, supplies, and services not covered by *Current Procedural Terminology* codes as well as modifiers that can be used with all levels of codes, developed by CMS; and III (eliminated December 31, 2003 to comply with HIPAA), local codes developed by regional Medicare Part B carriers and used to report physicians' services and supplies to Medicare for reimbursement

Hierarchical system: A system structured with broad groupings that can be further subdivided into more narrowly defined group or detailed entities

Home health resource group (HHRG): A classification system with 80 home health episode rates established to support the prospective reimbursement of covered home care and rehabilitation services provided to Medicare beneficiaries during 60-day episodes of care

Home health services: Items and services furnished to an individual—provided on a visiting basis in a place of residence used as the individual's home—under the care of a physician by a home health agency under a plan established and periodically reviewed by a physician

Hospice program: A public agency or private organization primarily engaged in providing care and services to individuals considered to be "terminally ill" with a life expectancy of 6 months or less

Hospital information system (HIS): The comprehensive database containing all the clinical, administrative, financial, and demographic information about each patient served by a hospital

Hospitalization insurance (Medicare Part A): A federal program that covers the costs associated with inpatient hospitalization as well as other healthcare services provided to Medicare beneficiaries

Independent consultant: An individual who works as a contractor to provide coding services to healthcare facilities

Information: Factual data that have been collected, combined, analyzed, interpreted, and/or converted into a form that can be used for a specific purpose

Information modeling: The use of clinical code sets with application software to create information that is meaningful to the end user

Inpatient coder: A person who codes inpatient medical records in an acute care hospital setting

Insurance code mapping: The methodology that allows a hospital to hold more than one CPT/HCPCS code per chargemaster item

Item description: An explanation of a service or supply listed in the chargemaster

Job sharing: A work schedule in which two or more individuals share the tasks of one full-time or one full-time-equivalent position

Late charge: A charge that has not been posted within the healthcare facility's established bill hold time period

LCD: *See* **Local coverage determination**

Level I of CPT: *See* **CPT Level I**

Level II of CPT: *See* **CPT Level II**

Local coverage determination (LCD): Coverage rules, at a fiscal intermediary (FI) or carrier level, that provide information on what diagnoses justify the medical necessity of a test

Long-term care hospital (LTCH): A healthcare facility that has an average length of stay greater than 25 days, with patients classified into distinct diagnosis groups called LCS-DRGs; prospective payment system for LTCHs was established by CMS and went into effect beginning in 2002

LTCH: *See* **Long-term care hospital**

Master patient index (MPI): A list or database created and maintained by a healthcare facility to record the name and identification number of every patient who has ever been admitted or treated in the facility

Medical Outcomes Study Short-Form Health Survey: A patient survey that reflects the patient's disease and symptom intensity to characterize the total burden of the disease

Medicare Part A: *See* **hospitalization insurance**

Medicare Part B: *See* **supplemental medical insurance**

MEDPAR database system: *See* **Medicare Provider Analysis and Review database system**

Medicare Provider Analysis and Review (MEDPAR) database system: A database containing information submitted by fiscal intermediaries that is used by the Office of the Inspector General to identify suspicious billing and charge practices

Minimum Data Set (MDS): The instrument specified by the Centers for Medicare and Medicaid Services that requires nursing facilities (both Medicare certified and/or Medicaid certified) to conduct a comprehensive, accurate, standardized, reproducible assessment of each resident's functional capacity

Multiaxial system: A system that can classify an entity in several different ways

Multiservice contractor: A small company that provides coding services or services related to coding

National Association of Children's Hospitals and Related Institutions (NACHRI) classification: A classification of congenital and chronic health conditions that uses disease progression factors for case-mix analysis

National coverage determination (NCD): The equivalent of LCDs at the national level. *See* **Local coverage determination (LCD)**

Needs assessment: A procedure performed to determine what is required, lacking, or desired by an employee, a group, or an organization

Nomenclature: A recognized system of terms used in a science or art that follows pre-established naming conventions; a disease nomenclature is a listing of the proper name for each disease entity with its specific code number

Nosology: The branch of medical science that deals with classification systems

Office of the Inspector General (OIG): The office through which the federal government established compliance plans for the healthcare industry

Optical image-based system: A health record system in which information is created initially in paper form and then scanned into an electronic system for storage and retrieval

Outcomes management: The process of systematically tracking a patient's clinical treatment and responses to that treatment, including measures of morbidity and functional status, for the purpose of improving care

Outcomes measurement: *See* **outcomes management**

Outpatient coder: An individual responsible for assigning ICD-9-CM and CPT/HCPCS codes to ambulatory surgery or emergency department cases

Outsourcing: The hiring of an individual or a company external to an organization to perform a function either on-site or off-site

Parents and children: A name for exploding charges wherein the parent is the item that explodes into other items and appears on the bill

Pending: A condition during which a facility waits for payment after a bill is dropped

Physician champion: An individual who assists in educating medical staff on documentation procedures for accurate billing

Pointer: An item that has no dollar value and no code attached to it that is mapped to two or more items with separate charges

Principal diagnosis: The disease or condition that was present on admission, was the principal reason for admission, and received treatment or evaluation during the hospital stay or visit

Probationary period: A period of time in which the skills of a potential employee's work are assessed before that person assumes full-time employment

Process improvement team: An interdepartmental task force formed to redesign or change shared processes and procedures

Productivity bonus: A monetary incentive used to encourage employees to improve their output

Pull list: A list of requests for records to be pulled for review during the audit process

Reimbursement: Compensation or repayment for healthcare services

Rejection: The process of having a submitted bill not accepted by the payer, although corrections can be made and the claim resubmitted

Relative weight (RW): 1. A multiplier that determines reimbursement 2. A measure of the resource intensity or clinical severity of a specific group of patients based on a specific case-mix methodology

Request for proposal (RFP): A type of business correspondence asking for very specific product and contract information that is often sent to a narrow list of vendors that have been preselected after a review of requests for information during the design phase of the systems development life cycle

Resource Utilization Groups, Version III (RUG-III): A case-mix–adjusted classification system based on Minimum Data Set assessments and used by skilled nursing facilities

Retrospective coding: A type of coding that takes place after the patient has been discharged and the entire health record has been routed to the health information management department

Revenue code: A three- or four-digit number in the chargemaster that totals all items and their charges for printing on the form used for Medicare billing

Risk adjustment: Any method of comparing the severity of illness of one group of patients with that of another group of patients

Secondary diagnosis: A statement of those conditions coexisting during a hospital episode that affect the treatment received or the length of stay

Service bonus: A monetary reward given to long-term staff in recognition of their skills and commitment to the organization

Service-line coder: A person who excels in coding one particular service line, such as oncology or cardiology

Sign-on bonus: A monetary incentive used by a facility to encourage a candidate to accept employment

Skilled nursing facility (SNF): A long-term care facility with an organized professional staff and permanent facilities (including inpatient beds) that provides continuous nursing and other health-related, psychosocial, and personal services to patients who are not in an acute phase of illness but who primarily require continued care on an inpatient basis

Soft coding: A process in which a coder reviews medical documentation and provides a CPT/HCPCS code for encounters that require analysis to justify the highest level of specificity from the documentation

Structured query language (SQL): A fourth-generation computer language that includes both DDL and DML components and is used to create and manipulate relational databases

Superbill: The office form used for physician office billing that is initiated by the physician and states the diagnoses and other information for each patient encounter

Supplemental medical insurance (Medicare Part B): A voluntary medical insurance program that helps pay for physicians' services, medical services, and supplies not covered by Medicare Part A

Telecommuting: A work arrangement (often used by coding and transcription personnel) in which at least a portion of the employee's work hours is spent outside the office (usually in the home) and the work is transmitted back to the employer via electronic means

Unbundling: The practice of using multiple codes to bill for the various individual steps in a single procedure rather than using a single code that includes all of the steps of the comprehensive procedure

Undercoding: A form of incomplete documentation that results when diagnoses or procedures are missing that should be coded

Upcoding: The practice of assigning diagnostic or procedural codes that represent higher payment rates than the codes that actually reflect the services provided to patients

Vocabulary mapping process: A process that connects one clinical vocabulary to another

Weight: The numerical assignment that is part of the formula by which a specific dollar amount, or reimbursement, is calculated for each diagnosis-related group or each ambulatory payment classification

Work-imaging study: A technique used to analyze the coding time required of full-time employees (FTEs) compared with established productivity standards

Zero balance: The result of writing off the balance of an account, which closes off the account and ends the days in accounts receivable

Index

(continued on next page)

Look for These **Quality AHIMA Publications** at **Bookstores, Libraries,** and **Online**

- *Applying Inpatient Coding Skills under Prospective Payment*
- *Basic CPT/HCPCS Coding*
- *Basic ICD-9-CM Coding*
- *The Best of In Confidence*
- *Calculating and Reporting Healthcare Statistics*
- *Clinical Coding Workout: Practice Exercises for Skill Development*
- *Coding and Reimbursement for Hospital Inpatient Services*
- *Coding and Reimbursement for Hospital Outpatient Services*
- *CPT/HCPCS Coding and Reimbursement for Physician Services*
- *Documentation for Acute Care* (Book and CD)
- *Documentation for Ambulatory Care*
- *Documentation and Reimbursement for Behavioral Healthcare Services*
- *Documentation and Reimbursement for Long-Term Care* (Book and CD)
- *Documentation and Reimbursement for Home Care and Hospice Programs*

- *Effective Management of Coding Services*
- *Electronic Health Record*
- *Essentials of Healthcare Finance* (Workbook)
- *Health Information Management*
- *Health Information Management Technology*
- *Health Information Management Compliance* (Book and CD)
- *HIPAA in Practice*
- *ICD-9-CM Diagnostic Coding and Reimbursement for Physician Services*
- *ICD-9-CM Diagnostic Coding for Long-Term Care and Home Care*
- *ICD-10-CM and ICD-10-PCS Preview* (Book and CD)
- *Pocket Glossary of Health Information Management and Technology*
- *Principles of Healthcare Reimbursement*
- *Quality and Performance Improvement in Healthcare*
- *Statistical Application for HIM Coding and Reimbursement for Hospital Outpatient Services*

More Information

For details and easy ordering, visit **www.ahima.org/store**.

For textbook content questions, contact **publications@ahima.org** or (800) 335-5535.

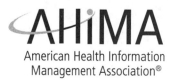

AHIMA
American Health Information
Management Association®

Kick Your Future into High Gear Today by Joining

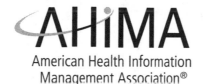

AHiMA
American Health Information
Management Association®

The American Health Information Management Association (AHIMA), the name you can trust in quality healthcare education, has represented the interests of HIM professionals since 1928.

We have been at the forefront of change in healthcare, anticipating trends, preparing for the future, and advancing careers. AHIMA membership affords you a vast array of resources including:

- **An Award-winning** *Journal of AHIMA*
- **HIM Body of Knowledge**
- **Virtual Communities of Practice**
- **Leadership Opportunities**
- **Latest Industry Information**
- **Continuing Education**
- **Advocacy**
- **e-HIM® Practice Guidance Reports**

This list just touches on the benefits of AHIMA membership. To learn more about the benefits of membership or how to renew your membership, just visit **www.ahima.org/membership**, or call **(800) 335-5535**.